A PRACTICAL HANDBOOK
OF PSYCHIATRY

Publication Number 907
AMERICAN LECTURE SERIES®

A Publication in
The BANNERSTONE DIVISION *of*
AMERICAN LECTURES IN CLINICAL PSYCHIATRY

Editor
GORDON L. MOORE, M.D.
Department of Psychiatry and Clinical Psychology
Mayo Clinic
Rochester, Minnesota

A Practical Handbook of Psychiatry

Edited by

JOSEPH R. NOVELLO, M. D.

Department of Psychiatry
University of Michigan Medical School
Ann Arbor, Michigan

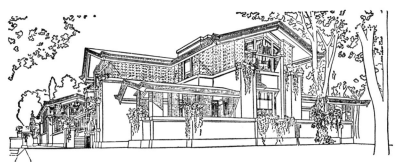

CHARLES C THOMAS • PUBLISHER
Springfield • Illinois • U. S. A.

Published and Distributed Throughout the World by
CHARLES C THOMAS • PUBLISHER
Bannerstone House
301–327 East Lawrence Avenue, Springfield, Illinois, U.S.A.

© *1974, by* CHARLES C THOMAS • PUBLISHER
ISBN 0-398-02868-0
Library of Congress Catalog Card Number: 73-7518

Printed in the United States of America

CC-11

Novello, Joseph R
    A practical handbook of psychiatry.

    (American lecture series, publication no. 907. A monograph in the Bannerstone
division of American lectures in clinical psychiatry)
    1. Psychiatry—Handbooks, manuals, etc. I. Title.
[DNLM: 1. Mental disorders. WM100 P893 1973]
RC454.N676   616.8'9'00202   73-7518
ISBN 0-398-02868-0

To Toni

CONTRIBUTORS

Gail Barton, M.D., M.P.H.
Clinical Assistant Professor of Psychiatry
University of Michigan Medical School
Research Associate in Community Mental Health, School
of Public Health
University of Michigan

Ronald M. Benson, M.D.
Instructor of Psychiatry
University of Michigan Medical School
Assistant Director, Child Analytic Study Program

Lynn W. Blunt, M.D.
Clinical Director, Center for Forensic Psychiatry
Ann Arbor, Michigan

Arlin Brown, M.D.
Resident in Psychiatry
University of Michigan Medical School

A. Keith W. Brownell, M.D., F.R.C.P. (C)
Instructor of Neurology
University of Michigan Medical School

Robert L. Hatcher, Ph.D.
Clinical Instructor of Psychiatry
University of Michigan Medical School

Clifford C. Kuhn, M.D.
Formerly Chief Resident in Psychiatry
University of Michigan Medical School

Naomi E. Lohr, Ph.D.
Assistant Professor of Psychology, Department of
Psychiatry
University of Michigan
Lecturer, Psychology Department
University of Michigan

David W. Pearson, M.A., M.D.
Resident in Psychiatry
University of Michigan Medical School

M. Joseph Pearson, M.D.
Clinical Instructor of Psychiatry
University of Michigan Medical School

H. J. Schulte, M.D.
Resident in Psychiatry
University of Michigan Medical School

Dean Schuyler, M.D.
National Institute of Mental Health
Clinical Research Branch, Depression Section

Michael J. Short, M.D.
Resident in Psychiatry
University of Michigan Medical School

Dennis Walsh, M.D.
Resident in Psychiatry
University of Michigan Medical School

Arthur R. Williams, Ed.D.
Formerly Clinical Assistant Professor of Psychiatry,
School of Medicine
West Virginia University

S. J. Wilson, M.D.
Fellow in Forensic Psychiatry
Department of Psychiatry (Legal Psychiatry Section)
University of California at Los Angeles, School of
Medicine

Jesse H. Wright, M.D.
Chief Resident in Psychiatry
University of Michigan Medical School

Raymond F. Zeh, Jr., M.D.
Resident in Psychiatry
University of Michigan Medical School

FOREWORD

Most of us, upon reflection, are likely bemused when the word practical appears in a book title. Certainly none of us would wish to expend our limited time reading a professional book that is impractical. Nor would we expect a serious physician to consciously write an impractical text, although I suppose some inadvertently have. To those of an intellectual bent, the word practical in the title might indicate a tome of lesser sophistication. To many, practical implies ordinary. The dictionary is kindly disposed to this word. Such phrases appear as "adapted or designed for actual use," "useful," "inclined toward or fitted for actual work." These latter definitions eminently describe this book.

Doctor Novello and colleagues have not deviated from the implication of their title. This is a useful book fitted to help psychiatrists do their actual work. It will be particularly useful to those who are beginning in psychiatry—but I suspect many with years of experience will also find it a handy reference. This book was designed to bring, in synopsis form, much of that information which always seems to elude us, just when we need it most, that is, in the turmoil of our daily work.

Psychiatrists in a multitude of practice situations, who are very practical people, will be the final judge of the practicality of this book. My speculation is they will find it "designed for actual use in actual work."

Gordon L. Moore, M.D.

PREFACE

The best way to introduce the reader to the purpose, plan and scope of this book is to begin at the beginning: sometime in 1970, when, as a first year resident in psychiatry, I discovered the need for a practical, concise handbook of the type that I had previously relied upon in surgery, medicine, pediatrics and other medical specialties. Those handbooks had served me well as a medical student, as an intern and in the military. Yet, to my surprise and disappointment, I found that there was nothing quite similar available in psychiatry.

There were two basic choices—the standard psychiatric reference books which were encyclopedic in both subject matter and physical bulk and a few paperback handbooks that were simply mini textbooks, condensations of the usual textbook type of information. While I valued these as sources of in-depth information and utilized them for that purpose, they did not answer my need for a quick, practical source of clinical information that would help me out on the firing-line in my day to day work with the kinds of patients that I was seeing in my residency.

I checked with other residents in psychiatry and they agreed. I checked with medical students, residents in various medical specialties and even practicing psychiatrists and they agreed too. We needed something new.

Thus, Part One (A Guide to Clinical Practice) was born.

The guiding principles for Part One were few but concise. It should contain a maximum of clinically-useful information with a minimum of verbiage, in a format that was brisk and readable. It was not to be a textbook nor a mini textbook; it was to be a handbook in the sense of the existing medical handbooks, an immediate source of sound, practical information for use on the firing line by psychiatrists, other medical practitioners and medical students. Additionally, it should be of use to nonmedical mental health workers who often require quick access to psychiatric information.

Part Two of this handbook (A Guide to Continuing Education) grew out of a different set of frustrations. As I moved along in my training I found that, in addition to information on patient care, I also required information that was directly related to my own psychiatric training. I wanted to know about reading lists and about journals in psychiatry. I was interested in knowing more about training opportunities in some of the subspecialities. I wondered about board certification in psychiatry. While I was usually able to find the answers to my questions, it took hours and sometimes days. If only all of this material was collected in one place! I found that fellow residents and even trained psychiatrists also wished there was a single common source for all of this information. Part Two is so designed.

Part Three (The Psychiatrist's Address Book) is an effort to pull together, in one concise volume, addresses of professional organizations and institutions related to psychiatry. These are addresses frequently required by psychiatrists in their professional correspondence. Psychiatrists that practice in an institutional setting have access to the several different volumes in which these addresses appear. Others are not so fortunate. The address book aims to bring this information within the reach of all.

Obviously, a project like this is not accomplished by one individual alone. I am indebted to a great many people without whose help this handbook would not have been possible:

Dr. Peter A. Martin, Clinical Professor of Psychiatry at the University of Michigan was the first to encourage this effort and he remained a source of sound advice and counsel from beginning to end.

Several other individuals from the Department of Psychiatry, University of Michigan, have contributed ideas and thoughtful criticisms: Dr. Albert J. Silverman, Chairman of the Department; Dr. Edgar Draper, Director of Training;

and Dr. Saul Harrison, Director of Training in Child Psychiatry.

It has been a pleasure being on the same team with Mr. Payne Thomas and Dr. Gordon Moore. They were great assets at several points along the way.

Many other individuals who assisted directly are cited in the text. This includes various authors and publishers who extended permission for their material to be republished in this volume and other individuals who provided up-to-the-minute information about training programs in psychiatry (Chapter XII).

I am particularly indebted to the eighteen contributing authors. These colleagues worked with enthusiasm and cooperation. Their creative touches are evident throughout the book and they deserve much credit for our finished product. Finally I would like to acknowledge two individuals who worked long and hard on this project: Miss Margaret Givens who assisted in the voluminous correspondence and typed much of the manuscript and Mrs. Josie DeMaso who provided the secretarial skill in preparing the final manuscript and who assisted in proofreading and in preparation of the index.

Joseph R. Novello

AN OPEN LETTER TO THE READERS
OF THIS HANDBOOK

It is the hope of the editor and the contributing authors that this handbook will fill the real need for a compact and practical source of psychiatric information for our colleagues.

Because it is your professional needs that we aim uniquely to serve, we intend to be responsive to your suggestions in any future edition of this work. We invite your reactions and criticisms. We look to you as a source of continuing enrichment and maturation for this handbook.

What things should be changed? How? What things, not included, should be added? What should be deleted?

We look forward to your reply.

Address correspondence to:

Joseph R. Novello, M.D.
Department of Psychiatry
University Hospital
Ann Arbor, Michigan 48104

NOTICE

In reference to somatic treatment (psychotropic drugs, convulsive therapy, etc.) the authors have been careful to recommend dosages and procedures that are consistent with responsible medical literature and that conform to the practices of the general psychiatric and medical community. However, because standards of usage do change, the clinician is advised to consult manufacturers' product information, especially when new or infrequently-used drugs or procedures are employed.

CONTENTS

Part One

A GUIDE TO CLINICAL PRACTICE

Part Two

A GUIDE TO CONTINUING EDUCATION

Part Three

THE PSYCHIATRIST'S ADDRESS BOOK

A PRACTICAL HANDBOOK
OF PSYCHIATRY

PART ONE

A GUIDE TO
CLINICAL PRACTICE

Chapter I

DIAGNOSIS AND CLASSIFICATION IN PSYCHIATRY

THE CONTROVERSIES, BOTH philosophical and practical, that are raised by any attempt to systematically classify the various clinical entities encountered in psychiatric practice are legion. To summarize the various points of view is beyond the purpose and scope of this handbook. For a historical overview of this topic the reader is referred to Brill, H., Classification in Psychiatry, in *Comprehensive Textbook of Psychiatry* (Freedman, A. and Kaplan, H. (Eds.), Baltimore, Williams and Wilkins, 1967.)

In this chapter (Table I-I) the reader is presented with the current, official diagnostic system in use in the United States, *Diagnostic and Statistical Manual of Mental Disorders,* Second Edition (American Psychiatric Association). Whatever its inherent strengths and flaws, this system is the most widely-used and widely-accepted reference of psychiatric diagnosis available in this country.

In addition, the reader is provided four supporting articles that deal with common diagnostic problems; they are designed to aid the psychiatrist in establishing an accurate diagnosis.

Diagnosis of Schizophrenia contains an outline of the many secondary symptoms encountered in schizophrenia with an emphasis on their relative diagnostic weight (Table I-II) and information on differential diagnosis of the schizophrenic

5

subtypes (paranoid, catatonic, etc.) as compared to various other psychiatric disorders (Table I-III).

Differential Diagnosis: Organic Psychosis vs. Functional Psychosis provides practical guidelines for distinguishing these two fundamental entities (Table I-IV).

The next article offers tips in the differential diagnosis of the five major classes of drug abuse (hallucinogens, CNS stimulants, CNS depressants, marijuana, narcotics) and three psychiatric entities (acute schizophrenia, acute mania, hallucinosis) that are easily confused with drug intoxications (Table I-V).

The fourth supporting article is entitled, Differential Diagnosis of Four Psychiatric Entities: Conversion Symptom, Hypochondriasis, Somatic Delusion, Malingering. These conditions are commonly encountered in psychiatric practice and often present difficulties in differential diagnosis. Table I-VI compares and contrasts these entities.

In addition to this chapter, the reader may refer to other sections of the handbook for assistance in diagnosis. Chapter III (Aids to Diagnosis in Psychiatry) presents several rating scales that are useful diagnostically. Chapter VII (Psychiatry in Medicine) outlines common problems in differential diagnosis that exist between psychiatric and medical disorders. Chapter VIII (Neurology for Psychiatrists) distinguishes between common neurological syndromes and certain psychiatric conditions. Chapter X (The Psychiatrist's Role in the Diagnosis and Treatment of Drug Abuse) presents a concise summary of the present drug abuse picture and offers a step-by-step guide to diagnosis.

DIAGNOSTIC AND STATISTICAL MANUAL OF MENTAL DISORDERS, SECOND EDITION (DSM-II)
(With permission, American Psychiatric Association)

The second edition of the *Diagnostic and Statistical Manual of Mental Disorders* (DSM-II) was prepared by the Committee of Nomenclature and Statistics of the American Psychiatric Association. It was published in 1968 and represents the current official psychiatric nomenclature to be used in the United States.

The manual is based on the International Classification of Diseases, Eighth Revision (ICD-8) which is a product of the World Health Organization. In certain circumstances, however, there are classifications listed in DSM-II that are used only in the United States. In the tables that follow, these are marked by an asterisk (*).

In addition to the four-digit numbered codes appearing in the first column of the tables, DSM-II provides for fifth digit qualifying phrases as follows:

Section II
.x1 Acute
.x2 Chronic

Section III
.x6 Not psychotic now

Sections IV through IX
.x6 Mild
.x7 Moderate
.x8 Severe

All disorders
.x5 In remission

In this chapter DSM-II (Table I-I: *Diagnostic and Statistical Manual of Mental Disorders,* Second Edition) is presented in its entirety. In most cases the descriptive information is summarized for the sake of brevity. The interested reader may refer to the official manual published by the American Psychiatric Association for further information. (Copies by request: Publications Office, A.P.A., 1700 18 St., N.W., Washington, D.C. 20009)

DIAGNOSIS OF SCHIZOPHRENIA

The diagnosis of schizophrenia can be a difficult clinical problem. In general, the rate of concurrence between any two psychiatrists is only 75 percent for the disorder.

The classic, primary symptoms described by Bleuler are still of paramount importance:

1. Disturbance of Association
2. Disturbance of Affect

TABLE I-I

DIAGNOSTIC AND STATISTICAL MANUAL OF MENTAL DISORDERS, SECOND EDITION

Code	Diagnosis	Description
		I. MENTAL RETARDATION
310.	Borderline	IQ 68 to 85
311.	Mild	IQ 52 to 67
312.	Moderate	IQ 36 to 51
313.	Severe	IQ 20 to 35
314.	Profound	IQ under 20
315.	Unspecified	Intellectual functioning has not or cannot be evaluated precisely but which is clearly subnormal
With each:	**Following or associated with**	
.0	Infection or Intoxication	Examples: Rubella, Syphilis, Kernicterus, Lead Poisoning, etc.
.1	Trauma or Physical Agent	Examples: Prenatal anoxia, Birth Injury, etc.
.2	Disorders of Metabolism, Growth, or Nutrition	Examples: Tay-Sach's, Niemann-Pick's, PKU, Porphyria, etc.
.3	Gross Brain Disease (postnatal)	Includes all diseases and conditions associated with neoplasms. Also degenerative brain diseases.
.4	Unknown Prenatal Influence	Existed prior to birth but no definite etiology Examples: Anacephaly, Craniostenosis, Congenital hydrocephalus, etc.
.5	Chromosomal Abnormality	Examples: Mongolism, etc.
.6	Prematurity	Birth weight below 5.5 pounds and/or gestational age of less than 38 weeks and who do not fit into any preceding category.
.7	Major psychiatric disorder	Following severe psychosis in early childhood.
.8	Psychosocial (environmental) deprivation	No evidence of organic disease but severe environmental deprivation.
.9	Other condition	Other not listed above.
		II.A. ORGANIC BRAIN SYNDROME, PSYCHOTIC
	Senile and Presenile Dementia	
290.0	Senile dementia	Impairment of: Orientation, memory, comprehension, calculation, judgment, etc. Labile affect. Occurs with senile brain disease.
290.1	Presenile dementia	Cortical brain disease (Alzheimer's, Pick's, etc.).

Alcoholic Psychosis

291.0	Delirium tremens	Delirium, coarse tremors, visual hallucinations.
291.1	Korsakov's psychosis	Disorientation, confabulation, **memory deficit, peripheral neuropathy.**
291.2	Other alcoholic hallucinosis	Not elsewhere classifiable. Must distinguish from schizophrenia.
291.3	Alcohol paranoid state	Usually chronic male alcoholics. Excessive jealousy and delusions of infidelity by spouse.
291.4 *	Acute alcoholic intoxication	With psychotic manifestations (i.e. do not confuse with simple drunkenness).
291.5 *	Alcoholic deterioration ·	Chronic brain syndromes caused by alcohol not meeting criteria for Korsakov's.
291.6 *	Pathological intoxication	Acute brain syndrome after minimal intake.
291.9	Other alcoholic psychosis.	All varieties not classed above.

Psychosis Associated with Intracranial Infection

292.0	General Paralysis	Signs and symptoms of parenchymatous syphilis of nervous system. Usually positive serology.
292.1	Syphilis of CNS	Includes all other varieties of psychosis attributed to intracranial infection by Spirocheta pallida. Has features of **OBS.**
292.2	Epidemic encephalitis	No cases since 1926; von Economo's encephalitis.
292.3	Other and unspecified encephalitis	Where possible, indicate the precise infecting agent.
292.9	Other intracranial infection	All acute and chronic infections not syphilis or encephalitis. Such as: meningitis, brain absess, etc.

Psychosis Associated with Other Cerebral Condition

293.0	Cerebral arteriosclerosis	May be impossible to differentiate from senile and presenile dementia.
293.1	Other cerebrovascular disturbance	Includes: cerebral thrombosis, cerebral embolism, hypertension, decompensated cardiac status.
293.2	Epilepsy	Used only for idiopathic epilepsy. Attack may take form of hallucinations, fears, violence.
293.3	Intracranial neoplasm	Include primary and metastatic tumors.
293.4	Degenerative diseases of CNS	Includes degenerative diseases not listed previously.
293.5	Brain trauma	Develops immediately after severe head injury, or brain surgery. Also posttraumatic chronic brain disorders.
293.9	Other cerebral condition	If not included above, or more precise diagnosis not possible.

TABLE I-I Continued

Code	Diagnosis	Description
Psychosis Associated with Other Physical Condition		
294.0	Endocrine disorder	Psychosis associated with endocrinopathies (Pancreas, thyroid, pituitary, adrenal, etc.).
294.1	Metabolic and nutritional disorder	Includes: Pellagra, avitaminosis, and metabolic disorders.
294.2	Systemic Infection	Examples: Severe pneumonia, typhoid fever, malaria, acute rheumatic fever.
294.3	Drug or poison intoxication	Includes psychedelic drugs, hormones, heavy metals, gases and other intoxicants. Does not include alcohol.
294.4	Childbirth	Diagnosis of exclusion, i.e. this excludes all other psychoses which may arise during pregnancy and postpartum and which, if possible, should be specifically diagnosed.
294.8	Other and unspecified physical condition	Any not included above or undiagnosed.
II.B. ORGANIC BRAIN SYNDROME, NONPSYCHOTIC		
309.0	Intracranial infection	Includes all OBS without psychosis. Diagnosis specifically as per code.
309.13 *	Alcohol (simple drunkenness)	
309.14 *	Other drug, poison or systemic intoxication	
309.2	Brain trauma	
309.3	Circulatory disturbance	
309.4	Epilepsy	
309.5	Disturbance of metabolism, growth, or nutrition	
309.6	Senile or presenile brain disease	
309.7	Intracranial neoplasm	
309.8	Degenerative disease of CNS	
309.9	Other physical condition	
III. PSYCHOSES NOT ATTRIBUTED TO PHYSICAL CONDITIONS LISTED PREVIOUSLY		
Schizophrenia		
295.0	Simple	Slow, insidious, progressive social withdrawal and mental deterioration. Less dramatically psychotic than other forms. Little or no progression.

295.1	Hebephrenic	Disorganized thinking, unpredictable giggling, silly and regressive behavior. Delusions and hallucinations, if present, are transient and not well organized.
295.2	Catatonic	Excited: excessive, even violent, motor activity. Withdrawn: Stupor, mutism, negativism, waxy flexibility. Sometimes vegetative state.
.23 *	; excited type	
.24 *	; withdrawn type	
295.3	Paranoid	Persecutory or grandiose delusions, often with hallucinations. Excessive religiosity. Behavior often aggressive and consistent with delusions. Personality disorganization not as great as with two previous types. Use of projection. Three subtypes: hostile, grandiose, hallucinatory.
295.4	Acute schizophrenic episode	Acute onset. Often recovery within weeks. Usually followed by recurrence. In time may become catatonic, hebephrenic or paranoid. Acute onset distinguishes from simple type.
295.5	Latent	Symptoms of schizophrenia but no history of psychotic episode. Other names: borderline schizophrenia, incipient, prepsychotic, pseudoneurotic.
295.6	Residual	Patients showing signs of schizophrenia but after psychotic episode are no longer psychotic.
295.7	Schizo-affective	Mixture of schizophrenic symptoms with pronounced elation or depression.
.73 *	; excited	
.74 *	; depressed	
295.8 *	Childhood	Develops before puberty. Autistic, atypical behavior. Failure to develop own identity. Gross immaturity.
295.90 *	Chronic undifferentiated	Mixed symptoms. Definite picture of schizophrenic thought, affect, behavior but not classifiable elsewhere. Chronic.
295.99 *	Other schizophrenia	Any type not previously described.

III. PSYCHOSES

Major Affective Disorders

| 296.0 | Involutional melancholia | Onset of mood not related to precipitating event; therefore, distinguished from psychotic depressive reaction and depressive neurosis. Impaired reality testing is due to disorder of mood. Involutional period. Worry, anxiety, agitation, insomnia. Guilt and somatic preoccupation may be delusional. No previous episode. |

TABLE I-I Continued

Code	Diagnosis	Description
296.1	Manic-depressive illness, manic	Manic episodes only. Elation, talkative, flight of ideas, accelerated speech and motor activity. Brief depression possible but not true depressive episodes.
296.2	Manic-depressive illness, depressed	Depressed episodes only. Mood and motor retardation. May observe guilt, hypochondrical or paranoid ideation.
296.3	Manic-depressive illness, circular	History of at least one manic episode and one depressive episode.
296.33 **	Manic-depressive, circular, manic	
296.34 **	Manic-depressive, circular, depressed	
296.8	Other major affective disorder	Include mixed manic-depressive where manic and depressive symptoms appear almost simultaneously. (Not including Psychotic depressive reaction or Depressive neurosis.)
Paranoid States		Delusion is the central abnormality.
297.0	Paranoia	Extremely rare. Gradual development of elaborate paranoid system often proceeding from logical misinterpretation of actual event. Usually not interfere with rest of patient's thinking or personality.
297.1	Involutional paranoid state	Delusion formation in involutional period. Absence of the thought disorder typical of schizophrenia.
297.9	Other paranoid state	
Other Psychoses		
298.0	Psychotic depressive reaction	Precipitated by real life event. No past history of same.
	IV. NEUROSES	
300.0	Anxiety neurosis	Free-floating anxiety extending to panic. Frequent somatic symptoms. Distinguish from normal fear (realistic) and phobia (unrealistic, object-related).
300.1	Hysterical neurosis	Involuntary psychogenic loss or disorder of function. Symptoms begin and end suddenly in emotionally-charged situations and are symbolic of the underlying conflict. Can often be modified by suggestion alone. Use subtypes below.

300.13 *	_____; conversion type	Special senses or voluntary nervous system involved (blindness, anosmia, paralyses, etc). Belle indifference. Often secondary gain present (sympathy, relief from responsibility, etc.) (Malingering, by contrast, is done consciously.)
300.14 *	_____; dissociative type	Alterations in consciousness or identity. Such as amnesia, somnambulism, fugue, multiple personality.
300.2	Phobic neurosis	Intense fear of object or situation that the patient consciously recognizes as no real danger to him.
300.3	Obsessive compulsive neurosis	Persistent intrusion of unwanted thoughts, urges or actions that patient is unable to stop. Ruminations, rituals. Anxiety if interrupted.
300.4	Depressive neurosis	Excessive depression due to internal conflict or identifiable loss.
300.5	Neurasthenic neurosis	Chronic weakness, easy fatigability. Symptoms are genuinely distressing, without secondary gain (unlike hysterical neurosis). Differs from depressive neurosis in moderateness of depression and chronicity of course.
300.6	Depersonalization neurosis	Feeling of unreality and estrangement from self, the body parts, or surroundings. Do not use if condition is part of some other disorder such as situation reaction. Brief depersonalization experience not necessarily a symptom of illness.
300.7	Hypochondriacal neurosis	Preoccupation with body and fear of disease. Fear not delusional (psychotic) but persists despite reassurance. Differs from hysterical conversion and psychophysiological disorder in that there is no actual impairment of function.
300.8	Other neurosis	Specific disorders such as writer's cramp and other occupational neuroses.

V. PERSONALITY DISORDERS AND CERTAIN OTHER NONPSYCHOTIC DISORDERS

Personality Disorders

| 301.0 | Paranoid | Unwarranted suspicion, excessive self-importance, jealousy, envy, hypersensitivity tendency to blame others. |
| 301.1 | Cyclothymic | Alternating elation (ambition, warmth, enthusiasm) and depression (worry, pessimism, low energy). Not readily attributable to external circumstances. |

TABLE 1-1 Continued

Code	Diagnosis	Description
301.2	Schizoid	Shyness, over-sensitivity, seclusiveness, avoidance of close, competitive relationships. Autistic thinking without loss of reality testing: daydreaming, rich fantasy life. React to events with apparent detachment. Inability to express ordinary aggressive feelings.
301.3	Explosive	Gross outbursts of rage, verbal or physical. Strikingly different from patient's customary behavior and he may be repentant later. Excitable. Over-reactors. If amnesic for the event diagnosis is hysterical neurosis.
301.4	Obsessive-compulsive	Rigid, overconscientious, overdutiful, inhibited, unable to relax.
301.5	Hysterical	Self-dramatization which is attention-seeking and often seductive. Excitable, instable, overreactivity. Self-centered, immature, vain, usually dependent on others.
301.6	Asthenic	Easy fatigability, low energy level, lack of enthusiasm, incapacity for enjoyment, oversensitive to stress.
301.7	Antisocial	Grossly selfish, callous, irresponsible, impulsive. Lack of guilt. Unable to learn from experience and punishment. Repeatedly in conflict with society although repeated legal or social offenses alone not sufficient to make this diagnosis. Low frustration tolerance. Blame others or offer plausible rationalizations for their behavior. Incapable of significant loyalty.
301.81 *	Passive-aggressive	Aggressiveness expressed passively by obstructionism, procrastination, intentional inefficiency, stubbornness. Reflects hostility which person feels he dare not express openly. Often expression of resentment at failure to find gratification from person or institution upon which he is overdependent.
301.82 *	Inadequate	Ineffectual responses to emotional, social, intellectual and physical demands. Patient seems neither physically nor mentally deficient but manifests inadaptability, ineptness, poor judgment, instability, lack of physical or emotional stamina.
301.89 *	Other specified types	

Sexual Deviations

302.0	Homosexuality	Persons whose sexual interests are directed toward:
302.1	Fetishism	1. Objects other than people of opposite sex
302.2	Pedophilia	2. Sexual acts not usually associated with coitus
302.3	Transvestitism	3. Coitus performed under bizarre circumstances (necrophilia, pedophilia, sexual sadism, fetishism, etc.).
302.4	Exhibitionism	
302.5 *	Voyeurism	Persons may find their practices distasteful but are unable to substitute normal sexual behavior.
302.6 *	Sadism	
302.7 *	Masochism	Diagnosis not appropriate for persons who deviate because normal sexual objects are not available to them.
302.8	Other sexual deviation	

Alcoholism

303.0	Episodic excessive drinking	Intake is great enough to damage physical health, personal or social functioning; or, if it is a prerequisite to normal functioning. Alcoholism present. Intoxicated at least four times per year, i.e. person's coordination or speech is impaired or behavior is clearly altered.
303.1	Habitual excessive drinking	Alcoholism present. Intoxicated more than 12 times per year or under influence of alcohol more than once per week, even though not intoxicated.
303.2	Alcohol addiction	Direct or strong evidence of dependence Direct: Withdrawal symptoms Presumptive: Inability to go one day without drinking.
303.9	Other alcoholism	

Drug Dependence

304.0	Opium and derivatives	Evidence of habitual use or clear need for the drug.
304.1	Synthetic, morphine-like analgesics	Addiction or dependence on drugs other than alcohol, tobacco, ordinary caffeine, beverages. Medically prescribed drugs also excluded if it is medically indicated and intake is proportionate to the medical need.
304.2	Barbiturates	
304.3	Other hypnotics, sedatives, tranquilizers	
304.4	Cocaine	Withdrawal symptoms not necessary for diagnosis.
304.5	Marihuana, hashish	
304.6	Other psycho-stimulants	
304.7	Hallucinogens	
304.8	Other drug dependence	

TABLE I-I Continued

Code	Diagnosis	Description
	VI. PSYCHOPHYSIOLOGIC DISORDERS	
305.0	Skin	Neurodermatitis, pruritis, hyperhydrosis, etc.
305.1	Musculoskeletal	Tension headache, back ache, myalgia, etc.
305.2	Respiratory	Asthma, hyperventilation, hiccoughs, etc.
305.3	Cardiovascular	Migraine, paroxysmal tachycardia, hypertension, etc.
305.4	Hemic and lymphatic	
305.5	Gastrointestinal	Peptic ulcer, gastritis, ulcerative colitis, constipation, etc.
305.6	Genitourinary	Dysmenorrhea, dyspareunia, impotence, etc.
305.7	Endocrine	Specify the disturbance.
305.8	Organ of special sense	Exclude conversion reactions.
305.9	Other type	
	VII. SPECIAL SYMPTOMS	
306.0	Speech disturbance	The psychopathology is manifested by a single specific symptom.
306.1	Specific learning disturbance	
306.2	Tic	Example: Anorexia nervosa under feeding disturbance (306.5).
306.3	Other psychomotor disorder	Do not use these diagnoses if the symptom is result of organic ill-
306.4	Disorders of sleep	ness or other mental disorder.
306.5	Feeding disturbance	
306.6	Enuresis	
306.7	Encopresis	Example: anorexia nervosa due to schizophrenia is not included
306.8	Cephalalgia	here.
306.9	Other special symptoms	
	VIII. TRANSIENT SITUATIONAL DISTURBANCES	
		Transient disorders of any severity, including psychosis. Occur in persons without apparent underlying mental disorders. Acute reaction to overwhelming stress. Symptoms recede as stress diminishes. If not, another diagnosis indicated.
307.0 *	Adjustment reaction of infancy	Example: Separation from mother resulting in crying spells, withdrawal, loss of appetite, etc.

307.1 *	Adjustment reaction of childhood	Example: Birth of sibling resulting in enuresis, attention-getting behavior, etc.
307.2 *	Adjustment reaction of adolescence	Example: Temper outbursts, brooding, etc.
307.3 *	Adjustment reaction of adult life.	Example: Fear in military combat. Suicidal gesture associated with unwanted pregnancy, etc.
307.4 *	Adjustment reaction of late life.	Example: Withdrawal, resentment following forced retirement, etc.

IX. BEHAVIOR DISORDERS OF CHILDHOOD AND ADOLESCENCE

		Describes disorders that are more stable, internalized, and resistant to treatment than situational disturbances but less so than psychoses, neuroses, and personality disorders.
308.0 *	Hyperkinetic reaction	Characteristic manifestations: overactivity, inattentiveness, shyness, feeling of rejection, overaggressiveness, timidity, delinquency. Overactive, restless, distractible, short attention span. Classify as organic if due to OBS.
308.1 *	Withdrawing reaction	Inability to form close relationships, seclusive, detached, shy, sensitive, timid. If stabilizes may later be diagnosed as schizoid personality.
308.2 *	Overanxious reaction	Chronic anxiety, excessive and unrealistic fears. Insomnia, nightmares. Immature, self-conscious, lacking in self-confidence, inhibited, approval-seeking, apprehensive. Exaggerated autonomic responses.
308.3 *	Runaway reaction	Escape from threat by running away. Often steal furtively. Immature, timid, feel rejected and friendless.
308.4 *	Unsocialized aggressive reaction	Overt covert disobedience, quarrelsome, physical and verbal aggression, vengeful, temper tantrums, destructive, solitary stealing, lying, hostile teasing.
308.5 *	Group delinquent reaction	Has acquired values and behavior of delinquent peer group to whom patient is loyal.
308.9 *	Other reactions	Steal, skip school, stay out late, shoplift, etc; specify other reactions.

X. CONDITIONS WITHOUT MANIFEST PSYCHIATRIC DISORDER AND NON-SPECIFIC CONDITIONS

| Social Maladjustment Without Manifest Psychiatric Disorder | These individuals are psychiatrically normal but encounter severe enough problems to warrant psychiatric consultation. |

TABLE I-I Continued

Code	Diagnosis	Description
316.0 *	Marital maladjustment	Conflict in marriage.
316.1 **	Social maladjustment	Culture shock or conflict arising from divided loyalties to two cultures.
316.2 **	Occupational maladjustment	Grossly maladjusted in work.
316.3 **	Dyssocial behavior	Not classifiable as antisocial personality but are predatory and follow more or less criminal pursuits.
		Examples: Dope peddlers, racketeers, dishonest gamblers, prostitutes.
		Other.
317 *	Nonspecific conditions	After psychiatric exam no preceding disorder is found.
318 **	No mental disorder	Not to be used if a disorder is in remission.

XI. NON-DIAGNOSTIC TERMS FOR ADMINISTRATIVE USE

Code	Diagnosis	Description
319.0 *	Diagnosis deferred	
319.1 **	Boarder	
319.2 **	Experiment only	
319.9 **	Other	

3. Ambivalence
4. Autism

The "4A's" were considered by Bleuler to be virtually pathognomonic for schizophrenia, yet their presence or absence cannot be entirely relied upon when attempting to evaluate a patient.

Spitzer and Endicott (*Schizophrenia*, New York, Medcom, Inc., 1971) point out, for example, that there are some cases in which none of the 4A's can be demonstrated, but the presence of some practically pathognomonic *secondary* symptoms clearly establishes the diagnosis.

The following tables, adapted from the work of Spitzer and Endicott, are presented to aid the reader in making the diagnosis of schizophrenia with greater precision.

Table I-II (Diagnostic Value of Different Symptomatology in Schizophrenia) outlines both primary and secondary features of schizophrenia and suggests the amount of diagnostic importance or weight that should be attached to any particular symptom.

Table I-III (Major Differential Diagnoses of Schizophrenia Subtypes) contrasts the most common subtypes of schizophrenia (paranoid, catatonic, etc.) with certain other nonschizophrenic entities that, under certain conditions, may be confused with schizophrenia.

DIFFERENTIAL DIAGNOSIS:
ORGANIC PSYCHOSIS VS. FUNCTIONAL PSYCHOSIS
A. KEITH W. BROWNELL, M.D.

The psychiatrist who is faced with the problem of distinguishing organic psychosis from functional psychosis stands at the crossroads of medicine, neurology, and psychiatry. He must in the course of performing a careful psychiatric examination, be cognizant of the cardinal features of the organic psychoses and, in some settings, he may be required himself to perform a general medical and neurological examination.

Table I-IV (Differential Diagnosis: Organic Psychosis vs. Functional Psychosis) provides general guidelines for dis-

TABLE I-II
DIAGNOSTIC VALUE OF DIFFERENT SYMPTOMATOLOGY
IN SCHIZOPHRENIA
(Reprinted with permission: *Schizophrenia,* Medcom, Inc., New York, 1971)

Symptom	Definition	Diagnostic Weight
A. Symptomatology practically pathognomonic of schizophrenia. When present, the diagnosis is extremely likely.		
Flat affect	Generalized impoverishment of emotional reactivity. Impassive face, monotous voice.	Very common in schizophrenia. Distinguish from shallow affect of organics and hysterics, and constricted affect of obsessional personality.
Thought disorder	Tendency of the associations to lose their continuity so that thinking becomes confused, bizarre, incorrect and abrupt.	Very common in schizophrenia. Most diagnostic when found in a setting of clear consciousness. Distinguish from looseness of associations as found in manic states, and from dull intelligence and poor education.
Delusions of influence or passivity	Delusional belief that thoughts, moods or actions are controlled or mysteriously influenced by other people or by strange forces.	Unusual in schizophrenia but present in no other condition.
Hallucinations of thoughts being broadcast or spoken aloud.		Unusual in schizophrenia but present in no other condition.
Delusions that everyone knows what the patient is thinking.		Unusual in schizophrenia but present in no other condition.
Specific catatonic symptoms Rigidity Waxy flexibility Posturing	Maintenance of a rigid posture against efforts to be moved. Maintenance of postures (e.g., if arm is raised, patient wlll leave it elevated). Voluntary assumption of inappropriate or bizarre postures.	Occasionally seen in schizophrenia, particularly during acute catatonic episodes or in regressed patients who have been hospitalized for many years. Similar behavior is sometimes associated with organic brain disease.
B. Symptomatology seen in schizophrenia and rarely in other conditions. When present the diagnosis is very likely.		
Apathy	Lack of feeling, interest, concern or emotion.	Common in schizophrenia. Of diagnostic value only if not due to depressive syndrome.

TABLE I-II Continued

Symptom	Definition	Diagnostic Weight
Inappropriate affect	Affect which is incongruous in light of situation or content of thought.	Common in schizophrenia. Rule out manic, hysterical or organic disorder.
Autism	Persistent tendency to withdraw from involvement with the external world and to become preoccupied with ideas and fantasies, illogical and in which objective facts tend to be obscured, distorted or excluded.	Common in schizophrenia. Rule out identification with a cultural subgroup which has deviant beliefs, as well as temporary withdrawal and preoccupation with fantasy life.
Catatonic stupor	Marked decrease in reactivity to environment and reduction of spontaneous movements and activity. Patient appears unaware of nature of surroundings, but generally is very aware.	Common in catatonic schizophrenia. Rule out organic brain disease, depressive disorder or hysteria.
Neologisms	Invention of new words.	Unusual in schizophrenia, but practically nonexistent in other conditions. Very suggestive of schizophrenia when accompanied by indifference to being understood.
Catatonic excitement	Apparently purposeless and stereotyped excited motor activity not influenced by external stimuli.	Rule out manic or hysterical excitement which is more purposeful and responsive to external stimuli.
Bodily hallucinations	False sensory impression experienced in the body. Example: Patient feels electricity is being sent through him.	Rare in schizophrenia. Very diagnostic when associated with persecutory delusions.
Auditory hallucinations	False sensory impression of sound.	Common in schizophrenia. Most diagnostic when voices. Unusual but present in affective psychoses and organic psychoses, particularly alcoholic hallucinosis.

C. Symptomatology commonly seen in schizophrenia and other conditions. When present the diagnosis is likely.

Delusions	Conviction in some important personal belief which is almost certainly not true and is resistant to modification.	Rule out organic and other functional psychoses. In affective psychoses the content of the delusion is in harmony with the disordered mood. Bizarre, incomprehensible or fragmentary delusions are more suggestive of schizophrenia.

TABLE I-II Continued

Symptom	Definition	Diagnostic Weight
Hallucinations	Sensory impression in the absence of external stimuli; occurs during the waking state.	Rule out organic and functional psychoses. When patient exhibits an inadequate emotional reaction, it suggests schizophrenia.
Inappropriate or bizarre behavior.	Behavior that is odd, eccentric or not in keeping with the situation.	Rule out organic and functional psychoses. The more incomprehensible the behavior, the more likely is schizophrenia.
Extreme social isolation	Avoidance of contact or involvement with people.	Also common in alcoholism, schizoid personality and depressive illnesses.
Markedly unstable interpersonal relationships.	Relationships with relatives, friends and associates tend to be stormy and ambivalent. Minor difficulties lead to anger and disruption of the relationship.	Also common in hysterical and paranoid personalities. The more chaotic the history of relationships, the more suggestive of schizophrenia.
Ideas of Reference	Detection of personal reference in seemingly insignificant remarks, objects or events. May be of sufficient intensity to be a delusion. Example: Patient interprets a person's sneeze as a message.	Rule out other psychoses. Occasionally seen in suspicious people who are not otherwise psychotic.
Poor academic and occupational adjustment		Present in all other conditions. Is more suggestive of schizophrenia when variable over period of time and there is a marked discrepancy between level of functioning and background or previous achivements.
Excessive concern with body symptoms	Includes preoccupation with real or imagined physical appearance; fears of becoming ill; health rituals.	Rule out depressive illness and hypochondriacal neurosis. Bizarre or incomprehensible complaints or beliefs are suggestive of schizophrenia.

TABLE I-III

MAJOR DIFFERENTIAL DIAGNOSES OF SCHIZOPHRENIA SUBTYPES
(Reprinted with permission: *Schizophrenia*, Medcom, Inc., New York, 1971)

Schizophrenia Subtype	*Differential Diagnosis*
Paranoid	1. Involutional paranoid state 2. Paranoia 3. Amphetamine-toxic psychosis 4. Paranoid personality
Simple	1. Schizoid personality
Childhood	1. Behavior disorders of childhood and adolescence 2. Withdrawing reaction
Schizoaffective	1. Manic-depressive, manic 2. Psychotic depression 3. Cyclothymic personality
Latent	1. Severe neurosis 2. Severe personality disorder
Catatonic	1. Retarded depression
Chronic undifferentiated	1. Chronic organic brain syndrome 2. Chronic use of stimulants or hallucinogens
Acute schizophrenic episode	1. Severe transient situational disturbance 2. Acute organic brain syndrome

tinguishing organic psychosis from functional psychosis. In addition, the reader may refer to Chapter VIII, Neurology for Psychiatrists; Chapter VII, Psychiatry in Medicine; and Chapter X, The Psychiatrist's Role in the Diagnosis and Treatment of Drug Abuse.

DIFFERENTIAL DIAGNOSIS:
FIVE MAJOR TYPES OF DRUG ABUSE (HALLUCINOGENS, CNS STIMULANTS, CNS DEPRESSANTS, MARIJUANA, NARCOTICS) VS. ACUTE SCHIZOPHRENIA, ACUTE MANIA, HALLUCINOSIS

H. J. SCHULTE, M.D.

Acute intoxication by either of the five most commonly abused classes of drugs (hallucinogens, CNS stimulants, CNS depressants, marijuana, and narcotics) may mimic certain psychiatric disorders, most notably acute schizophrenia, acute mania, and hallucinosis.

TABLE I-IV

DIFFERENTIAL DIAGNOSIS:
ORGANIC PSYCHOSIS vs. FUNCTIONAL PSYCHOSIS

	Organic Brain Syndrome	*Functional Psychoses*
1. Etiology	a. Trauma b. Metabolic (hypoglycemia, diabetes, liver disease, thyroid disease, chronic lung disease, etc.) c. Toxins (alcohol, amphetamines, hallucinogens, digitalis, etc.) d. Encephalitis e. Convulsive disorders f. Vitamin deficiencies g. Dementia (presenile and senile) h. CNS tumors	a. Schizophrenia b. Involutional melancholia c. Manic-depressive psychosis d. Paranoia e. Involutional paranoid state f. Psychotic depressive reaction
2. Past History	Positive for trauma, drug ingestion, metabolic disease, recent infection, exposure to toxins, etc.	Frequently positive for previous psychiatric disease; psychiatric disturbance in early mother-child relationship.
3. Family History	May be positive in case of metabolic disease, dementia, infections, etc.	Frequently positive for psychopathology but of little diagnostic value.
4. Precipitating Factors	Ingestion, infection, trauma, failure to take anti-convulsants, etc.	Environmental stress
5. Level of consciousness	More likely to be impaired	Unlikely to be impaired
6. Orientation to time, place and person	Frequently impaired	Not impaired unless delusional
7. Recent memory	Frequently impaired	Not usually impaired unless delusional distortion
8. Repetition of lists of numbers forward and backward	Frequently impaired	Not usually impaired
9. Remote memory	Less impaired	Not usually impaired
10. Proverb interpretation	Frequently impaired	Varies from not impaired to bizarre
11. Similarities and differences	Frequently impaired	Varies from not impaired to bizarre
12. Nominal aphasia	Frequently present	Absent
13. Constructional apraxia	Frequently present	Absent

TABLE I-IV Continued

	Organic Brain Syndrome	Functional Psychoses
14. Catatonia	Unlikely	More likely
15. Hallucinations	Most frequently visual	Most frequently auditory
16. Focal Neuro- logic Signs	May be present	Absent
17. Asterixis	May be present	Absent
18. Primitive Reflexes (suck, snout, grasp)	May be present	Absent
19. Laboratory values	May be abnormal	Normal
20. EEG	Usually abnormal	Normal

With the present day prevalence of drug abuse, the differential diagnosis of these entities has become a commonplace clinical problem for the psychiatrist. Obviously, correct diagnosis in these cases is crucial to disposition and treatment planning.

Table I-V (Differential Diagnosis: Five Major Types of Drug Abuse vs. Three Psychiatric Entities) outlines certain diagnostic criteria to aid the psychiatrist in this task.

For further information on the five classes of drug abuse referred to in this table, the reader is referred to Chapter X, The Psychiatrist's Role in the Diagnosis and Treatment of Drug Abuse.

References

Krupp, M. A.; Chatton, M. J.; *et al.: Current Diagnosis and Treatment.* Los Altos, California, Lange Medical Pub., 1972.

Zarafonetis, C. J. D. (Ed.) : *Drug Abuse: Proceedings of the International Conference.* Philadelphia, Lea and Febiger, 1972.

DIFFERENTIAL DIAGNOSIS OF FOUR PSYCHIATRIC ENTITIES: CONVERSION SYMPTOM, HYPOCHONDRIASIS, SOMATIC DELUSION, MALINGERING

JOSEPH R. NOVELLO, M.D.

Psychosomatic complaints are common to many types of patients. The psychiatrist encounters such phenomena in

TABLE I-V

DIFFERENTIAL DIAGNOSIS: FIVE MAJOR TYPES OF DRUG ABUSE VS. THREE PSYCHIATRIC ENTITIES

	Hallucinogen Intoxication	CNS Stimulant Intoxication (Amphetamines)	CNS Depressant Intoxication (Sedative-Hypnotics)	Marijuana Intoxication	Narcotic Intoxication (Heroin and other opiates)	Acute Schizophrenia	Acute Mania	Hallucinosis
History:	Ingestion of hallucinogen.	Ingestion or I.V. use. Prior use, often in spurts (days-weeks) leading to a crash.	Often used in suicidal attempts. May be taken in successive doses; person unaware of amount ingested.	Ingestion or Inhalation.	Previous heorin or other drug use. Variability in street sample strength may lead to inadvertent overdose.	Previous psychotic episode. Often unusual, bizarre or seclusive type people. May have ingested an hallucinogen which precipitates a prolonged reaction.	History of excessive mood swings.	Preceding period of alcohol spree, followed by withdrawal. Also after use of amphetamines, cocaine or volatile hydrocarbons (glue).
Course:	Onset in ½ hour; duration depends on substance: 3 to 12 hours. Secondary effects may last longer.	Dose and route dependent. Some symptoms may persist for months after abstinence.	Onset sudden; lasts from a few hours to a few days depending on drug used.	Onset in 15 to 30 minutes. Dose dependent.	Onset sudden. Persists for 4 to 8 hours. Methadone intoxication persists for 8 to 12 hours.	Onset gradual; or may be relatively abrupt. Person remains disturbed longer.	Onset gradual, remains disturbed longer.	Onset gradual, often preceded by period of apprehension. Variable course depending on drug taken in previous history: hours with glue, a week with amphetamine, days with alcohol.

Behavior:	Variable: from withdrawal to eruptive. Reality distortion may lead to accidents, suicide, homicide.	Dose-dependent. Hyperactive outbursts possible (assault, suicide). Repetitive, pointless activities.	Ranges from drowsiness to coma. Acts drunk; in stimulating environment it can act as a transient stimulant.	Ranges from drowsiness (nodding) to coma with overdose. Restless, irritable during early withdrawal.	Variable. Often preoccupied and/or emotionally labile.	Extremely hyperactive and very talkative. Unable to complete tasks.	Unpredictable. Potentially violent or self-destructive.
Thought:	Confusion about reality. Usually oriented to person, time, place. Chronic abuse can lead to difficulty with memory and concentration.	Racing associations which seem to make sense. Oriented in mild intoxication. Amphetamine psychosis (Chronic users) appear like paranoid schizophrenia.	Depressive preoccupation possible; mild to moderate confusion and disorientation generally dulled.	During high; thought processes obtunded. In early withdrawal preoccupation with obtaining next dose.	Disorder in logical thinking. Concrete thinking; associations may be bizarre, loose, tangential.	Racing associations, make sense but tangential, irrelevant. Oriented.	Thoughts of persecution and danger. May be disoriented.
Affect:	Highly labile. Panic reaction or bliss. Depends on environment and previous psychological makeup.	Labile. Early euphoria proceeds to anxious, tense. Blunting occurs.	Generally dulled.	Euphoria during high stage. As withdrawal progresses, tense, anxious.	Highly labile. Inappropriate to the situation.	Tense, anxious, euphoria.	Depends on delusional content: fear, rage, panic, quietness.

TABLE I-V Continued

	Hallucinogen Intoxication	CNS Stimulant Intoxication (Amphetamines)	CNS Depressant Intoxication (Sedative-Hypnotics)	Marijuana Intoxication	Narcotic Intoxication (Heroin and other opiates)	Acute Schizophrenia	Acute Mania	Hallucinosis
Hallucinations	All sensory modalities, mostly visual; not part of environment. May see body image distortions.	Dreamlike. Can be recognized as unreal.				Usually auditory, often related to reality.	Not pronounced.	Usually vivid, auditory.
Delusions	Paranoid preoccupation. Fear of going insane or may think body is changing in bizarre fashion.	About real-life issues; e.g. "police are following me."		Rare; paranoia can occur.		Bizarre, religious, magical or fantasy.	Ideas of grandeur and omnipotence.	Delusions are not systematized but may be consistent with real events; e.g. criminal record and police after him.
Laboratory		Serum, urine assay for amphetamine.	Serum level of barbiturates.		Opiates in urine.			

(Table I-V adapted from Krupp, 1972 and Zarafonetis, 1972)

many settings ranging from the patient who voluntarily seeks psychotherapy because of a physical complaint to evaluation of the more involuntary patient who steadfastly maintains that his symptom is entirely on a physical basis in spite of over-whelming evidence to the contrary.

The continuum of psychosomatic complaints stretches across the entire diagnostic landscape of psychiatry. Patients may range from *normal* (anxiety or fear associated with bona fide medical illness) to *neurotic* (hysterical conversion symptoms, hypochondriasis) to *character disorder* (malinger-ing) and even to *psychosis* (somatic delusion). To make matters even more complex, the differences are not always absolute. For example, it is not uncommon to find many hysterical traits in malingerers or to discover near-conscious dramatic play acting in the hysterical patient.

Definitions:

1. Conversion Symptom: A symptom that originates in the mind but is expressed and experienced as a physical symp-tom. An unacceptable idea, wish, or fantasy is defended against by "conversion" into a bodily symptom. The choice of the specific symptom is based upon its suitability to represent symbolically the particular idea, wish, or fan-tasy that is incapable of being fulfilled. The resulting conversion has four aims: (1) to permit expression of the forbidden wish, nevertheless, in a disguised form that is not recognizable by the patient, (2) to impose punishment through suffering and thereby atone for the guilt associated with the wish, (3) to remove the patient from a threaten-ing or disturbing life situation, (4) to provide a new mode of relating i.e. the sick role as a medical patient, a role that is sanctioned by society. The conversion symptom, therefore, is adaptive in that the patient successfully blocks from awareness the unacceptable wish (primary gain) and, at the same time, enjoys a substitute gratifica-tion as a medically ill person (secondary gain). The con-version symptom is working most effectively, therefore,

TABLE I-VI

MAJOR DIFFERENTIAL FEATURES OF CONVERSION SYMPTOMS, HYPOCHONDRIASIS, SOMATIC DELUSION, AND MALINGERING

	Conversion Symptoms	Hypochondriasis	Somatic Delusions	Malingering
1. Physical Appearance of Patient	Often stylish bordering on the garrish. Seductive, appealing, in spite of potentially serious medical symptom.	Usual forelorn, sad sack appearance.	From relatively normal appearance to bizzare.	Unremarkable.
2. Sex of Patient	Usually female.	Male or female.	Male or female.	Males appear to predominate.
3. Mannerisms of Patient	Calls attention to self in dramatic or provocative manner. Histrionic quality to history-giving. May be seductive.	Tired, run-down appearance. Slow movements. Appear drained of energy. Not engaging, dramatic or seductive. Appears genuinely fearful.	Often agitated, bizarre, psychotic mannerism. May be disoriented, hallucinating.	Concerned about symptom but unfriendly, distant, suspicious, secretive. May appear grim and even hositle.
4. Social-Economic-Educational Level of Patient	The most bizarre conversion symptoms (hysterical blindness, paralysis, etc.) are generally limited to lower social classes. Other less bizarre symptoms (pain, hyperventilation, dysphagia) are seen in all societal levels.	Not limited to any particular socioeconomic group.	Not limited to any particular socioeconomic group.	Many successful malingerers have paramedical backgrounds (RN's, aides, corpsmen, etc.) that allow them to simulate known diseases.
5. Suggestibility	Generally high, especially among lower socioeconomic groups that lack psychiatric sophistication.	Reassurance, suggestion, patently fail to afford relief.	Delusion is product of primary process thinking. Reassurance, suggestion fail.	Suggestion does not work with this class of patient.

6. Psychiatric Diagnostic Category of Patient	Hysterical personality; hysterical neurosis, conversion type; may be seen in other basic personality types as well.	Originally Freud considered it one of the actual neuroses. At this time it is not included specifically in the official diagnostic compendium (USA). Generally thought to be closely related to neurasthenia. Can be included under psychophysiologic nervous system reaction.	Psychotic; usually schizophrenia, paranoid type. May see in organic psychosis especially with hallucinogens, amphetamines.	Character disorders; often sociopathic, passive-aggressive.
7. How the Patient Comes to Medical Attention	Few self-referred patients with conversion symptoms are genuinely motivated for cure. Seeking the sick-role and the resulting 2° gain is important in the dynamics of the symptom formation in the first place.	Self-referred patient genuinely believes he is suffering serious or fatal disease. His alarm takes him from one physician to another.	Rarely self-referred. Usually brought by relative or friend who is aware that patient is psychotic. Often emergency basis.	Often sent to physician after claiming privileges in institutional setting on basis of being sick (military, prisons, industry, etc.); personal injury litigation, compensation; prolonging convalescence after a bona-fide illness or injury; insanity plea by accused criminals.
8. Attitude Toward Physician	Hungry for attention, especially some sort of praise. Will, to this end, praise and idealize the physician; this continues only as long as the physician, in turn, gives the patient admiration and perpetuates the myth of the patient being physically ill.	Dependence, usually relate to physician as unquestioned authority figure until he reports a negative workup. Then go to another physician.	Patient is consumed by his symptom and psychosis, no significant relationship to physician. May be tremendously frightened.	Hostile, suspicious. More sociopathic individuals are apt to adopt fawning praise of the physician and to convince physician that he is rarely sick and does not like to bother busy MD's, etc.

TABLE I-VI continued

	Conversion Symptoms	Hypochondriasis	Somatic Delusions	Malingering
9. Attitude of Physician Toward Patient	Physicians, especially those vulnerable to fantasies of omnipotence etc., may fall prey to these patients, especially if patient is of the opposite sex. At first these patients have a most appealing or seductive charm. Later they are seen as demanding or manipulating.	Physicians quickly identify these patients as crocks. Most MD's shun these patients and, by many conscious and unconscious means, succeed in alienating them.	Most medical physicians recognize the psychosis immediately and refer to psychiatrist on emergency basis.	Physicians generally have high index of suspicion for malingering and probably overdiagnose it (mistaking conversion and hypochondriasis often). Disdain, hostility.
10. Type of symptom	Wide range. Most bizarre include conversion blindness, seizures, coma, syncope, aphonia, paralysis, gait disturbances. Other common symptoms include conversion pain, hyperventilation, weakness, fatigue, dysphagia, globus hystericus, urinary symptoms, dyspareunia.	Most common general symptom is fatigue, malaise. Other symptoms are likely to be vague. Also, overconcern, i.e. insignificant findings such as skin blemishes, sebaceous cysts, etc.	Usually very bizarre: ("My eyes are falling out," "My foot is on fire," "My hand is turning to jello") etc.	Wide range. Likely to closely resemble a classic textbook version of an illness or injury. Some patients go to extreme of pricking finger and placing drop of blood in urine, factitial ulcerations, etc.
11. Manner In Which The Symptom Is Reported	Matter-of-factly; la belle indifference; may feign concern but it lacks genuine quality.	Alarm and concern.	Usually tremendous fear.	Concern. Physician should listen closely for a pay off i.e. if patient thinks MD is unaware of what he really wants, patient may add: "And, of course, I can't work today"...or something of the sort.

12. Consistency of Symptom with Anatomical Fact, Physiology, or Known Medical Illness	Some symptoms (stocking-glove anesthesia, etc.) are patently bizarre and impossible on physical basis. Others may be in realm of bona-fide medical symptom but careful questioning usually uncovers some inconsistencies. Diagnosis, therefore, usually possible by history alone.	The concern is usually centered upon a bona-fide medical symptom that requires examination.	Bizarre, psychotic symptoms, little or no relation to real medical symptomatology.	Most likely to closely resemble a classic textbook description of a real illness or injury.
13. Chronicity of the Symptom	Tend to be acute and time-limited for any particular symptom but patient usually has history of having had several conversion symptoms of various types in the past. May experience sporadic recurrence of the same symptom.	Tends to chronicity.	Acute.	Acute. Determined by some environmental factor (avoid work, lawsuit, etc.)
14. Primary Gain (i.e. Symptom exists primarily to block from conscious awareness an unacceptable wish)	Present. A hallmark of conversion.	Cannot be as aptly demonstrated as in conversion symptoms. Patients often masochistic, turning of aggression against the self.	Symptom may be metaphorically related to an unconscious conflict but is not crucial to causation of the symptom as in conversion. No primary gain in the usual sense from the symptom itself as in conversion.	Not a factor. Munchausen's syndrome is complex and is probably more on intrapsychic basis than customary malingering.

TABLE I-VI continued

	Conversion Symptoms	Hypochondriasis	Somatic Delusions	Malingering
15. Secondary Gain (i.e. adopts medically "sick" role which may have certain benefits, i.e. removes from stress, manipulate others, and is socially acceptable.)	Present. A hallmark of conversion.	Not as flagrant as in conversion. Is a more established life-role as sick.	Not a factor.	Is the primary motivation for the symptom production.
16. Symptom Precipitated by Psychological Stress	Present. A hallmark of conversion.	Not as apparent as in conversion, since symptom production is not acute.	Psychosis (as in acute schizophrenia) may be precipitated by stress but symptom itself follows later.	Psychological stress plays minimal part.
17. Environmental Factors	Although environmental stress may be present, the crucial conflict is intrapsychic and ultimate diagnosis is made on psychodynamic basis.	May be important but the major conflict is intrapsychic.	Drug-taking in organic psychosis. Also toxins, medical illness, etc. Stress may be a factor in schizophrenia.	Symptom is elaborated in order to get something from the environment. This aspect must be closely examined in diagnosis. Any manipulation? Litigation? Is patient an addict after narcotics?, etc.
18. Attitude Toward Further Diagnostic Procedures	Generally compliant but no eagerness to get to the bottom of it. May stress his ability to live with the symptom.	Patient's great concern leads to eagerness for diagnosis and treatment. Patient's attitude: "I can't go on like this."	Acute psychosis may interfere with patient's ability to cooperate.	Suspicious. May resist, particularly if patient believes that further testing may unmask his ruse.

19. Attitude Toward Suggestion of Psychiatric Referral	The most highly-defended patients will resist. Some will get angry at the suggestion and leave the first medical physician for another; (this may be repeated several times). Requires skillful and emphatic referral technique on part of physician.	If handled skillfully by physician these generally complaint-sufferers will agree to referral especially if their disease is given a scientific-sounding name. (At last they have something and are going to receive treatment.)	Will accept easily if suggestion is made with reference to helping patient and allaying his overwhelming fear.	Will resist unless he has gone beyond point of no return (as in compensation case or personal injury suit); then will accept, grudgingly.
20. Attitude Toward Consultant Psychiatrist	Even those who follow-through with visit to psychiatrist will resist therapeutic efforts. If symptom is working well i.e. firm 1° gain (no anxiety) and gratifying 2° gain, likelihood of patient wanting therapy is very poor. When either begins to crumble, patient becomes more motivated for psychotherapy. Recapitulation of familiar mode of relating: Charm, drama, seduction, etc.	Long-suffering appearance. Doubtful, yet hopeful, of cure.	Acute psychosis may interfere with patient's ability to cooperate in extended interview but he is driven to talk of his delusion.	Hostile, uncooperative. Sociopaths may be clever and appear genuinely concerned.

TABLE I-VI continued

	Conversion Symptoms	Hypochondriasis	Somatic Delusions	Malingering
21. Cardinal Features of Diagnosis	1. Symptom produced by psychological stress. 2. Therapeutic uncovering of the dynamic determinants of the particular symptom choice. 3. Primary and secondary gain. 4. La-belle indifference. 5. Hysterical personality. 6. Symptom inconsistent with anatomical, physiological possibilities.	1. Overconcern regarding a real (but often vague) symptom. 2. Depressed, apathetic appearance in contrast to hysteric; but no psychosis as in somatic delusion. 3. Usually long-established life-style and not seeking obvious gain as in malingering.	1. Existence of psychosis. 2. Bizarre complaints.	1. Patient must be always on guard, which is very difficult. Hospitalize patient and arrange for him to be observed unobtrusively. He may well let down his guard (As the crippled patient with low back pain who bounds out of bed to get a cigarette as soon as his door is closed.) 2. Substituting a placebo and eliciting patient's response is not a reliable diagnostic test of malingering (conversion hysterics and some hypochondriacs are notably suggestable and may react with symptom alleviation on this basis). Also, this leads to further mistrust and alienation. 3. Diagnosis may be difficult. Consultant may have to proceed to diagnosis of exclusion after first ruling out all other entities. Even then diagnosis may be somewhat uncertain. Ultimate diagnosic clue is if patient himself admits that he is indeed malingering; not often encountered.

if the patient is free of anxiety and this accounts for the customary indifference to the symptom itself, no matter how dramatic it might be (la belle indifference).

2. Hypochondriasis: The chronic habit pattern of physical complaints. Hypochondriacal patients exhibit somatic overconcern, exaggerated reporting of bodily sensations and physical complaints no matter how trivial. Typically, the patient believes these symptoms to be manifestations of serious or grave illnesses. This is often encountered in masochistic characters, psychodynamically representing a returning of agression against the self.

3. Somatic Delusion: Bizarre physical complaints elaborated by psychotic patients. Not generally a difficult diagnostic problem because of the patently delusional quality of the complaint (stomach "exploding," "insects under the skin," etc.).

4. Malingering: The conscious simulation of illness or injury with the intent to deceive. The malingerer usually has something to gain by being sick, i.e. the accused criminal feigning insanity as a defense, personal injury suits, compensation cases, military settings where the person may want to avoid further active duty or to avoid an undesirable assignment. Successful malingering requires careful knowledge of the injury or illness being feigned. The symptom, unlike the three cases above, may therefore closely approximate the textbook description. Munchausen's Syndrome is a special form of malingering; these people are so-called hospital hoboes who present themselves in clinics and emergency rooms often simulating serious, acute illness. They submit eagerly to dangerous diagnostic procedures and even major surgery but typically flee the hospital if their ruse is about to be discovered.

Table I-VI (Major Differential Features of Conversion Symptoms, Hypochondriasis, Somatic Delusion, and Malingering) is designed to aid the psychiatrist in the diagnosis of these four entities.

References

Abse, D. W.: *Hysteria and Related Mental Disorders.* Baltimore, Williams and Wilkins, 1966.

Engel, G. L.: Conversion Symptoms. In MacBryde, C. M. (Ed.) : *Signs and Symptoms: Applied Physiology and Clinical Interpretation.* Philadelphia, Lippincott, 1969.

Fenichel, O.: *The Psychoanalytic Theory of Neurosis.* New York, Norton, 1945.

Freedman, A. M. and Kaplan, H. I.: *Comprehensive Textbook of Psychiatry.* Baltimore, Williams and Wilkins, 1967.

Hinsie, L. E. and Campbell, R. J.: *Psychiatric Dictionary.* New York, Oxford University Press, 1970.

Chapter II

GENERAL PSYCHIATRIC EVALUATION

THE SINGLE MOST IMPORTANT diagnostic tool utilized by the psychiatrist is his own skillful technique in clinical interviewing. This skill, of course, comes through years of formal training and experience. While this handbook cannot be a substitute for the expertise that comes only through such experience, it does aim, in this chapter, to provide the psychiatrist with some useful guidelines that will assist him in organizing and conceptualizing the data that he gathers in the psychiatric interview.

The Psychiatric History and Mental Status Exam serves as a check-list of the items that are generally required in a complete psychiatric evaluation.

The second article, Assessment of Ego Function, provides a framework for conceptualizing the data. It approaches the material from the perspective of ego-psychology.

Mechanisms of Ego Defense is an article that adds another dimension to the psychiatric evaluation. It provides two separate systems for considering the defensive or coping mechanisms of the ego.

The fourth article, The Psychoanalytic Assessment, is an overview of the psychoanalytic schema of psychological growth and development. It is a handy reference for psychiatrists who prefer to base their conceptualizations upon the dynamic, psychoanalytic foundation. As presented, it can be used for children, adolescents, or adults.

The final article, Sullivan's 15 Questions Regarding the

Initial Psychiatric Interview, is based upon the work of Harry Stack Sullivan. It lists 15 questions that he suggested every psychiatrist ask himself after he has conducted an initial interview. If all can be answered adequately, the psychiatrist can be certain that he has performed a skillful, thoroughly professional evaluation.

THE PSYCHIATRIC HISTORY AND MENTAL STATUS EXAMINATION

JOSEPH R. NOVELLO, M.D.

The following outline is intended as a reasonably complete compendium of the kind of data that is required in the psychiatric history. In many cases the examiner will not require such a detailed history from the patient. In these cases the examiner may adapt the outline to his own special needs. Similarly, the outline may be adapted for use with both inpatients and outpatients by making suitable deletions and additions.

1. Patient's Name: Date:
2. Patient's Registration Number:
3. Name of Dictating Physician:
4. Referral Source
   (list address for ease of future correspondence)
5. General Introduction: A short, concise statement of the problem and the circumstances surrounding the patient's referral or hospitalization. List both the manifest (obvious) reasons for referral and the examiner's assessment of any latent (hidden) reasons. Also include identifying data: patient's name, age, sex, race, marital status, occupation, and other pertinent information.
6. Informant (s) :
   a. How reliable is the source?
   b. List any documents that are available as sources of information.
7. Previous Emotional Disability
   a. Hospitalizations
   b. Outpatient treatment and type (including tranquilizers by personal physician)

    c. Past emotional disability for which patient did *not* seek treatment
8. Present Emotional Disability
    a. Detailed discussion of present situation and precipitants
9. Biographical Data
    a. Date of birth, place of birth
    b. Prenatal History
       1. Was the patient planned for and desired by his parents?
       2. Illegitimacy?
       3. Any medical complications of the pregnancy?
       4. Any significant events during the pregnancy that might have altered the parents' attitude toward the child at birth?
    c. Neonatal History
       1. Features of labor and delivery
       2. Any hypoxia or trauma at birth?
    d. Earliest Memory
       1. Patient's recollection of his earliest memory. Describe content and affect in detail. May also include earliest memory of mother, earliest memory of father, happiest memory, saddest memory, etc.
    e. Childhood History
       1. Patient's overall feeling about what his childhood was like.
       2. What kind of child was the patient?
       3. Family situation, i.e. describe constellation
       4. Mother, describe re: relationship with the patient
       5. Father, describe especially re: relationship with patient
       6. Parental Relationship: i.e. what was the parents' marriage like?
       7. Siblings: description, relationships
       8. Other significant adults
       9. Other significant peers
      10. Motor milestones, especially important in cases of organicity

11. Feeding: any difficulties in feeding (possibly disturbed infant-maternal relationship)
12. Sleep: describe sleep pattern, especially any changes at six months, one year. What was reaction of parents if infant awoke crying? i.e. feed him, cuddle him, take him into parental bed?
13. Separation from mother in early infancy. At what age? For how long? Describe circumstances. Who cared for infant during the absence? Describe this person.
14. Recurrent dreams, nightmares. Describe.
15. Toilet training
16. Bed wetting, soiling
17. Speech problems
18. Tics
19. Tantrums
20. Illnesses, hospitalizations
21. Discipline: How? By whom? Successful?
22. Living arrangements in home? Describe especially the number of bedrooms, how occupied.

f. School History
1. How was it? What did patient like about it? Not like about it?
2. Grades, honors
3. Extracurricular activities
4. Friends
5. Teachers: describe general or specific relationships with teachers
6. Discipline: was patient a discipline problem?

g. Family History
1. Mother, current description: what has been her primary influence on patient?
2. Father: current description, influence, etc.
3. Siblings: current description, influence, etc.
4. History of emotional problems in any family member.
5. Significant or traumatic events in family life, especially loss of a loved one; patient's age at the time and his reaction to the event.

  6. Family's expectations for patient
  7. If more detailed information is required see Evaluation for Family Therapy, Chapter V.
h. Friends
  1. A description of the place of friends in the patient's life, past and present
  2. Sex preference in choosing friends
  3. With what kind of person is the patient most (least) comfortable?
  4. Attitude toward competition
i. Dating History
  1. Frequency, pattern, etc.
j. Sexual History
  1. Experience
  2. Masturbation, especially masturbatory fantasies
  3. Attitude of parents toward sex
  4. Attitude toward own body
  5. Which erogenous zone (s) gives the patient most pleasure
  6. Homosexual contact, fantasies
  7. If more detailed information is required, see Evaluation of Sexual Dysfunction, Chapter IV.
k. Marital History
  1. Previous divorce, separations
  2. Current marriage: describe
  3. Spouse: describe. Why did patient choose him/her for mate?
  4. What usually argue about
  5. Children: any problem children
  6. Psychiatric treatment: spouse or children
  7. If more detailed information required, see Evaluation for Marital Therapy, Chapter V.
l. Work History
  1. Present job, duration of employment, likes and dislikes
  2. Previous jobs: describe
  3. Ever fired? Why has patient left previous jobs?
  4. Relationship with bosses, co-workers
m. Military History

    1. Rank/rate at entry and discharge
    2. Attitude, relationships, etc.
    3. Type of discharge
    4. Disciplinary action? Describe.
n. Police Record
    1. Arrests, charges
    2. Contacts with police that did not actually result in arrest.
o. Accidents
    1. Accident prone?
p. Past Psychiatric Treatment
    1. Why, when, where, by whom, what type of treatment
    2. Patient's attitude and evaluation of that treatment
    3. What transference existed?
q. Alcohol and Drug Use/Abuse
r. Religion, "Philosophy of Life"
s. Favorite past time, hobbies
t. Future Plans
u. The Personified Self (from Sullivan, 1954)
    1. How does the patient handle stress, anxiety?
    2. What does the patient usually worry about?
    3. What does the patient think of self?
    4. What does the patient consider his strong points and weak points?
    5. What does the patient like (not like) about himself?
    6. What does the patient want to change?
v. Most Pleasant Experience
    1. Describe in detail the most pleasant experience that the patient has ever enjoyed.
w. Least Pleasant Experience
    1. Describe in detail the least pleasant experience that the patient can recall.
x. Influential People
    1. What person, living or dead, does the patient believe has been the best (and worst) influence on him. Why?
y. Other

      l. Anything to add that was not covered and that the patient thinks the interviewer should know about.

10. Past Medical History
    a. Significant medical/surgical illness
    b. Hospitalizations
    c. Surgical operations
    d. Allergies
    e. Current medication (s) , if any
11. Physical Examination
12. Psychiatric Examination
    a. General appearance, attitude, behavior
        1. Physical description (include posture, gait, grooming)
        2. Dress
        3. Eye contact
        4. Facial expression
        5. Motor activity
        6. Nonverbal communication
        7. Speech (intensity, pitch, accent or special mannerisms)
        8. Degree of cooperation
    b. Stream of Mental Activity and Thought Process
        1. Reality testing
        2. Major *content* of patient's productions. Include hallucinations, delusions, ideas of reference, obsessions, general theme of patient's conversation.
        3. Disruptions in *process* of communication. Consider such items as:
            a. Affective interference (depression, excitement, etc.)
            b. Attention span
            c. Spontaneity of narration
            d. Inhibition
            e. Blocking
            f. Prolonged reaction time
            g. Avoidance
            j. Flighty disassociation
            k. Fragmentation
            l. Memory
            m. Autism
            n. Neologisms, slang associations
            o. Perseverations,

      h. Resistance   p. Confabulation

      i. Loose association   echolalia

  c. Patient's major mechanisms of ego defense (see section in this chapter for detailed description of mechanisms of ego defense)

  d. Emotional Reaction

    1. Type, intensity, appropriateness

  e. Mental Status Examination

Strictly speaking the patient's mental status unfolds throughout the course of the entire interview. The psychiatrist draws inferences as he conducts a skillful, essentially unstructured interview. There is some data, however, that must be obtained by direct questioning. This material is outlined below under the heading of mental status examination.

Some of the questions used in this particular examination are drawn from the Wechsler Adult Intelligence Scale (WAIS). The author has found them useful because they are supported by research, wide usage, and are scorable. The reader may choose to alter his own examination from the one below. The important thing, however, is for each psychiatrist to have a routine mental status test available to him. He will then be assured of a complete and consistent examination in every case and he will, with experience, be able to judge the responses of any particular patient against the standards that apply to the examination.

    1. Orientation: time, place, person

    2. Delayed recall, early in the examination the patient should be given several items to remember. At the end of the examination, he is asked to name the items.

      a. blue-green-pink

      b. Chicago-Denver-Miami

    3. Similarities: (increasing order of abstraction). Ask in what ways are the following items similar or alike:

      a. orange-banana

   b. apple-baseball
   c. bicycle-airplane
   d. pencil-newspaper
   f. fly-tree
4. Proverbs (increasing order of abstraction)
   a. People in glass houses should not throw stones
   b. Every cloud contains a silver lining
   c. A stitch in time saves nine
   d. A rolling stone gathers no moss
   e. One swallow does not make spring
5. Digits Forward (to be repeated immediately)
   a. 5—8—2
   b. 6—4—3—9
   c. 6—13—9—4—12
   d. 2—7—16—9—23—11—26
6. Digits Backward (to be repeated immediately)
   Adds ability to integrate and synthesize to simple recall.
   a. 6—9—4
   b. 7—2—8—6
   c. 14—7—34—9—16
7. Serial 7's: (unobtrusively time the patient with a wrist watch and count his mistakes, i.e. 90 secs/ 1, etc.)
8. Fund of Knowledge
   a. Colors in U.S. flag
   b. Where is Egypt?
   c. U.S. presidents since 1900
   d. Capital of Italy
   e. Direction and distance to Los Angeles
   f. What is the Koran?
   g. Who wrote Faust?
   h. What is the apocrypha?
9. Vocabulary
   a. Bed   e. Tirade
   b. Assemble   f. Impale
   c. Sanctuary   g. Travesty
   d. Perimeter
10. Insight and judgment

  a. Does patient recognize his emotional disability?
  b. What does patient think is wrong?
  c. What does patient want to do about it?
  d. Are patient's future plans realistic?
13. Psychological Testing (Summarize the pertinent findings from psychological testing)
14. Diagnosis: Use DSM-II coding (Chapter I)
15. Prognosis
16. Dynamic Formulation
  a. Review of following features (from Wolberg, 1968)
    1. Symptom (s)
    2. Precipitating factor (s)
    3. Mechanisms of ego defense employed
    4. Immediate conflicts activated in the present disorder
    5. Underlying personality structure
    6. Related repressed conflicts originating in childhood
17. Summary of Hospital Course (Brief summary of hospital course if patient was treated on inpatient basis.)
18. Plans
  a. Describe optimal disposition for patient in terms of treatment and goals; also consider need of family, environmental and/or community intervention.
  b. Alternative planning
  c. If patient is hospitalized, refer to Chapter VI, Hospital Psychiatry, re: criteria for admission, treatment planning and criteria for discharge.

References

Sullivan, H. S.: *The Psychiatric Interview.* New York, Norton and Company, 1954.

Wechesler, D.: *Wechesler Adult Intelligence Scale.* New York, The Psychological Corporation, 1955.

Wolberg, Lewis T.: *Techniques of Psychotherapy.* New York, Grune & Stratton, 1968.

ASSESSMENT OF EGO FUNCTION

The psychiatric evaluation may assume various forms. One instrument frequently utilized for the collection and organization of data is the Egospsychological Assessment. In this framework the examiner focuses upon the patient's ego functioning and carefully evaluates each of the several ego components.

The following outline is adapted from the work of Bellak (By permission, Bellak, L., Loeb, L.: *The Schizophrenic Syndrome.* New York, Grune and Stratton, 1969.) Twelve distinct ego functions are described. Each function is defined below, its component factors are described, and the various disturbances associated with defects of each of the twelve functions are listed.

The twelve ego functions include:

I. Reality Testing
II. Judgment
III. Sense of Reality of Self
IV. Drive Regulation and Control
V. Object Relations
VI. Thought Processes
VII. Adaptive Regression In the Service of the Ego (ARISE)
VIII. Defensive Functioning
IX. Stimulus Barrier
X. Autonomous Functioning
XI. Synthetic—Integrative Functioning
XII. Mastery—Competence

I. Reality Testing
   A. Definition: The capacity of the organism to distinguish between ideas and percepts, to distinguish between inner and outer stimuli.
   B. Component Factors:
      1. Accuracy of perception (includes orientation to time and place and interpretation of external events).
      2. Accuracy of inner reality testing (psychologic-mindedness and awareness of inner states).
   C. Disturbances:
      1. Perceptual distortion, projection, delusion, hallucination, disorientation in time, place, and person, deja vu, deja reconnu, perceptual vigilance, low awareness of inner psychological reactions.

II. Judgment
  A. Definition: The capacity to determine the type of behavior that is appropriate, given an accurate perception of the situation.
  B. Component Factors:
    1. Awareness of likely consequences of intended behavior (e.g. anticipating probable dangers, legal culpabilities and social censure, disapproval or inappropriateness).
    2. Extent to which manifest behavior reflects the awareness of these likely consequences.
  C. Disturbances
    1. Oblivious to severe dangers to life and limb, unrealistic appraisal of consequences of actions, fails to learn from previous experiences.

III. Sense of Reality of Self
  A. Definition: Capacity to perceive self as a separate entity in the environment.
  B. Component Factors:
    1. The extent to which external events are experienced as real and as being embedded in a familiar context.
    2. The extent to which the body (or parts of it) and its functioning and one's behavior are experienced as familiar and unobtrusive and as belonging to (or emanating from) the individual.
    3. The degree to which the person has developed individuality, uniqueness, and a sense of self and self-esteem.
    4. The degree to which the person's self representations are separated from his object representations.
  C. Disturbances:
    1. Alienation, hypnagogic and hypnopompic hallucinations and stage fright, emotional isolation as a result of obsessive defenses, deja vu.

2. Depersonalization, derealization, dream-like states, trances, fugues, major dissociations, world destruction fantasies, identify diffusion.

IV. Drive Regulation and Control

A. Definition: The capacity to appropriately control the expression of drive derivatives; the degree to which aroused drives affect behavior.

B. Component Factors:

1. The directness of impulse expression (ranging from primitive acting out through neurotic acting out to relatively indirect forms of behavioral expression).

2. The effectiveness of delay and control, the degree of frustration tolerance, and the extent to which drive derivatives are channeled through ideation, affective expression, and manifest behavior.

C. Disturbances

1. Temper outbursts, habit and conduct disorders, lack of frustrative tolerance, acting out.

2. Tendencies toward homicide or suicide, impulsivity.

3. Drive-dominated behavior, chronic irritability and rage, catatonic excitement and rigidity, manic excitement, depressive psychomotor retardation, accident proneness, parapraxes, lack of sphincter control, nailbiting, tics, excessive control of impulse.

V. Object Relations

A. Definition: Capacity to relate to others, particularly to significant others.

B. Component Factors:

1. The degree and kind of relatedness to others (taking account of withdrawal trends, narcissistic self-concern, narcissistic object choice or mutuality).

2. The extent to which present relationships are adaptively or unadaptively influenced or patterned upon older ones and serve present mature

aims rather than past immature ones.

3. The degree to which the person perceives others as separate entities rather than as extensions of himself.

4. The extent to which the person can maintain object constancy (i.e. sustain relationships over long periods of time and tolerate both the physical absence of the object, and frustrations, anxiety, and hostility related to the object).

C. Disturbances

1. Withdrawal, detachment, narcissistic overinvestment of self, cannibalistic symbiotic-dependent attachments.

VI. Thought Processes

A. Definition: Comprised of the subfunctions of memory, concept formation, attention, concentration, anticipation.

B. Component Factors:

1. The adequacy of processes which adaptively guide and sustain thought (attention, concentration, anticipation, concept formation, memory, language).

2. The relative primary-secondary process influences on thought (extent to which thinking is unrealistic, illogical, and/or loose).

C. Disturbances

1. Magical thinking, autistic logic, condensations, attention lapses, inability to concentrate, memory disturbances, concreteness, primary process manifestations and primitive thought processes as described by Freud, Piaget, and others.

VII. Adaptive Regression in the Service of the Ego (ARISE)

A. Definition: Capacity to relinquish well-formed secondary processes to allow for creative utilization of more primitive modes of thinking.

B. Component Factors:

1. First phase of an oscillating process: Relaxation of perceptual and conceptual acuity (and other

ego controls) with a concomitant increase in awareness of previous preconscious and unconscious contents.

2. Second phase of the oscillating process: The induction of new configurations which increase adaptive potentials as a result of creative integrations.

C. Disturbances

1. Extreme rigidity in character structure and thinking where fantasy and play are difficult or impossible; uneveness in shifting from passivity to activity.

2. Regression of any ego function produces anxiety and disruption of functioning, lack of creativity, stereotyped thinking, intolerance of ambiguity.

3. Prejudice and sterility of thought.

4. If first phase predominates, overideational thinking, pseudo-intellectuality, pseudo-artistic tendencies, eccentricity.

VIII. Defensive Functioning

A. Definition: Capacity to control the emergence of anxiety or other dysphoric affect that may conflict with superego or reality demands.

B. Component Factors

1. Degree to which defensive components adaptively or maladaptively affect ideation and behavior.

2. Extent to which these defenses have succeeded or failed (degree of emergence of anxiety, depression, and other dysphoric affects).

3. Note: Different defenses are important at different stages of development. The earlier the origin of a defense, the more pathological, e.g. projection and denial which affect relationship to reality. Assessment must be directed not only to the type of defense but also to its relative stability or lability.

C. Disturbances
1. Parallel to loss of synthetic function, e.g. repression fails and leads to primary process emergence and patient fails to hold together; secondary inability to concentrate, memory impaired, efficiency impaired.
2. Probably because too much energy is used at barrier function and not enough is left for adaptation, e.g. with failure of defense have overstimulation by stimuli and mood lability.
3. With progressive decompensation one can have the same content but a change of defense. Example: Character trait can decompensate to neurotic symptom; neurotic symptom can decompensate to psychotic symptom. The process is reversed with compensation.

IX. Stimulus Barrier
A. Definition: Capacity to integrate external sources of stimulation which are irrelevant to ongoing behavior in such a fashion that the behavior remains adaptive.
B. Component Factors
1. Upper and lower threshold for, sensitivity to, or awareness of stimuli impinging upon various sensory modalities (primarily of external nature but also including pain).
2. Nature of response to various levels of sensory stimulation in terms of the extent of disorganization, avoidance, withdrawal, or active coping mechanisms employed to deal with them.
C. Disturbances
1. Easily upset by bright lights, loud sounds, temperature extremes, pain, resulting in withdrawal, physical symptoms, or irritability.
2. Thresholds over high: Person is oblivious to nuances, underresponsive to environmental stimuli, impoverishment of aesthetic sensibilities.

X. Autonomous Functioning
A. Definition: Capacity to neutralize libidinal and

aggressive energy toward a noninstinctual mode.

B. Component Factors
  1. Degree of freedom from impairment of apparatuses of primary autonomy (e.g. functional disturbances of sight, hearing, intention, language, memory, learning, intelligence, motor function).
  2. Degree of freedom from impairment of secondary autonomy (e.g. disturbances in habit patterns, learned complex skills, work routines, hobbies, and interests).

C. Disturbances
  1. Functional blindness or deafness, catatonic postures, inability to feed, dress, or care for oneself.
  2. Disturbances of skills, habits and automatized behavior are readily interfered with by drive-related stimuli; greater effort must be expended to carry out routine tasks.

XI. Synthetic-Integrative Functioning
  A. Definition: Capacity to reconcile or to integrate discrepancies in attitudes, values, affects, behavior, and self representations.
  B. Component Factors
    1. The degree of reconciliation or integration of discrepant role conflicts.
    2. Degree of active integration (relating together) of psychic and behavioral events, whether or not they are contradictory.
  C. Disturbances
    1. Disorganized behavior, incongruity between thoughts, feelings and actions; absence of consistent life goal; poor planning; little effort to relate different areas of experience together.
    2. Fluctuating emotional states without appropriate awareness of the change, as in hysterics.
    3. Minor and major forms of dissociation, from parapraxes to amnesia, fugues, and multiple personalities.

XII. Mastery-Competence

A. Definition: Capacity for successful planning and mastery over environment.
B. Component Factors
  1. Competence: Performance in relation to existing ability to interact with and mastery of the environment.
  2. Sense of competence: Expectation of success, subjective aspect of performance.
C. Disturbances
  1. Chronic anticipation of failure (success syndrome), underachievement, inadequate personality.

MECHANISMS OF EGO DEFENSE

Careful evaluation of the individual's characteristic mechanisms of ego defense is necessary to any complete psychiatric evaluation. This assessment must take into account several factors:

1. Defense mechanisms (with a few exceptions) are unconscious phenomena. They are directed against instinctual impulses, wishes, and desires in an effort to ward off associated anxiety. The defense may be directed at (1) the aim of the impulse, (2) the amount of force or pressure which the impulse exerts toward gratification, or (3) the object of the impulse.

2. In making an assessment of an individual's style of ego defense, it is not enough to simply list the mechanisms of ego defense that he characteristically employs. The examiner must also describe the specific drives or derivatives against which the defense is erected. Is the defense directed against the aim? the pressure toward expression? the object? Is the defense employed in a more global fashion against drive activity and instinctual pleasure as such? How effective is the defense in warding off anxiety? What real gains might the defense actually accrue for the individual's personality structure? Finally, what price is paid by the individual for using a particular defense in terms of interference with ego function?

3. Definitions of various mechanisms of ego defense overlap somewhat. At times, more than one mechanism may be used to describe the same piece of behavior.

While several different systems for the classification of ego defense have been proposed, none is all inclusive.

In this section the reader is presented with two different classifications. The first lists the major mechanisms of ego defense that have been described in the psychoanalytic literature. The second outlines Wolberg's attempt to attach diagnostic importance to the different mechanisms.

I. Mechanisms of Ego Defense

1. Sublimation
2. Repression
3. Suppression
4. Negation
5. Reaction Formation
6. Making Reparation
7. Regression
8. Externalization
9. Projection
10. Denial
11. Introjection (identification, imitation, internalization, incorporation)
12. Avoidance, Withdrawal
13. Dissociation
14. Splitting of Objects
15. Undoing
16. Displacement
17. Isolation
18. Rationalization
19. Intellectualization
20. Idealization
21. Counterphobic Mechanisms
22. Aim Inhibition
23. Acting Out
24. Fantasy
25. Somatization
26. Identification with the Aggressor
27. Turning Aggression against the Self
28. Turning Passive into Active
29. Anticipatory Provocation
30. Passivity
31. Phobia

1. Sublimation

Definition: aim or object of instinct is changed, with subsequent gratification, classically thought to be the most adaptive and most economic defense mechanism in that impulse gratification results (anxiety-free) without expenditure of defensive energy.

Example: A man with exhibitionistic impulses becomes an actor, etc.

2. Repression

Definition: Unconscious, purposeful forgetting. Exclusion from awareness of internal impulse, or memory which would be painful if it reached conscious awareness. First defense described by Freud; the primary mechanism which is supported by all others. Economically is expensive in that counter-cathexis (defense) must be permanently expended against the undesirable impulse. Impoverishes personality development and creativity.

Example: Forgetting of names in everyday life to full blown amnesia for entire periods of time.

3. Suppression

Definition: Simply described as conscious repression, i.e. conscious, intentional exclusion of material from consciousness.

Example: Person makes conscious effort to forget about an embarrassing thing that happened.

4. Negation

Definition: Similar to suppression in being a conscious mechanism. Conscious denial of something that person wishes not to face.

Example: When asked by a psychiatrist if he has ever had homosexual impulses, a man says "No," while knowing full-well that he has indeed had such impulses.

5. Reaction Formation

Definition: The reversal of the aim or object of the undesirable impulse into its opposite. After a period of time may become a well-fixed character trait and can be quite adaptive in many cases.

Example: Man overwhelmed by hostile, anti-social impulses may become a policeman (defender of the peace). Person who despises someone may transform the impulse into excessive kindness.

6. Making Reparation

Definition: Related to reaction formation (and to undoing) but is more limited to specific events. Individual undoes a previous event by returning to the person to whom the undesirable impulse was directed and making amends. May be used by obsessives to defend against an affect that momentarily emerged and now must be undone.

Example: A man has an argument with his wife in the morning; in the evening he brings her a bouquet of flowers.

7. Regression

Definition: Person abandons a level of psychosexual adjustment which he has achieved and returns to an earlier and more infantile level.

Example: Simple example is regression of child upon birth of sibling; (i.e. if toilet trained may begin wetting again, etc.); more pathologic example is catatonic schizophrenia.

8. Externalization

Definition: An unacceptable wish or impulse is simply attributed to someone else. Commonly used.

Example: Person complains that someone else is a money-grubber, a sex fiend, devious, deceitful, etc.

9. Projection

Definition: What is externalized is returned to the self; primitive mechanism.

Example: Person says that "So-and-so has been saying that I'm a money-grubber, a sex fiend, devious, deceitful, etc."

10. Denial

Definition: Unconscious negation. Person refuses to believe what should be obvious. Denial may be (1) in word (he says something is not so), (2) in action (he acts as if it is not so), and/or (3) in fantasy (he fantasizes as though it is not so).

Example: A man has suffered a heart attack. When asked

about it he denies it (word) ; he engages in strenuous activities (act) ; and he daydreams about athletic prowess (fantasy) .

11. Introjection

Definition: The person incorporates into himself a desired trait belonging to someone else. In some ways, is the opposite of externalization.

a. Identification: Somewhat similar but with important differences. Tends more to be ego building and adaptive than introjection. Unconscious modeling upon some valued person or group. Is unconscious and can lead to permanent change.

b. Imitation: Is conscious. Appears like identification on the surface but is more transitory and does not imply permanent structural change.

c. Internalization: For practical purposes, is indistinguishable from introjection. Children internalize parental values.

d. Incorporation: For practical purposes is indistinguishable from introjection but generally implies a more primitive defense.

12. Avoidance, withdrawal

Definition: Restriction of ego resulting in removal from sources of anxiety. Is often preliminary to the erection of other defenses.

Example: Man threatened by overwhelming sexual desire avoids the office of a pretty secretary. (This may later lead to hyper-religiosity via reaction formation, aim-inhibition, etc.)

13. Dissociation

Definition: Splitting off of thought (s) and/or action (s) from conscious awareness.

Example: Some forms are useful, such as not bringing problems home from the office, others are more clearly pathologic as in dissociative states (fugue) , conversion hysteria, or schizophrenia.

14. Splitting of Objects

Definition: Person reacts to some people as though they

are all good and others as though they are all bad. Qualities of objects exist only in absolutes.

Example: Madonna-Prostitute Complex, i.e. man can have sex with a prostitute (bad) but must treat his wife (good) like a saint or Madonna.

15. Undoing

Definition: A kind of expiation. An act or thought which negates (undoes) or neutralizes something which previously occurred and was experienced as anxiety-producing.

Example: A man has a momentary idle thought of killing his wife; that night he brings her a gift. Typical in obsessive-compulsive disorders. Magical rituals are used to undo undesirable thoughts, presumed consequences, etc.

16. Displacement

Definition: Affect originally attached to one object is displaced onto another which is more innocuous and less threatening.

Example: A man is berated by his boss and is furious but does not express it. When he gets home he blows up at his wife over a trivial matter.

17. Isolation

Definition: (a) Isolation of affect implies that the affect associated with a particular thought or event is repressed; (b) Isolation of content implies that some links in the associative chain regarding content are repressed. The first leads to an unfulfilled, bland life; the second leads to gaps in reality testing, if carried to extremes.

Example: Person can speak of usually emotion-laden events in a detached, unfeeling manner because he isolates affect. Person succeeds in avoiding anxiety by blocking from awareness conflictual material that might arise if he allows himself to recall the true sequence of a particular event.

18. Rationalization

   Definition: The person elaborates rational and socially acceptable reasons to justify behavior that is unconsciously determined and/or to hide from himself or others the actual motives for his behavior.

   Example: Rather than face failure in a course, a student drops it saying that it wasn't important and he would have passed it anyway. Common mechanism. If excessive, may be component of obsessive-compulsive disorder.

19. Intellectualization

   Definition: Closely related to rationalization. Excessive use of intellect in order to avoid affective experience.

   Example: Person who is threatened by feelings and spontaneity relates to people on an intellectual basis. Adolescents especially may defend against their own aggressive drives by intellectualizing about evil-doers in the world, etc.

20. Idealization

   Definition: Person overestimates the positive qualities and underestimates the negative qualities of a desired object.

   Example: Woman previously conflicted over which dress to buy begins to idealize the chosen one in order to reassure herself and allay anxiety.

21. Counterphobic Mechanisms

   Definition: Person attempts to ward off anxiety connected with a certain activity by purposefully engaging in it.

   Example: Person afraid of heights may take up mountain-climbing. (Reaction formation is similar but usually is more global and takes on the appearance of a character trait; counterphobic mechanisms tend to be specific and constricted.)

22. Aim Inhibition

Definition: Person places a limit on instinctual demands and accepts a modified form of gratification.

Example: A boy decides to become a lab tech rather than a physician. A man desires a certain woman sexually but is frustrated and decides he wants her only as a friend instead.

23. Acting Out

Definition: Gratification of an unconscious impulse through action without being aware of the unconscious conflict.

Example: Woman in psychotherapy begins to have affairs that succeed in discharging anxiety; is resistant to treatment since these conflicts must be worked-through psychotherapeutically in order to be resolved.

24. Fantasy

Definition: Includes stories, dreams, daydreams. Anxiety is disguised. Gratification through wish and pleasurable elaborations.

Example: Normal, yet can be pathological if such activity displaces reality or hinders person's daily living.

25. Somatization

Definition: Expression of psychic conflict by production of a physical (somatic) symptom. Can be considered a defense since the primary gain associated with the symptom is avoidance of anxiety. In conversion hysteria the symptom itself is symbolic of the underlying conflict.

Example: Child may suffer paralysis of hand after masturbation. Hysterical blindness may occur after patient sees an event that is anxiety-producing, etc.

26. Identification with the Aggressor

Definition: Person introjects the aggressive characteristics of an anxiety object therefore transforming himself from the person who is threatened into the person who does the threatening.

Example: Boy who fears aggression from his father begins to identify with his father's aggressive qualities and assimilate them.

27. Turning Aggression against the Self

Definition: Person defends against anxiety by self-destructive acts. Includes accident-proneness and (more subtle form) moral masochism.

Example: Man blocks awareness of anxiety associated with an earlier argument with his wife by getting into a minor auto accident.

28. Turning Passive into Active

Definition: Person acts in anticipation of being acted upon.

Example: Patient may miss the last therapy session before the therapist's announced vacation. Girl breaks up with her boyfriend, feeling that he is about, in fact, to leave her.

29. Anticipatory Provocation

Definition: Provoking an anxiety-laden and powerful object into committing some act so that the person, by thus controlling the object, obtains mastery over it even though the person himself may actually suffer in the process. Can be seen often in passive-aggressive individuals.

Example: A soldier-recruit breaks a rule and makes a superior furious. Although he is subsequently punished, the soldier feels good because he was able to achieve mastery over the superior officer.

30. Passivity

Definition: The simple act of repressing impulses and remaining passive where activity would be a more appropriate mode can serve as an ego defense. Related to repression, withdrawal, reaction formation.

Example: A person frightened by aggressive impulses or other conflict in a certain situation may become unexplainably passive, bored, tired, and may even fall asleep.

31. Phobia

Definition: Related to externalization, displacement. Unreasonable, irrational fear of a person, place, or thing. The phobic object often represents a displacement.

Example: (Oedipal) boy who unconsciously fears and hates his own father may become suddenly phobic of dogs while his relationship to his father remains unaltered on the surface.

References

Fenichel, O: *The Psychoanalytic Theory of Neurosis*. New York, W. W. Norton, 1945.

Freud, A.: *The Ego and The Mechanisms of Defense*. New York, International Universities Press, 1946.

II. Wolberg Classification

(Wolberg Classification adapted from *Techniques of Psychotherapy*, (1968), Lewis T. Wolberg, with permission of Grune & Stratton Inc. Publishers, New York.)

Wolberg, in *The Technique of Psychotherapy*, (Grune & Stratton, New York, 1968) conceptualizes four levels of defense against anxiety:

1. Conscious efforts at maintaining control
2. Characterologic defenses
3. Repressive defenses
4. Regressive defenses

Wolberg points out that a neurosis consists of a number of component parts dynamically interrelated, shifting in manifestations and symptoms. The defenses, too, may shift and should not be considered fixed and static; while a person may stabilize at any of the four levels described above, it is more common to see a mixture of several defenses spanning one or more levels.

I. First Line Defenses: Conscious Efforts at Maintaining Control Through Manipulating the Environment.
Note: All persons utilize these mechanisms to some extent. Such defenses may be considered normal.

Defense	Example
1. Removing oneself from sources of stress.	A man irritated with work conditions may quit his job and find a less strenuous work situation.
2. Escaping into bodily satisfactions.	Overeating and excessive sexual indulgence may be employed as tension-relieving mechanisms.
3. Extroversion.	Plunging into hobbies, and recreational and social activities may divert the individual's attention from his inner problems.
4. Wish-fulfilling fantasies.	Indulging in daydreaming may act as a substitute gratification for unfulfilled impulses.
5. Suppression.	Willfully keeping painful ideas or impulses from awareness.
6. Rationalization.	Providing reality and social justifications for behavior motivated by inner needs.
7. Use of philosophic credos.	Adoption of codes of behavior and ethics to reinforce one's conscience, or to justify one's impulse indulgence.
8. Exercising self-control.	Forceful conscious inhibition of tension-producing impulses.
9. Emotional outbursts and impulsive behavior.	Gaining release of tension through emotional catharsis and by acting out.

Defense	Example
10. Thinking things through.	Arriving at a rational solution of one's problems by carefully weighing alternative courses of action.
11. Alcoholic indulgence.	Alcohol often serves as a means of reducing tension and of allowing emotional release. Excessive alcoholic intake may occur.
12. Use of drugs.	Minor tranquilizers and sedatives (barbiturates) may be employed to alleviate anxiety and tension, while stimulants (amphetamines) help to promote energy in situations where the person feels listless and inert. Narcotics (marihuana and opiates) and psychotomimetics (LSD) may also be used.

If the first line defenses fail, the individual may begin to employ second line defenses which involve a manipulation of his relationships with other people.

II. Second Line Defenses: Characterologic Defenses
    Note: If exaggerated can result in personality disorders.

A. Strivings of an interpersonal nature.

Defense	Example
1. Exaggerated dependency	immaturity
2. Submissive techniques	passivity
3. Expiatory techniques	masochism, asceticism
4. Aggressive techniques	sadism
5. Dominating techniques	controlling other people
6. Withdrawal techniques	detachment

B. Strivings directed at the self-image.

Defense	Example
1. Narcissistic strivings	grandiosity, perfectionism
2. Power impulses	compulsive ambition

If anxiety cannot be controlled with characterologic defense, or if the defenses, and the conflicts they create produce more anxiety, third line defenses may be employed. These consist largely of repressive defenses.

III. Third Line Defenses: Repressive Defenses.
    Note: May result in Neurosis.

A. General efforts directed at reinforcing repression.

Defense	Example
1. Reaction formations	Characterologic drives to oppose and repudiate inner drives; for example, ingratiation and passivity to oppose hostile, murderous impulses.
2. Accentuation of intellectual controls (with compensations and sublimations)	

B. Inhibition of Function

Defense	Example
1. Blunted apperception, attention, concentration and thinking.	
2. Disturbed consciousness (fainting, increased sleep, stupor)	Hysterical neurosis, dissociative type
3. Disturbed memory (antegrade and retrograde amnesia)	Hysterical neurosis, dissociative type
4. Emotional indifference	Neurasthenic neurosis

Defense	Example
or apathy (emotional inhibitions)	
5. Sensory disorders (hypoesthesia, anaesthesia, amaurosis, ageusia, etc.)	Hysterical neurosis, conversion type
6. Motor paralysis (paresis, aphonia) .	Hysterical neurosis, conversion type
7. Visceral inhibitions (impotence, frigidity)	Psychophysiologic disorders, etc. The functions of inhibition of the various cognitive, affective, autonomic and visceral aspects (No. 5, 6, 7) is to deaden the appreciation of repressed inner impulses, to keep any symbolic derivatives from awareness, and to prevent the expression in any kind of motor action of a forbidden impulse.

C. Other

Defense	Example
1. Displacement 2. Projection 3. Phobic avoidance	The impulse in No. 1 through 3 is displaced to an external object and then an attempt is made to repudiate the impulse by avoiding (or blaming) the object. Example: phobic neurosis.
4. Undoing 5. Isolation	These (No. 4 and 5) consist of a kind of magical neutralization of the offending impulse or its derivative through compulsive rituals and/or isolating it from affectual awareness. Example: obsessive compulsive neurosis.

IV. Fourth Line Defenses: Regressive Defenses
Note: May result in psychosis.

Defense	Example
1. Return to helpless dependency.	Failing to adjust at an adult level, the individual may attempt to invoke the protective parental agencies who ministered to him in his childhood by assuming the attitudes and behavior of a child. This regressive appeal is associated with a renunciation of adult responsibility.
2. Repudiation of, and withdrawal from reality.	Characteristic of withdrawal from reality are autistic thinking; disorders of perception (illusions, hallucinations) ; disorders of mental content (ideas of reference, delusions) ; disorders of apperception and comprehension; disorders of the stream of mental activity (increased or diminished speech productivity, irrelevance, incoherence, scattering, neologisms) ; disturbances in affect (apathy, inappropriate affect, depression, excitement) ; and defects in memory, personal identification, orientation, retention, recall, thinking capacity, attention, insight and judgment. The syndromes are in the form of schizophrenia, the development of which perhaps requires a constitutional predisposition.
3. Internalization of hostility.	Resultant, where certain constitutional factors are present, may

Defense	Example
	be psychotic depressive reactions; manic depressive illness, depressed type; and involutional melancholia.
4. Excited acting out.	Hostile, sexual, and other repressed impulses may be expressed openly in the course of a psychotic reaction. Representative syndromes here are manic depressive illness, manic type, and paranoid states.

The patient may manage to stabilize with fourth line defenses at the expense of reality, while possibly still retaining some of the other three lines of defense.

Syndromes never occur in isolation; they are always contaminated with manifestations of other defensive levels. As stress is alleviated or exaggerated, or as ego strengthening or weakening occurs, shifts in lines of defense upward or downward may occur, and changes in symptoms and syndromes will develop.

THE PSYCHOANALYTIC ASSESSMENT
RONALD M. BENSON, M.D.

The psychoanalytic model of psychological growth and development provides a conceptual framework for the assessment of psychological development and psychopathology. This article is designed to provide the psychiatrist with an overview of the psychoanalytic model that will be useful to him in evaluating patients. It reviews the various libidinal stages with reference to drive activity, self and object relatedness, dangers and interferences, primary mechanisms of ego defense, ego functioning, and deviations that may result in developmental arrests or the establishment of fixation points. Patients may be evaluated in reference to all of these parameters. The psychiatrist may then determine whether they have achieved phase dominance in each of the various libidinal stages. The psychoanalytic assessment may be applied to children, adolescents, and adults.

I. Early Infancy: Birth to Six Months
   A. The mental apparatus at birth is rudimentary and unstructured. During this developmental phase, the prototypic mechanisms and structures for later highly specific and organized mental functioning appear. This is largely a result of the maturation of the child's central nervous system, assuming at least a minimally satisfactory environment.
      1. Drives:
         a. The libidinal drive during early infancy is at the stage of primary narcissism, but by the end of this phase will have advanced to orality. Primary narcissism means that the object of the infant's drive is his own body and sensations, synthesized into a rudimentary, but very primitive, me.
         b. Aggressive drive: During most of this phase, this drive is at the stage of primary masochism. Once again, this means that the child's aggression is turned upon his own body.
      2. Self and object representations:
         No self or object representation exists in a newborn.
         a. Self representation: As this phase develops, gradually through awareness via proprioception and other bodily sensations there will begin to form the nucleus of a mental image of the self, or self representation.
         b. Object representation: Increasing ability to perceive, particularly during tension states will result in some rudimentary, fragmented, mental representations of a very transitory nature which will form the earliest basis of a representation of an object in the infant's mind.

3. Dangers:
   The early infant is always in danger of being overwhelmed by the strength of his own drives, need tension states from within, or excessively strong stimuli from the environment. Such overwhelming is the prototype of psychic helplessness or trauma. It is not only the child's psychologic but physiologic helplessness that leads to his vulnerability.
4. Coping mechanisms:
   a. Stimulus barrier
   b. Good enough mothering (Winnicott, 1953)
   c. Denial: Possibly noncathexis (nonattending) to painful stimuli is possible as an active process by the end of early infancy.
   d. Projection: By the end of this phase of development, the infant may have developed some capacity to consider unpleasant feelings as part of the nonself, leaving only pleasant ones as part of the self-system, though the self-object distinction is poor.
5. Ego functioning
   a. The responsive smile (Spitz, 1965) : The infant responds with a smile to the stimulus of a face, and this is an important event for further personal, social, and expressive development.
   b. Autonomous ego functions are developing at an astonishing rate. Increasing motor control, particularly of the trunk and limbs, coordination of the hand and mouth, and increasing reliance on the distance receptors occur.
6. Interferences: Major underfulfillment of the infant's needs at this stage are either incompatible with the continuation of life itself or result in major disruptions in personality development. Such a child may appear seriously retarded or have the picture of infantile autism (Kanner,

1944), childhood schizophrenia, or other serious deviant syndromes. Adult schizophrenics and paranoids may result from personality defects imparted during this developmental phase.

II. Later Infancy: Six Months To Eighteen Months
- A. This phase continues the rapid maturation of the central nervous system and the acquiring of basic mechanisms and skills, which form the foundation of personality functioning.
  1. Drives:
     - a. Libidinal: This drive is at the oral phase, with aims of incorporating the object of the drive (i.e. making it part of the self through a mental process analagous to alimentation).
     - b. The aggressive drive is oral-sadistic, with aims of biting, chewing, masticating, or destroying the object. Both of these drive positions are very primitive and often difficult for adults to conceptualize. The aims of the drives are contradictory, resulting in ambivalence.
  2. Self and object representations:
     - a. Self: To the degree that the infant has a mental conception of himself, it is as if he were omnipotent and grandiosely capable. He feels as if his wishes were the actual causal activator of desired responses rather than another's actions.
     - b. Object: The infant is aware, at least at times of need tension, of those aspects of another associated with the satisfaction of his needs. He is not aware of the other as a whole person, but only of that aspect of the object which fulfills the needs. In a shorthand way, this is often spoken of as the part object or sometimes as the breast.
  3. Dangers: The main danger, from the infant's point of view, during this phase is abandonment. As the object or part-object becomes increasingly

important, its absence becomes increasingly frightening and dangerous to the infant. Anxiety can reach traumatic levels. The anxiety occurring at this phase of development which can be seen as a remnant in adults is called separation anxiety.

4. Coping mechanisms:
   a. Introjection: This defense mechanism permits the infant to psychologically take in the object and make it part of the self system, thus protecting against the fear of separation from the object to a limited degree.
   b. Motility: The acquisition of the capacity to move toward or away from stimulus may protect the child from helplessness in the face of an external, unpleasant stimulus, or from being unable to reach a pleasurable one.

5. Ego functioning:
   a. Cognitive functioning increases rapidly during this phase, with the beginnings of speech, increasing capacity for motor activity, walking, and greater perceptual ability.
   b. Stranger anxiety: The infant's distress upon perceiving unfamiliar people occurs at about eight months, indicates greater perceptual discrimination of objects, but most importantly, is a sign that specific attachments to specific (primary) objects is occurring.

6. Deviations: Significant failure or interference with development at this stage are seen in the symbiotic problems of childhood as well as psychosomatic disorders of children and adults. Failure of mastery of conflicts at this phase of development may result in a tendency towards serious depressions in adults.

III. Toddler Phase: One Year To Three Years
   A. During this phase of development, the child will be principally involved in the task of separation-

individuation: (Mahler, 1968). That is to say, the child will be engaged in the psychological task of seeing himself as separate from, but related to, important objects in his environment. This involves not only psychological distancing but spatial distancing as well.

1. Drives:

   a. Libidinal: The libidinal drive at this phase is anal, with the aims of retaining and expelling. Concerns of the child of this phase of development may revolve around issues of controlling, messing, withholding, or the opposites of these.

   b. Aggressive: Anal-sadism. The aggressive drive is much in evidence during this phase of development and may be manifested in oppositional behavior, activity rather than passivity, and great struggles with the object, which frequently take the form of control battles. Once again, the opposing trends of this phase of retaining and expelling, withholding and giving are manifested by ambivalence in relation to the object.

2. Self and object representations:

   a. The self-representation at this phase of development is still grandiose and the infant conceives of his words and actions as endowed with magical ability to alter the state of the world. This is different from the former stage in that he feels that he must do something to alter the world; yet it is not the specific action, but the gesture and words themselves which are conceived of as doing the deed.

   b. Object representation: By this phase of development, a whole person is related to, rather than a part as in the previous phase. On the other hand, the person's actual qualities are not yet accurately perceived. Rather, the object is viewed as being just like the self and particularly the junior toddler expects that control over the object will be similar to the control which he has over his own body parts.

3. Dangers: The principal danger at this phase in development is the experience of having lost the object's affection and esteem. Since the distinction between self and object is not yet firm, this is equivalent to the child of this phase to losing his own esteem. It is a particularly painful state of shame and children in this phase of development, despite their need to be in control and their omnipotence, will capitulate to the object's wishes to avoid this painful sense of loss of love.

4. Coping mechanisms:
   a. The new mechanism *par excellence* of this phase of development is reaction formation. This means the replacement of a wish by its opposite. Thus, the child at this phase of development who wishes to be messy may replace this in consciousness by a desire to be extremely orderly and neat.
   b. Another mechanism newly developed at this phase is isolation, which involves keeping thoughts and feelings separate from one another so that relationships between them are not apparent.
   c. Undoing: This depends on the magical mental mechanism of making something that happens seem as if it did not happen. Therefore, the consequences of the original situation are no longer of concern.

5. Ego functioning: The child develops many skills at this phase of development, such as the capacity to play alongside other children, markedly increased use of speech and the beginnings of imagination and of empathy. Typically in this

phase of development, control over the musculature and particularly over the sphincters is
acquired. This phase is ushered in by the
acquiring of the constant mental representation
of the object and ends with a clear distinction
between the self and object. A major advance
in structuralization of the mind begins at this
phase of development with the beginnings of
superego development. The child acquires at
least in limited areas an inner conception of
what is right and what is wrong and has some
capacity to enforce prohibitions upon himself.

6. Deviations: Significant difficulties with successful
resolution of the conflicts of this phase of development are seen in children and adults in the
form of obsessive-compulsive neurotic disorders
and obsessive-compulsive character disorders.
The very common descriptive disorder, "passive-
aggressive personality," may stem from fixations
at this phase of development as well. Sado-
masochistic perversions also involve fixations
from this developmental phase.

IV. Nursery School Age: Two and one-half to Five and
one-half

A. During this important phase of development, the
child acquires many of the social skills which he
will need to function in school. He becomes much
more independent, both phenomenologically and
intrapsychically.

1. Drives:

a. Libidinal: The drive is now at the phallic-
oedipal level where the aims are to intrude,
thrust, and exhibit and possess. The objects
of the drives for the first time become multiple, so that while one parent, usually the
member of the opposite sex, is getting the
major portion of the libidinal drive, the other

is getting the major portion of the aggressive feelings. Thus a triangular situation occurs.

 b. Aggressive drive is at the phallic-sadistic level, where the emphasis is on competing, being one up and besting the object of the drive through being bigger, better, and in general superlative.

2. Self and object representations:

 a. Self-representation: Grandiosity in this phase is given up for a feeling of self-esteem and status by relationship with the object that is loved and idealized. There is clear separation between the self and the object so that it is closeness to the object and winning the object's affections which is important as a confirmation of the status of the self rather than as in the previous phase that the objects' presumed omnipotence is felt as part of the self.

 b. Object representations: The object is aggrandized, idealized, and loved or hated. It is clearly distinct from the self with actual qualities of its own.

3. Dangers: Castration anxiety, fear of damage to the self or particularly to the genitals, upon which functioning and intactness so much of the child's self esteem depends, is the major fear of this age.

4. Coping mechanisms:

 a. Fantasy and imagination take on a much more important role with the onset of this phase of development.

 b. Play has a conflict-resolving component and the use of symbolization is more prominent in play.

 c. The defense mechanism of displacement, that is, shifting the object of a drive, is very prominent and is seen in play extensively. For example, the child may have mock wars instead of having conflicts with the parent.

d. Avoidance of any anxiety-producing situation also becomes prominent.

e. Repression becomes obvious though the mechanism of repression probably has been available to the child at a much earlier time. However, here in particular, the exclusion from consciousness of conflict-producing wishes is most prominent and a massive repression will end the oedipal situation and lead to the internalization of the superego proper.

5. Ego development: Cognition improves greatly with the capacity of reading readiness, further ability to use symbols, and the beginning of pre-operational thought (Piaget). Structurally of particular importance is the internalization of parental values, attitudes and prohibitions which constitute the superego and which makes the child very much more independent of the actual presence of the parents. This also leads to conflicts being much more between intrapsychic agencies (i.e. id, ego, and superego) rather than between the child and his environment.

6. Deviations: The infantile neurosis is ubiquitous during this phase of development. This may involve transient evanescent symptoms resulting mainly from developmental conflicts peculiar to the age, or it may lead to more permanent symptomotology with conflicts from previous phases represented as well. Fixations at this point are frequent in those adults demonstrating hysterias and phobias.

V. **Grade** School Years: Five to Eleven

A. These are the so called latency years in which overt demonstrations of sexual interests are less apparent. Knowledge increases dramatically during this phase of development, and the child gains many new social, intellectual, and motor skills. Boys and girls tend to avoid each other and prefer the company of their own sex.

1. Drives:
   a. Libidinal: The libidinal drive during latency seems relatively weaker in comparison to the repressing and channeling forces. Therefore, direct drive expression of sexual wishes is less common, though there may be breakthroughs in masturbatory activity, exploratory games, etc. However, these are accompanied by severe guilt and are generally the result of temporarily increased drives or temporarily weakened ego states. The unconscious aim and objects of the drives are relatively unchanged, though there is some shift from the primary objects to peers.
   b. Aggressive drive: The aggressive drive may be manifested directly in competitiveness with the primary object, but to a far greater degree it is expressed through beginning sublimations and learning situations, games, particularly those of a competitive nature, and may be particularly manifested as hostility to those people or situations which threaten the repression of libidinal urges.
2. Self and Object representations:
   a. Self: Self-esteem and self-regard is, to a far greater degree, based on real accomplishment. Doing well in school, at games, and in other situations enhances self-esteem, while failure diminishes it. The child no longer sees himself as omnipotent and grandiose, but at times he will boastfully overestimate his capabilities. This has a much more defensive quality than formerly in that the child is more aware that these boasts do not represent reality.

    b. The idealization that formerly was invested in parents is now invested in other adults or peers in the child's environment. Teachers may be seen as totally wise and omniscient. Often the school principal becomes the recipient of this kind of fantasy. A typical constellation of fantasies develop about objects at this stage of development, the family romance in which the child develops some kind of fantasy indicating that his parents are not his real parents but he is the child of more exhalted parentage.

3. Dangers: The main threat to the child at this phase is not being able to control his impulses. Each failure in this regard with direct breakthrough of his impulses leads to a severe repudiation by his conscience (superego) with resulting guilt.

4. Coping mechanisms: The major addition to the defensive armamentarium at this phase of development is increasing use of ego skills. This can go in a number of directions, most adaptively is the use of sublimation, the attaining of new skills which allow partial gratification of the primitive impulse but at a much higher and socially acceptable level. The beginnings of intellectualizing occur during this phase, too; that is the capacity to shift from the primitive concern with sexual matters to a more distant, abstract, and symbolized concern with the impulse. Excuses are prevalent in the form of rationalizations.

5. Ego Functioning: The attainment of a certain degree of rationality and conceptual constancy becomes paramount in this phase of development. Thus the cognitive functions of the ego are hypertrophying during this phase of development. The child's knowledge, perception, memory are all increasing rapidly.

6. Deviations: The most commonly seen deviation of this phase of development is learning disorders, though the onset of neurotic symptoms may first appear here also. Impairments of development at this age may lead to severe intellectual handicaps or character problems in adults, though the latter would depend on fixations at earlier phases of development. Should earlier phases be traversed successfully and an interference occur here, the picture in an adult would be the absence of certain ego skills.

VI. Junior High School: Eleven to Thirteen
   A. This is the period of the acquisition of secondary sexual characteristics and rapid physical growth.
   1. Drives: Both the libidinal and aggressive drives at this phase of development undergo a marked increase in relative strength. The libidinal drive may become quite variable and fluid in regard to aim and object. The re-emergence temporarily of pregenital aims is common. The primary objects usually become highly cathected but defenses vs. the cathexis are quickly mobilized. Competitiveness with the parent of the same sex is markedly increased during this phase of development and is the representation of the aggressive drive position.
   2. Self and Object Representations: Fluidity in self and object representations is the major picture.
      a. The self-representation becomes disrupted at this phase of development by the rapid growth and the acquisition of secondary sexual characteristics. Problems in identity are frequent and competing representations of self are also frequent. For example one moment a highly grandiose conception of the self may appear while at another time a very deflated self-image may take its place. There

may be shifts in values and attitudes reflecting these changes.

b. Object representations also undergo dramatic shifts during this phase of development with the primary objects idealized and depreciated in a highly fluid way. Similar shifts may occur in relation to peers, teachers, and other authority figures.

3. Dangers: In this area also, fluidity and disruption of previously effective means of coping are seen. The junior high school child may try first one defensive posture and then another, but the clear cut defense organization which he may have exhibited before is no longer present. All of the former dangers become intensified. He may alternately experience extreme castration anxiety, separation anxiety, loss of the object's love, guilt, or shame.

4. Coping mechanisms: There may be a fluid shifting of defensive postures, defenses, and defense organizations during this phase of development. The previously established and relatively stable modes may not be effective during this rapid period of readjustment.

5. Ego Functioning: Again, fluidity is the order of the day. Previously well-established ego functions may temporarily be interrupted and there may be impairments of learning and skills formerly unaffected. There may be rapid shifts in values as the parents themselves and their internalized representation, the superego, are partially decathected.

6. Interferences: A failure to master conflicts at this stage of development will lead to delinquency, severe identity problems, or shifting pathologic pictures which one minute may appear to be neurotic, another moment characterologic, or even psychotic-like phenomena.

VII. High School: Fourteen through Eighteen

   A. These are the years of post pubertal consolidation. A number of tasks must be completed during this phase of development, including some direction of life's vocation, establishment of a sexual object, and more or less permanent removal from the primary objects.

      1. Drives: The normal aim of the libidinal drive becomes sexual union, and throughout this phase the object shifts from the primary object to the nonfamilial heterosexual object choice. The aggressive drive may be manifested in competitiveness for the sexual object in work and play. In the case of both the libidinal and the aggressive drives high levels of sublimation and neutralization become possible with the attainment of many new skills.

      2. Self and object representations: There may be a phase of a return to an aggrandizement of self and a highly narcissistic self-loving position which by the end of this phase gives way to a realistic appraisal of one's strengths and weaknesses, skills and deficiencies. Objects may be aggrandized and over-valued, particularly in the state of being in love, though by the end of the adolescent phase and the beginning of adulthood, a realistic perception of the object in relation to the self should have been acquired.

      3. Dangers: The course of adolescence is a gradual diminution of danger arising from infantile sources and a gradual recognition of the real dangers that confront one in life. The attainment of this realistic appraisal is relative with some youths accomplishing this more successfully than others.

      4. Coping mechanisms: From the preadolescent highly fluid shifts between aceticism, impulsivity, etc., there is a return to sublimation, neutraliza-

tion, and the use of realistic adaptations to obtain gratification of needs.

5. Ego Functioning: A gradual re-establishment of a more structuralized personality results, replacing the more fluid state of the early adolescent. Defensive organization, coping style, object choices, ethics, and cognitive styles will all be firmly established and their sum total is a more or less fixed personality. Increasing synthetic capacities of the ego are manifested in adaptations which at once meet the demands of reality, the drives, the conscience, and the executive functions of the personality.

6. Interferences: Adolescence represents the last chance in normal development to organize all of the previous traits, conflicts, fixations, styles, resulting from development up to this point into a cohesive well-functioning whole. To the degree that this is not possible during the adolescent phase of development there will be impairments in the choice of object and vocational adaptations and the ability to find satisfying recreational outlets. If previous conflicts are handled in a rigid, stereotypic, defensive fashion, the outcome will be fixed character pathology.

References

1. Blos, P.: *On Adolescence.* New York, The Free Press, 1969.
2. Freud, Anna: *Normality and Pathology in Childhood.* New York, International University Press, 1965.
3. Freud, S.: *Three Essays on the Theory of Sexuality,* (1905), Standard Edition. London, Hogarth Press, 1953.
4. Mahler, Margaret with Furer, M.: *On Human Symbiosis and the Vicissitudes of Individuation,* Vol. I. New York, International University Press, 1968.
5. Piaget, J. and Inhelden, B.: *The Psychology of the Child.* New York, Basic Books, 1969.
6. Spitz, R.: *The First Year of Life.* New York, International University Press, 1965.
7. Winnicott, D. W.: Transitional objects and transitional phenomena. *International Journal of Psychoanalysis, 34:* 89–97.

SULLIVAN'S 15 QUESTIONS REGARDING
THE INITIAL PSYCHIATRIC INTERVIEW

Harry Stack Sullivan (1954) viewed psychiatry as an interpersonal process and considered the psychiatric interview within the same theoretical and philosophical framework. The interview was conceptualized as a coming together of two people, one an expert in the field of interpersonal relations, and the other a designated patient. Sullivan considered it the psychiatrist's foremost task to be *of use* to the patient in clarifying his characteristic patterns of living. The psychiatrist applies his skills *for the benefit* of the patient.

Sullivan's concept of the psychiatric interview, therefore, goes beyond mere data collection. In fact, Sullivan would not consider such an approach psychiatric at all.

The foregoing material in this chapter presents the psychiatrist with various systems that aid in the collection, organization, and interpretation of data collected in the interview. Regardless of which system the psychiatrist employs, it is helpful to keep in mind some of Sullivan's basic philosophy regarding the psychiatric interview. This philosophy is summarized in the fifteen questions listed below. The psychiatrist might utilize them as a checklist on his own technique.

1. Do I have a good idea of how the consultation came to happen?
2. Do I have a fairly clear impression of the patient as a person?
3. Do I think that an adequate reason for the interview was elicited from, or told to, the patient?
4. Do I have a fairly clear idea of the impression made on the patient by the physician?
5. Do I have an adequate idea of how the patient came to be the person he is?
6. And in the course of which, he experienced an important difficulty in living?
7. And which difficulty in itself is a sufficient reason for seeking the help of a psychiatrist?

8. What do I believe is the major problem which currently troubles the patient?
9. What does the patient consider to be his major problem?
10. Was the comment or recommendation of the physician to the patient adequate and appropriate to the needs of the patient and the circumstances of the interview?
11. Was nothing said which would have been apt to be misunderstood by the patient, or otherwise to make trouble in subsequent treatment interviews?
12. Was the interview situation terminated in a suitable and useful fashion?
13. Am I certain that the patient derived a little benefit and no serious damage or discouragement from the interview?
14. Might the interview have tended to discourage the patient about the usefulness of psychiatry?
15. Did the interview show the patient that psychiatry might well be helpful to him?

References

Sullivan, H. S.: *The Psychiatric Interview.* New York, W. W. Norton and Company, 1954.

Chapter III

AIDS TO DIAGNOSIS
IN PSYCHIATRY

ALTHOUGH THE PSYCHIATRIST's basic and most fundamental tool in diagnostic assessment is his own clinical interview (Chapter II, General Psychiatric Evaluation), there are certain other aids available to him. These diagnostic aids can be valuable adjuncts but it must be stressed that they should be regarded as *adjuncts* and cannot replace the psychiatrist's own professional skills and judgment. In this respect they are analogous to laboratory tests in clinical medicine: results must always be evaluated in the context of the overall clinical picture.

The first article (Psychological Testing in Clinical Psychiatry) provides guidelines for the psychiatrist so that he may employ psychological testing most effectively in his practice. The various tests are described together with information concerning their inherent strengths and weaknesses.

Three psychiatric rating scales are also provided: The Brief Psychiatric Rating Scale (BPRS), the Self-Rating Depression Scale (Zung), and the Michigan Alcoholic Screening Test (Selzer). These are among the most effective and clinically useful scales currently available. As with psychological testing, these rating scales have certain inherent strengths and weaknesses. They add a quantitative element to psychiatric diagnosis but they do not provide information regarding dynamic formulation. They do not capture the essence of the individual patient and the nuances that are revealed in the customary psychiatric interview.

The final article (Barbiturate Interview) describes the technique of the barbiturate or Amytal® interview which, used appropriately, can be a valuable diagnostic instrument. Indications and contra-indications for its use are listed.

PSYCHOLOGICAL TESTING IN CLINICAL PSYCHIATRY
DAVID W. PEARSON, M.A., M.D.

I. The Clinical Psychologist

  A. Training

A clinical psychologist is a student of human behavior with extensive training in basic scientific methodology, psychological theory, personality theory and assessment. His academic and clinical training, which usually takes place in a university and/or psychiatric setting, gives him a broad background in research techniques, diagnostic work, and psychotherapy. Licensing is necessary in most states although there is little uniformity concerning requirements. Typically, in the clinical setting, the psychologist is called upon to assist in diagnostic evaluations, to do research, and to carry on psychotherapy.

  B. The use and abuse of psychological testing

A request for psychological testing should be looked upon much as any other consultation or laboratory test in medicine. In requesting a psychological consultation, the physician making the request should ask specific questions that he would like answered. Some typical questions asked of psychological testing are: Does this patient have the intelligence and the strength to use insight therapy? How well are his defenses working and how much does anxiety impair his intellectual functioning? Is there an organic factor underlying his present problems? What are the nature of this person's interpersonal relationships? Can he tolerate the stress of working closely with someone in therapy? Psychological tests are also used legally to determine mental retardation. Vocational testing and career planning are additional areas where psychological tests can help.

In the referral to psychology, questions are often asked

which are too vague or are not conceptualized clearly enough to enable a psychologist to know what is wanted. Such questions as: What are the general dynamics of this patient? Complete psychological examination on this patient. Please do a Rorschach on this patient. What is the personality configuration of this patient? What is going on with this guy and what is his IQ? are not specific enough to permit the psychologist to select those instruments which would best enable him to perform a meaningful evaluation. It must be remembered that any experienced clinical psychologist, having the results of a test battery, can write a book of many pages on the various characteristics of the patient's psychological functioning. The problem is selecting the material which will be most useful to the person requesting the testing.

In requesting psychological consultation it is necessary for the person making the referral to give as clearly as possible his own impressions of the patient and to describe where he hopes the psychologist will add information. This enables the psychologist to select the most useful instruments and to organize his report so as to best answer these questions. It is also important to remember that psychological tests are not magical sources of true knowledge and that there is no 100 percent accurate way of assessing homicidal potential, suicidal risk, or other impulsive acts on the basis of test protocols or any other sample of behavior. This is not to say that testing cannot be useful in the evaluation of such factors but it should not be considered a sure way of finding the truth. The psychologist's opinion in these areas, as in many others, should be considered as any other professional opinion, the best educated guess that can be made from the data, his experience, and the present state of the art. The referring person then considers the results in the context of the overall clinical picture, much as a physician weighs the importance of any one laboratory result in terms of the patient's overall condition.

C. What to tell the patient

In preparing the patient for psychological testing, depending upon his mental state and intelligence, it is wise to notify him that you are asking for a consultation from a psychologist. A brief explanation might go something like, "The psychologist will probably want to ask a few background questions and then will give you some tasks to do. The major purpose of the tasks is to help in understanding how you (the patient) see your world so that we (the diagnosticians) can be of greater help to you (the patient)." Some patients need reassurance that they will not be penalized for doing poorly or flunking. Obvious comparisons to school, depending upon the patient's experience, can be useful.

When the clinical psychologist sees the patient for diagnostic purposes, he usually plans on two or three testing sessions of two to three hours to give a full battery of tests. After a careful review of the referral information, the clinician selects the instruments that will best serve in evaluating those areas he feels important in understanding the patient's presenting problems and the questions asked in the referral.

Rarely will a clinical psychologist feel that one brief sample of behavior collected by only one instrument is enough. Usually he will integrate tests which tap personality functioning at different levels into a battery which will vary from patient to patient, depending upon the patient and the referral problem. For example, a typical battery for an adult might consist of the Bender-Gestalt, the Draw-a-Person, the WAIS, a 10 card TAT, and the Rorschach. By using such a battery the most observable level of ego functioning can be assessed, as well as such things as the patient's cognitive functioning, the quality of the patient's object relations, possible sources of conflict that might be causing the present symptom formation, ego weaknesses, possible ego defects, etc. Such a battery gives a fairly complete assessment of personality functioning and enables the experienced clinician to give useful additional information on nearly any question of diagnostic or psychotherapeutic relevance. It is important to remember that the usual goal of psychological testing is not to arrive at a label (i.e. Schizophrenic reaction, paranoid type 000.$\times$23) but to give a description of personality variables so that the patient's behavior can be understood and a meaningful treatment program can be formulated. The findings of the social worker, the psychiatric interviews and the report of the clinical psychologist should all be taken into consideration when formulating a treatment program for the patient.

II. Psychological Testing

Psychological tests have been devised to assess various aspects of ego functioning. One of the basic assumptions made in the use of psychologicals is that everything that a patient does reflects the patient's personality to some extent. The psychological report usually has some discussion of the patient's overt behavior, mannerisms, and reaction to the psychologist and the testing procedure.

All test data are considered samples of behavior. Most clinical tests involving clinical inference are administered individually rather than to groups of subjects so that motoric and affective responses can be noted. As in the psychiatric interview, verbal behavior is sampled in response to stimuli of varying concreteness. One end of a concreteness continuum is characterized by objective tests such as achievement tests, personality inventories, and aptitude tests. Here simple yes or no answers are required. In the middle of the continuum are the subtests of the Wechsler Intelligence Scales where the meaning of proverbs are asked, where similarities between two objects are requested, or where a story is made up to a series of pictured events. At the most abstract end of the concreteness continuum are the projective tests such as the Thematic Apperception Test where stories are constructed to pictures, the Rorschach where percepts are described in inkblots or the Draw-a-Person test where the patient draws a picture of a person and may make up stories to his own drawing. Tests used in any assessment are based upon clinical considerations as well as considerations of reliability and validity. There are cues on all testing data to check for malingering or cheating.

A. Intelligence Testing

1. Basic Considerations

Intelligence, for our purposes, will be defined as the "aggregate or global capacity of the individual to act purposefully, to think rationally, to learn, and to deal effectively with his environment." (Wechsler, D., *The Measurement and Appraisal of Adult Intelligence:* p. 7). Tests designed to assess intellectual abilities are categorized in two general ways: those assessing performance variables and those assessing verbal variables. Performance tests are usually tests of speed in putting something together, quickness in seeing a missing part of a picture, or ordering of a sequence of events. They are tests in which the use of language, aside from giving instructions, is minimized. On some performance tests, instructions are given nonverbally. People with poor English skills or who are otherwise culturally deprived do better on nonverbal tests.

Verbal tests are usually employed to measure the person's fund of knowledge, vocabulary, or memory. In verbal tests the use of language is required in both test content and response. Middle class people, particularly those with advanced education and relatively rich verbal background do best on these tests.

Results from intelligence tests are usually reported in the form of an IQ (Intelligence Quotient). This is defined as: $\dfrac{\text{M.A.}}{\text{C.A.}} \times 100 = \text{IQ}$ C.A. is chronological age, M.A. is mental age. The distribution of IQ scores within the total population is described in Table III-I.

It is important to realize that actual IQ is a relatively

TABLE III-I

Intelligence Classification of WAIS I.Q.'s

ages 16 to 75+ (actual)

(Wechsler, D. *The Measurement and Appraisal of Adult Intelligence:* p. 42)

Classification	I.Q.	Percent of Population Included
Defective	69 and below	2.2
Borderline	70 to 79	6.7
Dull–Normal	80 to 89	16.1
Average	90 to 109	50.0
Bright–Normal	110 to 119	16.1
Superior	120 to 129	6.7
Very Superior	130 and above	2.2

constant score in the adult between 20 and 50. However, in children and in the emotionally unstable adult, IQ's tend to vary. Early testing may well pick up the child who is in the lower IQ group, but it does not often identify the child with potentially superior abilities. Adults with inconsistent records are generally considered to have some intellectual impairment, either of an emotional or organic nature. This is not true for children and is one of the reasons why a good diagnostician will see a child a number of times to make sure of obtaining a true picture.

2. The Stanford-Binet

a. Age range: two years to sixteen years. Clinically the normative data is probably at its best in the child from four years to fourteen years.

b. Organization: Performance and verbal items are intermixed. The patient is started at a level where he will miss no items (basal mental age) and given tasks of increasing difficulty until he misses all tasks for a given year (ceiling age). In general there are six items for each year and for each item the patient passes he is given two months mental age credit. In the second and third year there are twelve tests and the child is given one month of mental age credit for each task passed.

c. IQ range: low 30's to low 170's.

d. Most recent revision: 1960 (stratified national sample of 4498 subjects).

3. The Wechsler Intelligence Scale for Children (WISC)

a. Age range: Five years to fifteen years. Clinically it is probably at its best from six years to early fifteen years.

b. Organization
1. Six verbal subtests:
   a. Information   d. Similarities
   b. Comprehension   e. Digit Span
   c. Arithmetic   f. Vocabulary
2. Six Performance subtests:
   a. Digit Symbol

    b. Picture Completion   e. Mazes

    c. Block Design   f. Object Assembly

    d. Picture Arrangement

The patient continues on any one subtest until he fails a certain number of items. Bonuses are given for speed of performance and level of abstraction on specific subtests. The raw scores from these subtests are converted to standard scores and are compared to the scores of the standardizing population.

    c. IQ range: mid 40's to mid 150's.

    d. Most recent revision: 1949 (stratified national sample of 2200 subjects).

    4. The Wechsler Adult Intelligence Scale (WAIS)

    a. Age Range: 16 to 75+. Clinically, it is probably at its best from sixteen to sixty-five.

    b. Organization:

      1. Six verbal subtests:

        a. Information   d. Similarities

        b. Comprehension   e. Digit Span

        c. Arithmetic   f. Vocabulary

      2. Five performance subtests:

        a. Digit Symbol   d. Picture

        b. Picture Completion   Arrangement

        c. Block Design   e. Object Assembly

The organization is the same as on the WISC. The patient continues on each subtest until a criterion of number-of-items-failed is reached. Bonuses are given for speed of performance and level of abstraction on specific subtests. Again, the raw scores from these subtests are converted to standard scores and are compared to the scores of the standardizing population.

    c. IQ range: low 40's to low 150's.

    d. Most recent revision: 1955 (stratified national sample of 1700 subjects).

    5. Other Intelligence Tests

    There are other tests for determining IQ that correlate highly with these IQ scores. The three tests outlined above are the ones most commonly used by clinical psychologists. There are abbreviated forms in which certain specific subtests are used when intellectual functioning is not the focus of evaluation. The sum of these selected subtests correlate highly with full scores and enables the clinician to use more time to focus on other specific questions.

In all of these tests of intelligence it is important to realize that IQ is only a number. People vary as much as five to seven points from day to day. When it was first introduced, IQ was seized upon with almost a religious fervor as an absolute means of differentiating those who can perform from those who cannot. However, even in his earliest writings Binet emphasized that the numerical results have little meaning unless the complete test performance is carefully evaluated and noted. IQ can be clinically misleading if it is not interpreted within the total context of the patient's social background and psychological functioning.

B. Personality Testing

Basic considerations: the Actuarial Approach vs. the Clinical Approach.

There are two broad approaches to the assessment of personality functioning. One position, the actuarial position, maintains that behavioral phenomena are too transient and there are too many observer variables in clinical evaluation. Proponents of this position use objective tests such as personality inventories. The second approach is the clinical one. Here careful note is made of the patient's responses throughout the testing. Note of any idiosyncratic behavior or response is made and described in the final formulation. Inferences drawn from test data, behavior, research on the tests, and the clinician's personal experience are all related in the final formulation.

1. The Actuarial Approach: the Minnesota Multiphasic Personality Inventory (MMPI)

The most frequently used personality inventory is the MMPI. The test consists of 566 statements about the way people feel about themselves. The patient is asked to check on an answer sheet whether he believes the statement pertains to him, is not like him or he does not know. The patient's responses can then be hand scored or computer scored. The patient's pattern of responses are compared to the responses of patients with known psychiatric illness and diagnosis. There are three scales to evaluate the reliability of the individual's responses. These, combined with the "K" scale, detect malingerers, liars, and false negative cases. There are nine clinical scales: (1) Hypochondriasis (Hs), (2) Depression (D), (3) Hysteria (Hy), (4) Psychopathic-deviate (Pd), (5) Masculinity-femininity interests (M-F), (6) Paranoia (Pa), (7) Psychasthenia (Pt), (8) Schizophrenia (Sc), (9) Hypomania (Ma). A tenth scale, the social introversion scale (Si) is on the profile but it has little clinical significance at this time.

Uses of MMPI:

    a. Not to be used for definitive diagnosis but only as an aid in the diagnostic process.

    b. Good screening device when large numbers of patients are to be seen and the sickest patients must be selected.

    c. Has been used in general medical setting to add a personality dimension to records kept on each patient.

    d. Research use, especially where large numbers of subjects are used.

  2. The Clinical Approach: The Bender Visual Motor Gestalt Test (Bender-Gestalt)

    a. Material: Nine 3 in $\times$ 5 in cards, each with one design on it.

    b. Task:

    To copy the designs as they are presented one at a time. There is no time limit. A memory trial may be used after the initial copy administration and obvious mistakes may be questioned.

    c. Data interpretation:

    As this is the simplest task in the psychological test battery, anxiety and certain defensive patterns can often be most clearly seen.

3. The Thematic Apperception Test (TAT)
   a. Material:
   30 pictures, each on a separate 11 in × 8½ in card. Each picture depicts a possible conflictual situation. Ten cards can be given to both males and females (the MF cards), ten cards are more oriented towards males (the M cards) and ten cards are oriented toward females (the F cards).
   b. Task:
   The patient is asked to make up a story to the picture with a beginning, a middle, and an end. He is asked to tell what the characters are thinking, feeling, and doing. The psychologist then presents the cards he has selected (usually eight to ten cards centered around the conflictual situations thought to be of importance to the patient). He writes down the patient's responses verbatim, both verbal and behavioral, and questions the subject further if clarification is needed.

4. The Rorschach Test (Rorschach)
   a. Material:
   Ten photographic plates, five of which are monochromatic, two are dichromatic and the last three are polychromatic.
   b. Task:
   Before he sees any of the cards, the patient is asked to report everything he will see on the cards. He is assured there is no right or wrong and that some people see this and others see that. Traditionally, any questions are answered and then the patient is handed the first card. One may initially question, encouraging further responses on the first card, but then there is no further verbal intervention on the part of the clinician until the patient has responded to all ten cards. Needless to say, this period is called free association period where all re-

sponses, both verbal and behavioral, are recorded verbatim and time taken to respond is noted. Originally, it was even recommended that the patient sit with his back to the clinician. The second part of the test, which involves a great deal of skill, is the inquiry. During the inquiry the psychologist attempts to elicit exactly what about the blot caused the patient to see what he saw. The clinician can then go on to ask the patient for further responses or even "test limits" by asking interpretation of specific aspects of the blot. Variation in administration may be determined by the patient's productions or by the clinicians theoretical convictions.

c. Data interpretation:
Various systems based upon:
1. The part of the ink blot included in the response; the space or shaded area.
2. The form level of the response, how good or how bad the response is.
3. The effects of shading, and/or color on the response.
4. The effects of movement in the response (human, animal, inanimate).
5. The content category of the response (animal, human, plant, clothing).
6. Is the response unique or one commonly given by subjects on a particular card?

Normative values are available on all of the above categories and there are other systems used less universally. Scoring systems are devised as a means of evaluating the structure of thought and perception; the intactness of ego functioning, the defensive tactics, and the severity of the anxiety experienced from underlying conflicts. Some clinicians depend primarily upon the content of the responses for their use of the Rorschach, but it is generally thought that the structural variables also deserve consideration.

5. The Draw-a-Person Test

a. Materials:
   A pencil (No. 2) with an eraser and four pieces of 11 in $\times$ 8½ in plain white paper.
b. Task:
   1. The patient is asked to draw the best picture of a person he can. No further comments are made.
   2. After the first drawing is completed, the patient is asked to draw the best picture of a person of the opposite sex from his first drawing that he can.
   3. A third and a fourth drawing can be suggested if only heads are drawn. The psychologist takes careful note of how the drawing is done, what is erased and any spontaneous comments. (Comments about the kind of persons the patient has drawn are sought and the patient may be asked to make up a story about his drawings.).
c. Interpretation of the data:
   Position of the figure, line quality, elaboration in the drawing, heaviness of line, clothing, sex of the first drawing, position of the paper and other idiosyncracies are noted. These appear independent of drawing skills. (The first drawing is assumed to be the patient and conflictual areas are often clearly described in the story about each figure.) Correlations are made between this data and data gathered on other tests in the psychological test battery and inferences are drawn.

C. Testing for Organicity:
   It is often said that psychological testing can detect subtle indications of brain damage earlier than the relatively gross neurological examination. Frequently psychologists will add a paragraph to an already lengthy report suggesting that the results are not inconsistent with diffuse encephalopathy or an organic lesion. It is wise to pay attention to these cues

although often they are added for completeness sake. Ideally such patients should be evaluated by specially trained neuropsychologists, but all too few of them exist. There are special batteries of tests of psychological functioning which can often pick up signs of an early localizing lesion or of a diffuse process. However, in the hands of any but the expert, these tests can be misused and information can be misleading. It is particularly important to discuss any suggestions of organic lesions directly with the consulting psychologist.

References

Anastasi, Anne: *Psychological Testing.* New York, The MacMillan Company, 1954.

Freeman, Frank S.: *Theory and Practice of Psychological Testing,* Revised Edition. New York, Henry Holt and Company, 1955.

Rappaport, David; Gill, Merton M.; and Schafer, Roy: *Diagnostic Psychological Testing,* Revised Edition. New York, International Universities Press, Inc., 1968.

Schafer, Roy: *The Clinical Application of Psychological Tests.* New York, International Universities Press, Inc., 1948.

Wechsler, David: *The Measurement and Appraisal of Adult Intelligence,* 4th ed. Baltimore, The Williams & Wilkins Co., 1958.

BRIEF PSYCHIATRIC RATING SCALE (BPRS)

The Brief Psychiatric Rating Scale was initially designed to measure patient response to therapy. It has proven to be a useful instrument for this purpose, particularly in measuring response to drug therapy. The scale is widely used in both clinical practice and in psychiatric research.

An additional use of the scale is as an adjunct in differential diagnosis (syndrome scoring). The BPRS has revealed significant demographic variables that help distinguish agitated depression from retarded depression and thought disorder from paranoid disturbance.

Instructions

The BPRS is easy to use if the clinician familiarizes himself with the definitions of the sixteen rated items. The definitions must be accepted arbitrarily and employed consistently in order to maintain accuracy. Table III-II presents the BPRS in its entirety.

TABLE III-II

BRIEF PSYCHIATRIC RATING SCALE

(Reprinted with permission of John E. Overall, Ph.D. and Courtesy of Roche Laboratories)

ITEMS	Mark the column headed by the term which best describes the patient's present condition.	Not Present	Very Mild	Mild	Moderate	Moderately Severe	Severe	Extremely Severe
					RATINGS			
1. Somatic Concern	Degree of concern over present bodily health. Rate the degree to which physical health is perceived as a problem by the patient, whether complaints have a realistic basis or not.	0	1	2	3	4	5	6
2. Anxiety	Worry, fear, or overconcern for present or future. Rate solely on the basis of verbal report of patient's own subjective experiences. Do not infer anxiety from physical signs or from neurotic defense mechanisms.	0	1	2	3	4	5	6
* 3. Emotional Withdrawal	Deficiency in relating to the interviewer and to the interview situation. Rate only the degree to which the patient gives the impression of failing to be in emotional contact with other people in the interview situation.	0	1	2	3	4	5	6
4. Conceptual Disorganization	Degree to which the thought processes are confused, disconnected or disorganized. Rate on the basis of integration of the verbal products of the patient; do not rate on the basis of patient's subjective impression of his own level of functioning.	0	1	2	3	4	5	6
5. Guilt Feelings	Overconcern or remorse for past behavior. Rate on the basis of the patient's subjective experiences of guilt as evidenced by verbal report with appropriate affect; do not infer guilt feelings from depression, anxiety or neurotic defenses.	0	1	2	3	4	5	6

CATEGORIES

Table III-II (continued)

ITEMS	Mark the column headed by the term which best describes the patient's present condition.	Not Present	Very Mild	Mild	Moderate	Moderately Severe	Severe	Extremely Severe
* 6. Tension	Physical and motor manifestations of tension nervousness, and heightened activation level. Tension should be rated solely on the basis of physical signs and motor behavior and not on the basis of subjective experiences of tension reported by the patient.	0	1	2	3	4	5	6
* 7. Mannerisms and Posturing	Unusual and unnatural motor behavior, the type of motor behavior which causes certain mental patients to stand out in a crowd of normal people. Rate only abnormality of movement; do not rate simply heightened motor activity here.	0	1	2	3	4	5	6
8. Grandiosity	Exaggerated self-opinion, conviction of unusual ability or powers. Rate only on the basis of patient's statements about himself or self-in-relation-to-others, not on the basis of his demeanor in the interview situation.	0	1	2	3	4	5	6
9. Depressive Mood	Despondency in mood, sadness. Rate only degree of despondency; do not rate on the basis of inferences concerning depression based upon general retardation and somatic complaints.	0	1	2	3	4	5	6
10. Hostility	Animosity, contempt, belligerence, disdain for other people outside the interview situation. Rate solely on the basis of the verbal report of feelings and actions of the patient toward others; do not infer hostility from neurotic defenses, anxiety or somatic complaints. (Rate attitude toward interviewer under uncooperativeness.)	0	1	2	3	4	5	6

Table III-II (continued)

ITEMS	Mark the column headed by the term which best describes the patient's present condition.	Not Present	Very Mild	Mild	Moderate	Moderately Severe	Severe	Extremely Severe
11. Suspiciousness	Belief (delusional or otherwise) that others have now, or have had in the past, malicious or discriminatory intent toward the patient. On the basis of verbal report, rate only those suspicions which are currently held, whether they concern past or present circumstances.	0	1	2	3	4	5	6
12. Hallucinatory Behavior	Perceptions without normal external stimulus correspondence. Rate only those experiences which are reported to have occurred within the last week and which are described as distinctly different from the thought and imagery processes of normal people.	0	1	2	3	4	5	6
*13. Motor Retardation	Reduction in energy level evidenced in slowed movements. Rate on the basis of observed behavior of the patient only; do not rate on the basis of patient's subjective impression of own energy level.	0	1	2	3	4	5	6
*14 Uncooperativeness	Evidence of resistance, unfriendliness, resentment and lack of readiness to co-operate with the interviewer. Rate only on the basis of the patient's attitude and responses to the interviewer and the interview situation; do not rate on basis of reported resentment or uncooperativeness outside the interview situation.	0	1	2	3	4	5	6
15. Unusual Thought Content	Unusual, odd, strange or bizarre thought content. Rate here the degree of unusualness, not the degree of disorganization of thought processes.	0	1	2	3	4	5	6
16. Blunted Affect	Reduced emotional tone, apparent lack of normal feeling of involvement.	0	1	2	3	4	5	6

Total Pathology Score = Sum of all ratings

Five items (3,6,7,13,14) are marked by an asterisk (*). These are items of observable behavior. All other items refer to the patient's verbal responses.

The sum of all the ratings represents the total pathology score (TPS). By rating the patient at various points in therapy or during hospitalization, the psychiatrist is able to follow the clinical course quantitatively.

TOTAL PATHOLOGY SCORE (TPS)

The total pathology score for any particular patient is not an absolute diagnostic indicator. Patients suffering the same psychiatric disorder may have widely differing scores while patients with dissimilar diagnoses may have virtually the same total score. The total pathology score is most useful as an indicator of response to treatment and not as a diagnostic tool.

Nevertheless, TPS profiles have been established for thirteen major classes of functional psychosis. These profiles are useful as a general guideline.

	TPS
Chronic undifferentiated schizophrenic	32.5
Paranoia	34.0
Manic-depressive, manic	34.3
Simple schizophrenic	34.3
Paranoid state	39.6
Residual schizophrenic	46.6
Schizo-affective	46.6
Paranoid schizophrenic	48.7
Manic-depressive, depressive	49.6
Hebephrenic schizophrenic	51.1
Psychotic depressive	52.1
Acute undifferentiated schizophrenic	52.8
Catatonic schizophrenic	58.6

(Maximum possible score is 96 i.e. 16 $\times$ 6)

SYNDROME SCORING

Extensive work with the BPRS has revealed four syndromes that are mutually independent. Each syndrome consists of a different trio of items and each can be scored by simply adding the scores of the three items.

The four syndromes include:

Thinking Disturbance (Items 4,12,15)
Paranoid Disturbances (Items 10,11,14)
Withdrawal Retardation (Items 3,13,16)
Anxious Depression (Items 2,5,9)

The psychiatrist can utilize these clusters as an aid in differential diagnosis and treatment planning. For example, it is often difficult to distinguish the anxious patient from the patient with mixed anxiety and depression; yet it is important, in terms of prescribing drug treatment, to make this differentiation.

There are several other uses (clinical and research) of the BPRS. Many are summarized by Overall and Klett (1972).

References

Lorr, M.: *Inpatient Multidimensional Psychiatric Scale Manual,* Revised Ed. Palo Alto, California, Consulting Psychology Press, 1966.

Lyerly, S. B. and Abbott, P. S.: *Handbook of psychiatric rating scales (1950–1964).* U.S. Government Printing Office, 1966.

Overall, J. E. and Gorham, D. R.: The Brief Psychiatric Rating Scale. *Psychol Rep, 10:* 799, 1962.

Overall, J. E.: Standard psychiatric symptom description: The factor construct rating scale (FCRS). *Triangle, 8:* 178, 1968.

Overall, J. E. and Klett, C. J.: *Applied Multivariate Analysis.* New York, McGraw-Hill, 1972.

SELF-RATING DEPRESSION SCALE

The Self-Rating Depression Scale was developed by W. W. K. Zung, M.D., Associate Professor of Psychiatry, Duke University Medical Center. It is a useful and tested tool for quantitatively assessing the degree of depression felt by a patient.

The Scale is comprised of a list of twenty items that relate to specific characteristics of depression. The twenty items comprehensively delineate widely recognized symptoms of depressive disorders. Opposite the statements are four columns headed: None or A Little of the Time, Some of the Time, Good Part of the Time, and Most or All of the Time.

The patient is given the list of items and asked to put a check mark in the box most applicable to him at the time of the test. To obtain the patient's depression rating, each item (Numbers 1 through 20) is scored on a one through four point basis. This raw score is then converted to an index based on 100. The scale is so constructed that a low index indicates little or no depression and a high index indicates depression of clinical significance.

While some depressed patients volunteer little information, most will readily cooperate when asked to check the scale if told that this will help the doctor know more about them. The statements in the scale are worded in the everyday language of the patient. Occasionally a patient may ask how he should check item No. 5 because he is on a diet and therefore should not be eating as much as he used to; in this case the patient is asked to answer as if he were not on a diet. A patient who hesitates over item No. 6, about sex, may be asked does he enjoy being with people of the opposite sex. Questions usually indicate the patient's desire to cooperate with the physician.

Table III-III presents the Self-Rating Depression Scale in its entirety. Table III-IV is to be used for converting the raw numerical score to the SDS Index score.

MICHIGAN ALCOHOLIC SCREENING TEST

The Michigan Alcoholic Screening Test (MAST) was devised by Melvin L. Selzer, M.D., Professor of Psychiatry, University of Michigan Medical School. It provides a consistent, quantifiable interview instrument to detect alcoholism. A score of 5 is considered diagnostic of alcoholism. For maximum effectiveness it is useful to have arrest records available since this will lessen the incidence of *false negatives* if subjects choose to withhold this information from the interviewer.

Table III-V presents the MAST in its entirety.

TABLE III-III

*The Self-Rating Depression Scale**

	None or a little of the time	Some of the time	Good part of the time	Most or all of the time
1. I feel down-hearted and blue				
2. Morning is when I feel the best				
3. I have crying spells or feel like it				
4. I have trouble sleeping at night				
5. I eat as much as I used to				
6. I still enjoy sex				
7. I notice that I am losing weight				
8. I have trouble with constipation				
9. My heart beats faster than usual				
10. I get tired for no reason				
11. My mind is as clear as it used to be				
12. I find it easy to do the things I used to				
13. I am restless and can't keep still				
14. I feel hopeful about the future				
15. I am more irritable than usual				
16. I find it easy to make decisions				
17. I feel that I am useful and needed				
18. My life is pretty full				
19. I feel that others would be better off if I were dead				
20. I still enjoy the things I used to do				

©W. Zung, 1965

Scoring

Diagnosis	Mean SDS Index	Range
1. Normal Controls	33	25-43
2. Depressed (Out-patient)	64	50-78
3. Depressed (Hospitalized)	74	63-90

*Reprinted with permission: W. Zung, M.D. and courtesy of Lakeside Laboratories

TABLE III-IV

A Table for the Conversion of Raw Scores to the SDS Index

Raw Score	SDS Index	Raw Score	SDS Index	Raw Score	SDS Index
20	25	40	50	60	75
21	26	41	51	61	76
22	28	42	53	62	78
23	29	43	54	63	79
24	30	44	55	64	80
25	31	45	56	65	81
26	33	46	58	66	83
27	34	47	59	67	84
28	35	48	60	68	85
29	36	49	61	69	86
30	38	50	63	70	88
31	39	51	64	71	89
32	40	52	65	72	90
33	41	53	66	73	91
34	43	54	68	74	92
35	44	55	69	75	94
36	45	56	70	76	95
37	46	57	71	77	96
38	48	58	73	78	98
39	49	59	74	79	99
				80	100

TABLE III-V

Michigan Alcoholic Screening Test *

Points	Questions
2	* 1. Do you feel you are a normal drinker?
2	2. Have you ever awakened the morning after some drinking the night before and found that you could not remember a part of the evening before?
1	3. Does your wife (or parents) ever worry or complain about your drinking?
2	* 4. Can you stop drinking without a struggle after one or two drinks?
1	5. Do you ever feel bad about your drinking?
2	* 6. Do friends or relatives think you are a normal drinker?
0	7. Do you ever try to limit your drinking to certain times of the day or to certain places?
2	* 8. Are you always able to stop drinking when you want to?
5	9. Have you ever attended a meeting of Alcoholics Anonymous (AA)?
1	10. Have you gotten into fights when drinking?
2	11. Has drinking ever created problems with you and your wife?
2	12. Has your wife (or other family member) ever gone to anyone for help about your drinking?
2	13. Have you ever lost friends or girlfriends/boyfriends because of drinking?
2	14. Have you ever gotten into trouble at work because of drinking?
2	15. Have you ever lost a job because of drinking?
2	16. Have you ever neglected your obligations, your family, or your work for two or more days in a row because you were drinking?
1	17. Do you ever drink before noon?
2	18. Have you ever been told you have liver trouble? Cirrhosis?
5	19. Have you ever had delirium tremens (DTs), severe

Points   Questions

	shaking, heard voices or seen things that weren't there after heavy drinking?
5	20. Have you ever gone to anyone for help about your drinking?
5	21. Have you ever been in a hospital because of drinking?
2	22. Have you ever been a patient in a psychiatric hospital or on a psychiatric ward of a general hospital where drinking was part of the problem?
2	23. Have you ever been seen at a psychiatric or mental health clinic, or gone to a doctor, social worker, or clergyman for help with an emotional problem in which drinking had played a part?
2	**24. Have you ever been arrested, even for a few hours, because of drunk behavior?
2	**25. Have you ever been arrested for drunk driving or driving after drinking?
	*Negative responses are alcoholic responses **Two points for each arrest

*Reprinted with permission: Selzer, M. L.: The Michigan Alcoholic Screening Test: The Quest for a New Diagnostic Instrument. *Amer J Psychiat. 127*:12, 89-94, June 1971. Copyright 1971, the American Psychiatric Association.

BARBITURATE INTERVIEW
MICHAEL J. SHORT, M.D.

The barbiturate (or Amytal) interview is a useful psychiatric tool. The patient is interviewed during a controlled, barbiturate-induced twilight sleep. Conscious control is relaxed and repressed information is made more accessible to scrutiny. It must be emphasized, however, that neither Sodium Amytal nor sodium pentothal (the two most commonly-used agents) are truth serums. What the patient reveals may be fact, fantasy, or a mixture of both. The psychiatrist must evaluate the information with as much skill and sound clinical judgment as he would any other communication from the patient.

I. Indications for Use

  A. Conversion Reactions

    1. Includes amnesia, dissociative states, and sudden, dramatic conversion symptoms such as hysterical blindness that are precipitated by sudden emotion trauma.

    2. Information revealed may have therapeutic as well as diagnostic value.

    3. The patient may be helped by re-experiencing the event while under the influence of the drug or the therapist may choose to wait until a later time and work through the information when the patient is fully conscious.

  B. Elective Mutism

    1. The uses are similar to those described for conversion phenomena.

  C. Medico-Legal Uses

    1. Although courts do not allow barbiturate interviews as direct testimony, some courts do admit as evidence a professional opinion based on the interview.

    2. Uses include determining guilt or innocence of the patient or of another person when the patient is a victim or witness of crime.

    3. Even if not admissable in court, the barbiturate interview can be important to the (a) prosecutor in his decision whether not to prosecute; (b) the patient and his attorney in preparing a defense, especially if some piece of legally significant information is revealed.

  D. Confirmation of Subtle or Questionable Organic Brain Disease

    1. In the person with subtle or questionable organic brain disease a barbiturate interview reveals increased disorientation, memory deficit, and confabulation.

    2. The barbiturate infusion does not have this affect on the patient who is free of organic brain disease.

E. Adjunct to Psychotherapy

    1. Barbiturate interview may facilitate rapport, suggestibility and shorten the search for significant nuclear events.

II. Contra-indications

    A. Specific allergy to barbiturates.

    B. Significant heart, renal, or liver disease.

    C. Less severe ailments should be evaluated, risks, weighed, and appropriate precautions taken if the patient is to undergo the procedure.

III. Description of Drugs Used

    A. Sodium Amytal

        1. Is a hypnotic agent

        2. First relaxes, then produces drowsiness and eventually sleep.

        3. Drowsiness and sleep recede slowly. Therefore, dosage must be titrated carefully or patient will be put to sleep and the interview will be terminated prematurely.

        4. If used as described below, overdoses should result only in sleep.

    B. Sodium pentothal

        1. Is an anesthetic agent

        2. Has a narrow critical point between relaxation and clouding of consciousness, therefore dose must be titrated carefully.

        3. Is shorter acting than Amytal and frequent additional amounts may be required.

        4. Prolonged interviews are easier with pentothal than amytal because the effects wear off quickly and the patient can be titrated with frequent additional amounts.

        5. Caution: Pentothal may reduce respirations; overdose may produce anoxia. Monitor respirations closely.

IV. General Procedures
   A. Obtain written consent.
   B. If the interview is to be tape recorded, the patient should sign specific consent, documenting the uses to which the tape may be put.
   C. Patient should be accompanied by responsible adult if the procedure is done on outpatient basis.
   D. NPO for 12 hours.
   E. Patient is not to drive a car immediately following the procedure.
   F. State law or hospital practice may require the presence of an anesthetist or anesthesiologist.
   G. If anesthetist or anesthesiologist are not present, the psychiatrist must be trained in intubation and resuscitation techniques.
   H. Suitable emergency equipment, medication, and attendants should be available.
   I. Patient should be lying comfortably, preferably in hospital gown.
V. Method of Injection
   A. Start IV infusion with 500 cc normal saline or Ringer's lactate.
   B. It is easiest to use a stopcock and inject the medication through a permanently placed syringe. An alternative would be to inject the medication directly into the IV tubing.
   C. Direct injection into the patient's vein is cumbersome. The patient may move his arm, extravasating the medication.
   D. If using stopcock or injecting directly into IV tubing, be sure to shut off the IV flush solution above the level of the injection or the medication may reflux into the bottle.
   E. Flush solution should run at 10 to 30 drops/minute.
VI. Amytal Method
   A. Used as a 5 percent or 10 percent solution
      1. 5 percent solution $= 5$ cc H_2O added to 0.25 gm ($3\frac{3}{4}$ gr.) ampule of sodium amytal

B. Rate of infusion
  1. 2 cc/minute for 5 percent solution
  2. 1 cc/minute for 10 percent solution
  C. Average total dose = 0.2 to 0.4 gm
VII. Pentothal Method
  A. Do not use 10 percent solution
  B. Rate of infusion
  1. 2 cc/minute for 5 percent solution
  2. 4 cc/minute for 2.5 percent solution
  C. Total dose is slightly higher than Amytal
VIII. Conduct of Interviewer
  A. The interviewer must properly prepare the patient by allaying his fears about the procedure, real or imagined. The results are better, too, if the patient approaches the procedure in the spirit of a therapeutic alliance: the psychiatrist and himself working together for his own ultimate benefit.
  B. The conduct of the interviewer is crucial. He should be as confident, relaxed, and nonthreatening to the patient as possible.
  C. Begin by suggesting that the procedure will be soothing and relaxing; it will make talking easier and allow thoughts to flow more freely.
  D. While slowly injecting the medication, ask the patient to count backwards from 100. This allows the interviewer to judge the state of consciousness. Note slurred speech, and a slowing in the counting. This is when the interview begins.
  E. Start the interview by again establishing rapport. Then go on to neutral topics. Only after the cooperation of the patient is ascertained should the interviewer begin to gently probe for repressed material. In doing this, the interviewer should use all the tact and skill that he would use if the patient was fully conscious.
IX. Post-Interview
  A. After the interview is completed, allow the patient

to rest or sleep for one to three hours. The patient should be observed during this time, as per any postanesthetic period.

B. If the patient is to go back home after the interview he should be accompanied by a relative or other responsible adult. He should not drive.

References

Arieti, S. (Ed.) : *American Handbook of Psychiatry.* New York, Basic Books Inc., 1959.

Kolb, L. C.: *Noye's Modern Clinical Psychiatry.* Philadelphia, W. B. Saunders Co., 1968.

Chapter IV

SPECIAL EVALUATIONS IN PSYCHIATRY

THE PSYCHIATRIST IS CALLED UPON to perform many different types of clinical assessments. While it is true that his *modus operandi* will be quite similar from one type of evaluation to another, in that he relies fundamentally upon a sound, basic psychiatric interview as his primary instrument of data collection, it is also true that each particular type of consultation requires the psychiatrist to be aware of certain specific data, above and beyond what is customarily obtained in the routine psychiatric interview. If he fails to collect this special data, his evaluation will be incomplete at best.

For example, what specific questions, apart from the customary psychiatric interview, should be asked of the suicidal patient? the terminally-ill patient? the patient complaining of a sexual problem? the patient being evaluated for psychiatric competency to stand trial? the individual seeking psychiatric deferment from military service? For each of these special psychiatric evaluations and for many other such evaluations, the psychiatrist should be prepared to elicit the necessary special information from the patient. He must know what questions to ask and what tests to apply if he is to make an accurate diagnostic assessment and if he is to make suitable recommendations.

This chapter is designed to aid the psychiatrist in the arena of these special evaluations. Various types of evaluations were selected for inclusion in this chapter on the basis of two broad criteria: (1) the special evaluations that are most commonly referred to psychiatrists (the suicidal patient, the dying patient, sexual dysfunction, the adolescent patient, the child patient), and (2) certain other special evaluations about which little information exists in the current psychiatric literature (forensic evaluations, suitability for military service, evaluations for cosmetic surgery and transgender surgery).

EVALUATION OF THE SUICIDAL PATIENT

One of the most crucial evaluations that the psychiatrist must make is that of the potentially suicidal patient. Whether he encounters such a patient in his private practice setting or in the turmoil of a busy emergency room, life and death can virtually hang in the balance as he ponders the nature of his clinical intervention.

This section is designed to aid the psychiatrist in his evaluation of the suicidal patient. It is divided into four parts. Part One (The Suicidal Patient) offers some general guidelines. Part Two (Suicide Ideation Scale) provides a rating scale for use with the patient who talks or hints of suicidal ideation but has not yet made an attempt; it seeks to aid the psychiatrist in determining the probability that the patient will, indeed, attempt suicide. Part Three (Suicide Intent Scale) is for use with the patient who has already made an attempt at suicide; it seeks to distinguish the bonafide suicide attempt from the less serious attempt and will aid the psychiatrist in making suitable disposition of the case. Part Four (The Suicide Caller) deals with one of the most difficult of all clinical problems—the suicidal patient who calls on the telephone.

Part One: The Suicidal Patient
Dean Schuyler, M.D.

I. In evaluating the suicidal patient, consider demographic factors, motivational factors, clinical diagnosis and resources.

A. Demographic Factors: High Suicidal Risk (derived from population data and useful for general orientation purposes only).
1. Age (over 40)
2. Sex (male)
3. Marital Status (div., sep., wid.)
4. Living Condition (alone)
5. Employment Status (unemployed or retired)
B. Motivational Factors
(suicidal risk increases along a continuum based upon the quality of the person's motivation for the act.)
1. Lowest risk: Wishes to influence someone else's behavior and still survive.
2. Low intermediate risk: Wishes to influence someone else's behavior through death.
3. High intermediate risk: Wishes cessation or sleep, not death.
4. Highest risk: Wishes to escape an intolerable situation (intrapsychic or external) by death.
C. Clinical Diagnosis
1. The presence of clinical depression should alert the examiner to ask about current suicidal ideas and past suicidal behavior. The presence of a thought disorder should alert the examiner to explore the possibility of suicide based upon a hallucinated command or delusional belief.
D. Resources
1. If there is no significant other available to the patient, the risk of suicidal ideas being translated into action increases.
II. In Interviewing The Suicidal or Depressed Patient:
A. Ask about suicidal ideas even when the patient does not mention them spontaneously.
B. If ideation is present, use the Suicide Ideation Scale (Part Two) and then ask if the patient has formulated a plan.

    C. Ask if the patient has access to the lethal resources needed to carry out his plan.

    D. Use past suicidal behavior as a clue to future behavior. Patients motivated to die will, in general, increase the medical dangerousness of their actions. Those motivated to influence another's behavior usually up the ante (make a more medically dangerous attempt) if there has been no response to past behavior.

    E. Ask the patient what he believes will result from his death, and what effect he believes his death will have on significant others.

III. In Evaluating The Patient After He Has Actually Made A Suicide Attempt:

    A. Evaluate the medical lethality (seriousness) of the attempt (e.g. extent of injury, significant blood loss, loss of consciousness).

    B. Evaluate the psychological intent (motivation) of the patient.

        1. Carefully record the circumstance surrounding the suicidal behavior. Use the Suicide Intent Scale (Part Three).

        2. Ask about the patient's concept of the method's lethality (e.g. Did he do more or less to himself than he thought might be lethal?).

    C. Evaluate his state of consciousness prior to the suicidal act (clouded due to alcohol? to drugs?).

    D. Is he happy or sorry to be alive? What are his plans for the future?

IV. Management

    A. When in doubt about immediate suicide risk, *admit the patient.* The picture may clarify with additional history and interview data.

    B. Contact significant others so that they may add historical detail and be engaged in treatment planning.

    C. Contact the treating psychiatrist, if any.

    D. There is a poor rate of return on outpatient followup with suicidal patients. If there are no responsible people present with the patient and if there is no treating psychiatrist that can be reached, it is usually best to admit the patient, develop a therapeutic relationship, and later arrange for proper outpatient treatment.

E. Attend to countertransference feelings. The suicidal patient evokes in us the fear of our own death, anxiety related to dealing with a patient out of control and fantasies of rescue.

Part Two: Suicide Ideation Scale

This scale was developed by Aaron T. Beck, M.D., Professor of Psychiatry, University of Pennsylvania School of Medicine. It consists of 15 factors that should be investigated in evaluating the person who is considering suicide. The patient's responses are scored on a basis of 0–1–2 for each factor; 0 indicates negligible concern re: suicide potential, while a score of 2 would indicate greatest concern.

The scale has not yet been formally quantified, but Beck believes that a total score of 15 should be interpreted as severe suicidal risk.

> *A word of caution: This scale should be considered as a valuable clinical adjunct and aid in the accumulation and formulation of data. The score is not foolproof; it is not a substitute for a thorough, skillful psychiatric evaluation.*

1. Another's[1] report of patient's intent to attempt suicide
   0. No intent, or very slim chance
   1. Possibility, or will try under certain conditions
   2. Definite intent
2. Patient's report of own intent to attempt suicide
   0. Wants to live
   1. Is not sure, does not care, or it "waiting to see"
   2. Definitely wants to die
3. Patient's attitude toward living
   0. Gives good reasons for living

[1] family member or close friend

      1. Says reasons for dying equal or outweigh reasons for living

      2. Sees no reason for living

4. Patient's feelings about his suicidal thoughts

      0. Feels negative, frightened, or disturbed about them or ignores them

      1. Is in acute distress or is ambivalent about them

      2. Accepts or welcomes them

5. Specificity of ideation

      0. Has abstract and general thoughts (i.e. "I'm thinking of suicide") without visualizing specific events or circumstances related to suicide as: method, place, funeral, or results of death.

      1. Has thought of some specific events or circumstances related to the act of suicide.

      2. Has considered many specific events or circumstances related to the act of suicide.

6. Urgency of ideation

      0. No urgency; keeps his thoughts under control

      1. Is afraid he will be driven to do something he does not want to do, and/or wants someone to control him

      2. No longer makes any attempt to keep suicidal thoughts under control, and may in fact be carrying the thoughts into action

7. Time course of ideation

      0. Isolated and fleeting thoughts at well-spaced intervals

      1. Frequent isolated thoughts, periods of persistent thoughts (hours or more) at well-spaced intervals, or habitual thoughts

      2. Current and persistent thoughts, occupying the patient's mind in a manner he finds unusual

8. Patient's perception of sources of help and support

      0. Has numerous and reliable sources

      1. Sources exist, but are few or unreliable

      2. Has nowhere to turn

9. Seeking help

0. Has not sought help because he has not felt a need for it
1. Has sought help or is seeking help
2. Has not sought help because he does not want interference with his suicidal thoughts or plans
10. Preparations for death
    0. Has none
    1. None, but has thought about them
    2. Have been made or are under way
11. Suicide note
    0. Not thought about
    1. Considered, but not planned out or written
    2. Planned out or written
12. Method
    0. Not thought about
    1. Possibilities have been considered but no method picked out
    2. Has been definitely chosen
13. Means by which method will be put to use
    0. Have not been obtained or worked out (as, pills not purchased, type of pill not decided, means of hanging not decided)
    1. Have been obtained or worked out to some extent, but are not instantly accessible or ready to be put to use
    2. Are ready at a moment's notice
14. Plan
    0. Not thought about
    1. Possibilities being considered, but none is "definite"
    2. Definite plan worked out
15. Stage of plan
    0. Not ready to put into effect
    1. About to be put into effect
    2. Is nearing completion

(Reprinted, with permission, from Beck, A.T.: The Science and Art of Suicide Prediction. *Hospital Physician,* 7: 3: 54, 1971.)

Part Three: Suicide Intent Scale

This scale is for use with the patient who has already made a suicidal attempt. Such a patient is usually encountered in the emergency room. The psychiatrist is asked to evaluate the seriousness of the act. If the patient is no longer in medical danger when he is interviewed and will not be admitted to the medical-surgical unit, the major decision facing the psychiatrist is whether to admit the patient to the psychiatric unit or discharge him from the hospital.

This scale is presented in two sections. The first section consists of eight items that are relatively objective in nature and can be used in the emergency room to assess the seriousness of the patient's suicidal attempt. Like the Ideation Scale, this scale is still being perfected and firm quantifiable parameters have not yet been determined. Schuyler (one of the designers of the scale), however, believes that a score of 5 or greater on these first eight items indicates high intent.

The second section of the Intent Scale consists of 12 additional items. These factors have not yet been quantified and should not be scored. Nevertheless, the psychiatrist should consider all of them in reaching his own final evaluation of the seriousness of the suicidal intent.

> *A word of caution: This scale should be considered as a valuable clinical adjunct and aid in the accumulation and formulation of data. The score is not foolproof; it is not a substitute for a thorough, skillful psychiatric evaluation.*

Section One (To Be Scored)
    5 indicates serious intent
  1. Isolation
     0. Somebody present
     1. Somebody nearby or in contact (as by phone)
     2. No one nearby or in contact
  2. Timing
     ( ) Does not apply
     0. Timed so that intervention is probable
     1. Timed so that intervention is not likely
     2. Timed so that intervention is highly unlikely

3. Precautions Against Discovery and/or Intervention
    0. No precautions
    1. Passive precautions, as avoiding others but doing nothing to prevent their intervention (alone in room with unlocked door)
    2. Active precautions (as locked door)
4. Acting to Gain Help During/After Attempt
    ( ) Does not apply
    0. Notified potential helper regarding attempt
    1. Contacted but did not specifically notify potential helper regarding attempt
    2. Did not contact or notify potential helper
5. Final Acts in Anticipation of Death
    0. None
    1. Patient thought about making or made some arrangements in anticipation of death
    2. Definite plans made (changes in will, giving gifts, taking out insurance)
6. Degree of Planning for Suicide Attempt
    0. No preparation
    1. Minimal or moderate preparation
    2. Extensive preparation
7. Suicide Note
    0. Absence of note
    1. Note written, but torn up or note thought about
    2. Presence of note
8. Conceptions of Method's Lethality
    0. Patient did less to himself than he thought would be lethal or patient didn't think about it
    1. Patient wasn't sure or thought what he did might be lethal
    2. Act exceeded or equalled what patient thought was lethal

Section Two (Not to be scored)
    Responses listed in order of presumed seriousness
    a = least serious, c = most serious)
9. Overt Communication of Intent Before Act
    a. None

    b. Equivocal communication

    c. Unequivocal communication

10. Purpose of Attempt

    a. Mainly to change or manipulate environment

    b. Components of a and c

    c. Mainly to remove self from environment

11. Expectations Regarding Fatality of Act

    a. Patient thought that death was unlikely or did not think about it

    b. Patient thought that death was possible but not probable

    c. Patient thought that death was probable or certain

12. Seriousness of Attempt

    a. Patient did not consider act to be a serious attempt to end his life

    b. Patient was uncertain whether act was a serious attempt to end his life

    c. Patient considered act to be a serious attempt to end his life

13. Ambivalence toward Living

    a. Patient did not want to die

    b. Patient did not care whether he lived or died

    c. Patient wanted to die

14. Conception of Reversibility

    a. Patient thought that death would be unlikely if he received medical attention

    b. Patient was uncertain whether death could be averted by medical attention

    c. Patient was certain of death even if he received medical attention

15. Degree of Premeditation

    a. None; impulsive

    b. Suicide contemplated for three hours or less prior to attempt

    c. Suicide contemplated for more than three hours prior to attempt

16. Reaction to Attempt

    a. Sorry made attempt

b. Accepts both attempt and fact he is still alive

c. Regrets he is still alive

17. Visualization of Death

    a. Viewed as life-after-death or reunion with descendants

    b. Viewed as never-ending sleep or darkness

    c. Not visualized or thought about

18. Number of Previous Attempts

    a. None

    b. One or two

    c. Three or more

19. Consumption of Alcohol at Time of Attempt

    ( ) Does not apply

    a. Enough alcohol was ingested so patient was confused and did not know what he was doing at time of attempt

    b. Alcohol was ingested to get up enough nerve to make attempt

    c. Alcohol was taken to potentiate drugs ingested or other method used

20. Use of Drugs at Time of Attempt

    ( ) Does not apply

    a. Patient under the effect of a drug so he did not know what he was doing at time of attempt or not aware of full implications of attempt

    b. Drug used to free patient of inhibition so attempt could be made

    c. Drug used to potentiate and supplement method used

A. T. Beck, D. Schuyler, and I. Herman, "Development of Suicide Intent Scales," in H. L. Resnik, A. T. Beck and D. Lettieri, (Eds.) : *The Prediction of Suicide.* Philadelphia, Charles Press, 1972.

Part Four: The Suicide Caller

DEAN SCHUYLER, M.D.

Virtually every psychiatrist at some point in his career, will face the problems presented by the suicide caller. This is the person who calls by telephone to report that he is either

(1) contemplating a suicide attempt or (2) has already begun a suicide attempt (by ingestion, open gas jets, etc.).

Successful therapeutic intervention calls for skillful application of the principles outlined in Parts One, Two and Three with the addition of some special techniques listed below.

I. Basic Premise

The most basic fact to remember is that, in almost all cases, a suicide call is indicative of (at the very least) some ambivalence about dying; at the other end of the spectrum it may represent a very real will to live. On the other hand, the *bona fide* suicider has reached a resolute decision to end his life and will do it in planned isolation in most cases.

II. The psychiatrist should identify himself and ask how he can be of help.

III. If in doubt about what to say, and it appears as though the caller may precipitously hang up the phone, attempt to keep him talking by any means until the issues are clarified.

IV. Strive to establish helpful concern and rapport. Attempt to obtain the person's name, his location, and phone number only after a relationship is established.

V. Ask specific questions to evaluate suicide risk (See Parts One, Two, Three):

A. Age and sex

B. Mood (severity of depression)

C. History of previous suicidal behavior

D. Method planned and degree of readiness

E. Precipitant event, if any

1. Degree of interpersonal manipulation involved

F. Resources (spouse, children, relatives, friends)

1. Try to learn the whereabouts of these people so they may be contacted if necessary.

VI. Make specific recommendations after carefully assessing the seriousness of the suicidal communication.

A. No action: Caller has contacted psychiatrist mostly to unburden himself. No suicidal risk. Further contact unwarranted.

B. Advice: No immediate suicide risk. Make suggestions about possible help available to the patient: psychiatric clinic in morning, legal aid, etc. Be careful not to appear to be simply getting rid of the person by referring him elsewhere. It is often most helpful if he feels he can contact the same psychiatrist personally if necessary.

C. Action:

    1. Serious Suicide Risk: The person must be in-instructed to come to see the psychiatrist immediately. If his motivation is doubtful or if he lacks transportation, it is necessary to contact a friend or relative. In extreme cases it may be necessary to continue talking to the patient while someone else contacts the friend or relative on another phone. If no other person is immediately available to go to the suicidal patient, the police may be asked to assist.

    2. Suicidal Act Underway: If the person is calling to say that he has already ingested pills, etc., and the psychiatrist judges that the ingestion is of dangerous proportions, an ambulance and police should be dispatched.

References

Beck, A. T.: The science and art of suicide prediction. *Hospital Physician,* 7: 3: 54, 1971.

Beck, A. T.; Schuyler, D.; and Herman, I.: Development of Suicide Intent Scales. In Resnik, H. L., Beck, A. T., Lettieri, D. (Eds.): *The Prediction of Suicide.* Philadelphia, Charles Press, 1972.

Carter, R. E.: Some effects of client suicide on the therapist. *Psychotherapy: Theory, Research & Practice, 8:* 287–89, 1971.

Lester, G. and Lester, D.: *Suicide: The Gamble with Death.* Englewood Cliffs, Prentice-Hall, Inc., 1971.

Resnik, H. L. P. (Ed.): *Suicidal Behaviors.* Boston, Little Brown & Co., 1968.

Rubenstein, R.; Moses, R.; and Lidz, T.: On attempted suicide. *AMA Archives of Neurology and Psychiatry, 79:* 103–113, 1958.

Surman, O. S. and Lazare, A.: Management of the attempted suicide patient. *Medical Insight.* 1972.

PSYCHIATRIC EVALUATION OF THE DYING PATIENT
Joseph R. Novello, M.D.

One of the most difficult, yet potentially most rewarding, consultations that will be asked of a psychiatrist will be the request to see a dying patient.

Many such consultations will come from physicians who are asking either: (1) Should I tell him or not? or, (2) What kind of antidepressant should be used? At other times there will be other requests, implicit or explicit. Usually at the root of all such consultations is an uneasiness in the physician himself regarding his own attitudes toward death and a plea for an expert to do something.

The psychiatrist, then, must often begin by getting to know the referring physician and understanding as much as he can about what is being asked of him and why.

If the patient is hospitalized, the psychiatrist must similarly familiarize himself with the nursing staff and others in the patient's sphere. What are their attitudes? How do they see the patient? What are they asking? (See Psychiatric Consultation to Medical-Surgical Units, Chapter VII for more information on the process of consultation.)

I. Principles to Remember Before Seeing the Patient

Even before seeing the patient there are several things to be done if the psychiatrist is to make a meaningful consultation:

1. The formal request for consultation, especially if written on a routine form, contains only a small part of the information that the psychiatrist will need in order to make a meaningful evaluation and to be of use to the patient. It is like the tip of an iceberg.

2. Speak privately with the referring physician before seeing the patient. Get below the tip of that iceberg. Gather as much useful information as possible. This includes an impression of the referring physician himself, especially in terms of the probable relationship he has established with the referred patient.

3. Meet with nurses and ward staff. Collect information and impressions.

4. Read the patient's chart. Do not neglect the nurses' notes.

5. The question of to tell or not to tell is not germane. The question that the consultant psychiatrist should pose to himself is: "How do I share this knowledge with this dying person in as understanding, warm, and empathic manner as possible." Remember, as Dr. Elizabeth Kubler-Ross has taught in *On Death and Dying* (Macmillan Company, New York, 1969), most, if not all, dying patients know they are dying. Another useful rule of thumb is that the more people in the patient's sphere who "know the truth" (physicians, nurses, relatives, etc.) the more likely it is that the patient will also "know" regardless if nothing has been "said"; the patient will not mistake the implicit cues. The task of the psychiatrist is to evaluate the level of the patient's knowing, to be available to talk to him about it when he is able to face it and in the manner that he chooses.

6. The complaints of referring physicians often focus upon the patient's denial of his illness in any of several forms. Remember that the dying patient's need for denial is in direct proportion to the need for denial of those around him. If his physicians cheerily insist that everything is fine, the patient will usually play that game too. The same goes for nurses, relatives and friends. Conversely, if there are people in the patient's environment who do *not* need to deny his impending death he will be able to face it with them, if he is ready. It is not unusual for a patient to go all the way to his death denying it to those who themselves had a need to deny it and sharing his deep innermost thoughts and feelings with those who were able to overcome their own conflicts and be of comfort to the patient when he needed it most.

II. Interviewing the Patient

The next step is to get to know the patient. The meeting should be empathic and open-ended. The patient will reveal where he stands. Listen. Most people react to their impending death in the same way in which they have reacted to tragic news in the past. Deniers will deny. Confronters will confront. The psychiatrist should get to know the person he is interviewing. What are his characteristic strengths and weaknesses?

The interview should be private and unhurried. The psychiatrist gives the patient the message by his willingness to listen to whatever he has to say, that, when he is ready, the psychiatrist will be able to face it with him. Also, he should be implicitly assured that he will be allowed to keep his defenses up as long as he needs them. The psychiatrist is not there to club him over the head with the facts. Often this understanding and nonthreatening attitude on the part of the psychiatrist is all the patient needs in order to begin facing it and preparing himself for death.

Even so, the patient's first response may be tentative and couched in metaphor. The psychiatrist's "third ear" must be tuned-in.

It is useful to conceptualize the patient's psychological position in reference to the stages of death and dying that have been formulated by Dr. Ross. She has pointed out that there is a continuum of reactions that most patients go through during this most difficult of all periods in their life. Although there is overlapping and although not all patients can reach the end stage (a realistic acceptance of their fate) , the stages are useful in evaluation, especially in helping medical staff and relatives deal with the particular problems and crises associated with each stage in the process.

Stages of Death and Dying

(The following summary is adapted with permission of the Macmillan Company from *On Death and Dying* by Elizabeth Kubler-Ross, Copyright 1969 by Elizabeth Kubler-Ross.)

Stage I: Denial and Isolation

The patient's customary first reaction is: "No. It can't be me. There must be some mistake." If the need to deny is very great the patient may shop around for other physicians, sign out of the hospital, refuse initial treatment recommendations, etc.

It is important to realize that a certain amount of denial is normal and to be expected. It is used by almost all dying persons initially and then from time to time throughout their terminal illness. It is healthy in that it serves as a buffer to allow them the time to collect themselves and later mobilize less radical defenses.

THERAPEUTIC INTERVENTION (S) :

Respect the patient's early need for denial. Resist the impulse to force him to accept the truth. Medical physicians, especially, may be threatened by the patient who refuses to follow their treatment recommendations. This is their *own* special form of denial. The sensitive psychiatric consultant can also respect this and help the physician to understand.

Stage II: Anger

At this stage it is as if the patient has worked through his denial and is saying, So it is true after all, but why me?

This may be a difficult time for medical staff and relatives since the intense anger is usually displaced in many directions. Unreasonable demands, temper tantrums, and criticisms are common. Such statements as, The doctors (or nurses) don't know what they're doing, etc. are not uncommon at this time.

Dynamically, such acting out may be a way for the patient to reassure himself (and others) that he is still alive. He says, in essence, I am still alive. Don't forget it!

THERAPEUTIC INTERVENTION (S) :

A common response of the medical staff at this point is to either meet hostility with hostility or, by avoiding the patient, to express their hostility covertly. Both maneuvers have the same predictable result: The patient will become even angrier and more demanding.

The psychiatrist can be of great value at this point. The patient, more than ever, needs an empathic ear; he will appreciate a concerned and skillful listener and realize that he is still valued as a person, that he does not need to throw a temper tantrum in order to get attention.

The medical staff should be made to realize the nature of the displacement. There is no need for them to take the insults personally. They should learn that avoidance of or hostility toward the patient only exacerbates the problem. They will also learn more by what the psychiatrist *does* than by what he *says* at this stage. It is especially important for the consultant psychiatrist to spend time with the patient and not be turned off by his anger. The staff will then be able to learn from his example.

Stage III: Bargaining

At this point the patient attempts to bargain his fate. It is as if he says, "If God has decided to take me from this earth and no one is responding to my anger, maybe things will be better if I ask nicely."

This usually takes the form of a bargain with God. Such patients may promise a life dedicated to God in return for more time. It may also take the form of bargaining with physicians: "I will dedicate my body to science if you will do more to prolong my life." Such bargaining may be insistent and unreasonable and place increased stress on an already overburdened physician.

THERAPEUTIC INTERVENTION (S) :

It is important to try to understand the unique dynamics of the patient at this point. Often at the root of such bargaining with God is a sense of profound guilt; the guilt may be due to past sins, real or imagined. The psychiatrist's job at this point is to help the patient work through this guilt. The patient must be relieved of irrational fears and for the latent wish for punishment because of excessive guilt.

If the purely religious aspects of the situation are particularly significant at this point is often useful to arrange a visit by a clergyman, with the patient's cooperation. If this is done, if it is important of course, for psychiatrist and clergyman to be able to work together for the patient's benefit. If the psychiatrist has not worked with the particular clergyman previously, it is wise to meet with him before he sees the patient.

Stage IV: Depression

At this stage the consulting psychiatrist may come under pressure by referring physician, nursing staff, and even relatives to give him something to lift his spirits. The request, of course, is for antidepressant medication. Such a request, of course, grows out of the difficulties that staff or relatives *themselves* are facing. At this point they *may* need more help than the patient. Staff and relatives can be helped by thoughtful conversations with the consulting psychiatrist.

This type of intervention with patient and staff begins with an accurate assessment of the nature of the patient's depression.

Dr. Ross identifies two types of depression at this stage:

1. Preparatory depression
   A. In this type of depression, the patient is preparing for the impending loss of his own life.
   B. Therapeutic Intervention (s) : Allow the patient to express his sorrow openly. Although the patient may become withdrawn and silent, the psychiatrist can still be a great comfort by simply sitting silently with the patient, touching his hand, etc. Do not make the mistake of trying to cheer the patient up; to do so is inappropriate and serves to block the patient's preparation for his own death.
2. Reactive depression
   A. In this type of depression the patient is reacting to certain situational factors; such as the terminally-ill mother worrying about how her children are faring while she is in the hospital and what will become of them, etc.
   B. Therapeutic Intervention (s) : For this type of depression some environmental manipulation and cheering up is indicated. A social worker to take

care of home problems, for example, can dramatically relieve the patient of a great burden; and, in turn, free the patient to begin preparing for his own death, i.e. preparatory depression.

Stage V: Acceptance

The patient who is able to work through to this final stage before death has been able to put his house in order, to finally give up the struggle and enter a period of resting before the long journey. He is neither depressed nor angry about his fate; he accepts it.

While this is not a happy stage, it is not a hopeless giving up. There is something peaceful and dignified about it. Patients who unfortunately do not adequately work through the earlier stages cannot reach this final stage.

THERAPEUTIC INTERVENTION (S) :

Communication becomes more and more nonverbal. The patient may begin to methodically decathect family members, even to the point of asking certain ones not to visit any more. Consequently, it is often the family rather than the patient himself who needs most help at this point.

The most difficult task for the psychiatrist may be to distinguish the patient who has worked through to a realistic acceptance of his fate from the patient who becomes prematurely resigned to his death. This second patient may still have several months or more ahead of him with adequate treatment. If such a patient refuses his physicians' efforts to treat him, a consultation will likely go out to the psychiatrist to talk sense into the patient. Here the psychiatrist must use his skills to uncover the motives for the patient's unrealistic behavior and, if possible, help him work toward accepting treatment.

On the other hand, insisting upon further heroic treatment to the patient who has reached a quiet, dignified, and realistic acceptance of his imminent fate can be insensitive and inhumane. Such insistence usually grows from the physician's own need to prolong life and is more his problem than the patient's at this stage.

Hope

The physician should encourage a sense of hope throughout the patient's terminal course. It is not necessary to tell lies but even the patient's hope for a sudden miracle discovery in medicine that will cure him should be respected and allowed. Yet the physician should not insist upon hope-at-all-costs, especially once the patient reaches the stage of realistic acceptance.

EVALUATIONS AND PROCEDURES IN FORENSIC PSYCHIATRY

LYNN W. BLUNT, M.D.

Forensic psychiatry is that area of psychiatry which deals with the application of psychiatric principles to the criminal and civil justice systems.

I. Areas of Interest to the Forensic Psychiatrist.
A. Commitment Procedures:
1. Involuntary hospitalization and treatment. Laws regarding the commitment of mentally ill persons to hospitals for treatment are generally administered through the probate court. The criteria for commitment vary with the type of order and can be found in one's state mental health statutes.
2. Restoration to soundness of mind. Following commitment, an additional hearing for "uncommiting" a patient is usually required. Such hearings usually require an evaluation by two psychiatrists indicating that the patient is no longer mentally ill.
B. Civil Competency: A person's competency is assumed unless there has been some reason to raise the question. Sometimes the forensic psychiatrist is asked to evaluate a person regarding competency in regard to such questions as:
1. Ability to make contracts or transact other specific business.

2. To marry or divorce.
3. To make a will (testamentary capacity). In order to have testamentary capacity, it must be established that the testator, at the time he made the will:
   a. Understood at least in a general way the nature and location of his property.
   b. Knew who his heirs would normally be under the laws of his particular state.
   c. Had the capacity to understand that he was engaged in making a will that would divide his property upon his death.

C. Civil Law Procedures:
   1. Torts (damage suits). Evaluation and testimony may be required in order to give an opinion regarding cause and effect relationships between some behavior or an event and possible subsequent emotional trauma.
   2. Professional malpractice.

D. Family Law Procedures:
   1. Child custody in divorce proceedings.
   2. Adoption.

E. Juvenile Court Procedures:
   1. Psychiatric diagnosis.
   2. Treatability.
   3. Prognosis.
   4. Recidivistic potential.
   5. Dangerousness.
   6. Disposition.

F. Criminal Law Procedures:
   1. Competency to stand trial. Concern based on premise that the defendant should be mentally, as well as physically, present at his trial. See "Criteria for Competency to Stand Trial: A Checklist for Psychiatrists" in Chapter 13, *Readings in Law and Psychiatry* (Allen, Ferster, and Rubin). Generally, the defendant is deemed

incompetent to stand trial if, by reason of mental illness:

a. He is unable to understand the charge against him.

b. He is unable to understand his position in relation to the charge against him.

c. He is unable to cooperate in a reasonable and rational manner with defense counsel in his own defense.

2. Criminal irresponsibility. Specific legal tests for criminal irresponsibility are used in all states. In contrast to competency to stand trial, criminal irresponsibility applies to the mental state of the defendant at the time of the crime rather than at the time of trial. The specific tests used in a given state can be found in Chapter 11, "Mental Disability and the Criminal Law" in *The Mentally Disabled and the Law* (Brakel and Rock). The tests currently used include:

a. The M'Naghten (Right-Wrong) Test: "To establish a defense on the grounds of insanity, it must be clearly proved that, at the time of the committing of the act, the party accused was laboring under such a defect of reason, from disease of the mind, as not to know the nature and quality of the act he was doing; or, if he did know it, that he did not know he was doing what was wrong.

b. Irresistible-Impulse Test: Applies to a defendant who may know the nature and quality of his act and may be aware that it is wrong, but who, nevertheless may be irresistibly driven to commit a criminal act by an overpowering impulse resulting from a mental condition. This test is not used alone in any jurisdiction but is accepted in conjunction with the M'Naghten Right-Wrong Test in at least 15 states. Informally, this test is sometimes referred to as "The Policeman at the Elbow Test." That is, "If there were a policeman present, would the defendant have committed the act?"

c. The Product Rule (The New Hampshire and Durham Test) : "An accused is not criminally responsible if his unlawful act was the product of mental disease or mental defect.

d. The American Law Institute's Model Penal Code: (1) "A person is not responsible for criminal conduct if at the time of such conduct as a result of mental disease or defect he lacks adequate capacity either to appreciate the criminality of his conduct or to conform his conduct to the requirements of the law." (2) "The terms 'mental disease or defect' do not include an abnormality manifested only by repeated criminal or otherwise antisocial conduct. The terms 'mental disease or defect' shall include congenital and traumatic mental condition as well as disease."

3. Other professional opinion regarding a defendant including:

a. Psychiatric diagnosis.

b. Treatability.

c. Prognosis.

d. Recidivistic potential.

e. Bailability and escape potential.

f. Dangerousness.

g. Disposition.

G. Court Psychiatry: The courts themselves may have psychiatric clinics which may:

1. Perform evaluations in regard to any criminal law procedures.

2. Perform presentence evaluations and act as advisors to the court.

H. Prison and Institutional Psychiatry:

1. Evaluation and treatment of criminal offenders.
2. Training of mental health workers in forensic concepts.
3. Research in the interrelationship between psychiatry and the law.

See *Forensic Psychiatry* (Davidson) for a more complete discussion of the various forensic areas of interest.

II. Rudiments of the Forensic Evaluation.

Characteristically, requests to evaluate a patient in regard to a forensic matter are received from the attorney representing the person to be examined or, in the case of the criminal defendant, sometimes from the prosecutor. Rarely, one may be asked to testify in regard to a patient that he has evaluated or treated for another purpose.

A. The Initial Contact: Several areas should be covered and clearly understood prior to agreeing to accept a referral for forensic evaluation. These include:

1. The issues to be evaluated. One should be clear regarding what legal issue is involved and understand any particular legal test involved. The term legal test refers to previously established legal criteria now used as the basis in deciding a legal issue.
2. When the evaluation must be completed and the probable dates for testimony, if needed.
3. Request all collateral information. Ask that the attorney share all information that he has with you and, if possible, obtain past summaries of any medical or psychiatric treatment that might in any way be pertinent.
4. Discuss your fees. The psychiatrist's fee should never be dependent upon the opinion rendered. It is usually best to charge a flat hourly fee which includes the total time spent in reviewing past records, evaluating the patient, writing a re-

port, testifying, and traveling to and from court if this is required. If one has not previously had referrals from an attorney, it is prudent to ask for an advanced payment that would at least cover the estimated time to be spent in completing an initial report.

5. Make arrangements for interviewing the patient. Set up an appointment, or if the patient is incarcerated, request a court order authorizing the evaluation.

B. Interviewing the Patient:
1. Introduce yourself and inform him of the purpose of the evaluation. The patient has a legal right to know this.
2. Take notes to help assure accuracy in report writing, making special note of specific answers to important questions.
3. Be particularly aware of and attempt to resolve any conflicts between collateral information that you have and information obtained from the patient.
4. If you feel that psychological testing or other ancillary tests are necessary to form or confirm an opinion, discuss this with the referring attorney and assist in making arrangements if he approves.
5. Spend as much time as necessary to feel assured of your opinion. Arrange for additional interviews if necessary.

C. Post-Evaluation Conference:
1. Discussion of findings or discussion of your conclusions with the referring attorney prior to writing your report is important, particularly if your opinion is unfavorable to the attorney's case. In this situation the attorney may ask that a report not be written, since a copy could be demanded by the opposing counsel, with the court's approval, resulting in your being called as an adverse witness.

2. Report writing. Attempt to formulate clearly answers to questions posed by the referring attorney. Do not feel pressured to give a psychiatric opinion about an area which you are unable to evaluate. If you enumerate possibilities, admit your uncertainty. To do otherwise may well put you in a bind later when you are called to testify in the matter and find that you are unable to give any meaningful basis for your opinion when being examined. The report should be concise but give enough background information and data to support any conclusions that are finally made. In general, the report should include a paragraph on each of the following:

   a. Circumstances of the referral and a summary of the event that lead to the request for evaluation.
   b. Pertinent background information, including any past history that might have particular bearing on the matter at hand.
   c. A description of the evaluation, including the amount of time spent and where the evaluation was conducted.
   d. A discussion of your findings as they relate to the reason for referral.
   e. A statement of your final conclusions with special attention to answering any specific questions posed by the referring attorney, if possible. Include a specific psychiatric diagnosis if it is significant.
   f. Recommendations resulting from your evaluation, if indicated.

D. Confidentiality: Because of the legal issues involved, protection of the patient is particularly important.

   1. Never discuss the evaluation or your conclusions with anyone other than the attorney retaining

you unless authorized to do so in writing by the patient and his attorney.

2. Protect your records. Sometimes, even in the courtroom, opposing counsel will attempt to review them. This is not permitted except on order by the court. Be aware, however, that the judge will usually allow review of any records you use for reference on the witness stand.

III. Preparation and Presentation of Testimony.

A. Pretrial Conference: Once it is known that testimony is necessary, request a conference with the referring attorney if he has not already suggested this. At this time:

1. Agree on a time for your court appearance. Even though there are some limitations in scheduling due to the needs of the court, it is generally recognized that the physician's time is valuable. Proper planning can help avoid spending unnecessary time in the courtroom.

2. Discuss direct testimony. Review your evaluation with the referring attorney and assist in preparing questions which will best present your opinion and conclusions during testimony. You will have the most ideal time during this period of questioning by the referring attorney to clearly and completely state your opinion. You and the referring attorney should both know what questions will be asked and what the answers will be.

3. Anticipate cross-examination. Use the referring attorney's expertise to help predict what kinds of questions might be faced in cross-examination; discuss with him what your answers would be. Some particularly helpful techniques include:

a. Use a preceding clause to qualify yes or no answers to questions. For example, an answer of "Yes, but . . ." may be cut off by the attorney saying, "Thank you, doctor, that's all." Use of an initial phrase such as, "Because of . . . , yes" or "Except for . . . , no" will avoid this.

b. Handling unanswerable questions. If a yes or no answer is demanded without qualification, and it is not possible to give such an answer, it is proper to turn to the judge and say, "I cannot give a yes or no answer to that question. May I be allowed to explain?" Such a request usually will be honored.

c. Stalling for time. Sometimes more time to think about a question before answering would be beneficial. Requesting that the question be clarified or repeated, as if it was not initially understood, may be helpful in this regard. See *Coping with Psychiatric and Psychological Testimony* (Ziskin) for further samples and suggestions regarding cross-examination.

B. Presentation of Testimony:

1. Do your homework. Shortly before your court appearance, refamiliarize yourself with your records. Knowledge of basic facts such as dates, places, etc. without notes accentuates the appearance of being thoroughly familiar with the matter at hand. Avoid taking any notes or reports that conflict with your position to the witness stand since these can be seized by the opposing attorney. For example, the report of a psychologist that contains an opinion conflicting with yours could be used to aid opposing counsel in cross-examining you.

2. Dress neatly and conservatively. The formal atmosphere of the courtroom is no place for casual or untidy dress.

3. Appear in court promptly. Not only could tardiness be construed as contempt of court, but promptness implies courteousness and responsibility.

4. Taking the witness stand. When your name is

called, take the necessary records and walk confidently to a position in front of the court clerk. Raise your right hand and, after administering of the oath, answer, "I do." If the spelling is not obvious, spell out your name for the court stenographer and be seated in the witness chair.

5. Control nervousness. Use your anxiety to keep you more alert.
   a. Sit erect but comfortably.
   b. It may be helpful to draw upon your experience with the doctor-patient relationship and think of everyone in the courtroom as patients who are asking you to explain something to them.
   c. Often, it appears that the formality of being in court automatically becomes associated with being judged yourself. Always keep in mind, I'm not on trial. This is not to say that the value of your testimony is not going to be weighed by the judge and jury. It does say, however, that you are not being accused of any wrongdoing but are simply there to give the most well-supported and meaningful testimony you can in regard to the matter at hand.

6. Speak to the judge and jury.
   a. Remember that it is the judge and jury, if there is one, that will evaluate what you say.
   b. Observe the jurors and estimate their educational level and pick out those who appear most receptive to your testimony, frequently making eye contact with them while speaking but not to the point of ignoring others.
   c. Speak clearly and loudly enough for the furthest juror to hear without straining. Remember also that a stenographer must record what you say.

d. Avoid "psychiatric jargon," always making explanations in simple terms whenever possible.

e. Be polite to the judge. A positive attitude towards you by the judge is helpful in soliciting a positive response from the jurors. Always say, "Thank you, your Honor" at appropriate times.

7. Presenting professional qualifications. Prior to being accepted as an expert witness, one must present his professional qualifications to the court in initial direct examination. Never give your qualifications in a way which appears apologetic. For example, when asked to give his qualifications, one resident simply said, "I'm a fifth year resident." A statement such as, "I'm a psychiatrist, having completed three years of psychiatric residency approved by the American Board of Psychiatry and Neurology for board eligibility in psychiatry, and am presently a second year post-graduate fellow at . . ." would be much more impressive to a judge and jury.

8. Know when to be silent.

a. Never speak during time that an objection is being made by opposing counsel. Wait until permission is given by the judge to continue. If you are unsure of the question at that time, ask for it to be repeated.

b. Always respond only to the question asked. Do not volunteer additional information. For example, when asked, "Doctor, do you have an opinion?", answer, "Yes, I do."

9. Control anger. Expression of anger has no place on the witness stand. Opposing attorneys may purposely use techniques designed to upset the professional witness and bring forth anger, which casts an unfavorable shadow on the witness. It is difficult for a judge and jury to ac-

cept a witness's opinion about someone's emotions when he is unable to control his own.

10. Conduct following testimony:
    a. Never leave the witness stand until you have permission to do so by the judge.
    b. Control your affect. A broad-faced smile of triumph or an angry sullen look do not compliment your professional appearance.
    c. Leave the courtroom promptly unless you have also been retained as a psychiatric advisor by the referring attorney. Remaining in the courtroom makes it appear that you have a personal interest in the outcome of the case.

Although one can know "do's and don'ts" in giving testimony, there is no substitute for experience in gaining confidence. However, if one is well prepared and understands basic forensic concepts, the performing of a forensic evaluation and presentation of testimony may be a most rewarding and meaningful experience.

References

Allen, Richard C., *et al.* (Eds.) : *Readings in Law and Psychiatry.* Baltimore, The Johns Hopkins Press, 1968.

Brakel, Samuel J. and Ronald S. Rock: *The Mentally Disabled and the Law,* Rev. ed. Chicago, The University of Chicago Press, 1971.

Davidson, Henry A.: *Forensic Psychiatry, 2nd ed.* New York, The Ronald Press Co., 1965.

Ziskin, Jay: *Coping with Psychiatric and Psychological.* Beverly Hills, Law and Psychology Press, 1970.

PSYCHIATRIC EVALUATION OF FITNESS FOR MILITARY SERVICE

CLIFFORD C. KUHN, M.D.

The involvement of psychiatrists in the determination of an individual's fitness for military duty has been a controversial issue. Some psychiatrists have admittedly allowed their own political or philosophical biases to determine their recommendations. Nevertheless, psychiatry can perform a very important service to both the individual and the military establishment in this arena. Political or philosophical prejudice notwithstanding, the psychiatrist must perform an expert examination and base his recommendations on a consideration of what is best for the individual, the military, and ultimately for society. Very often what is best for one will also be best for the others. The psychiatrist must, therefore, know something about the needs and requirements of the military service just as he must understand the patient himself. He must also consider the wider societal implications of his recommendations.

The following outline is designed to aid the psychiatrist in making an intelligent and effective evaluation of an individual's fitness for military service.

I. Diagnostic Categories

Individuals who fit into certain diagnostic categories are consistently unable to function effectively within the military setting. The military service is bad for them and, similarly, they are a liability to the military. It is in the best interest of the individual, the military service, and society-at-large to prevent their induction into active military duty. The following diagnostic categories are at greatest risk in the military setting:

A. Schizophrenia and other psychotic disorders.

1. Paranoid individuals are especially likely to become dangerous to themselves and others at some time in a military setting.

2. The military considers these diagnoses to be medical illnesses, and as such, they qualify an individual for a medical deferment or discharge.

B. Personality or character disorders.

1. These individuals, especially those who fit the diagnosis of inadequate personality or those with a schizoid or borderline syndrome, are almost always going to have problems with military life, and when they arise, the military is

very likely to deal with them in a punitive manner. (Friedman, 1972).

2. The military considers these diagnoses to be
nonmedical and as such they qualify an individual for possible deferment or discharge ad-
ministratively as unsuitable or unfit.

C. Sexual Perversions

1. The military does not feel that individuals with
this diagnosis are desirable.

2. These disorders are considered nonmedical by
the military and, as with character disorders,
qualify an individual for an administrative deferment or separation.

D. Neurosis: In these cases the psychiatrist must base
his recommendations primarily on the severity of
the symptoms. Many neurotic individuals can function well in the military. Quite often military psychiatrists can be of great help to these individuals.

1. Obsessive-Compulsive: This disorder, if it is
of significant severity, has a particularly poor
prognosis in the service. Very few of these individuals survive the rigid demands of basic
training without some kind of decompensation.

2. All neuroses are considered medical disorders
by the military.

E. Drug Abuse: Although this symptom spans many
diagnoses, an individual can qualify for deferment
or discharge on the basis of drug abuse alone.

1. Abuse of LSD: From the point of view of the
military, the documented (admitted) use of this
substance on one occasion constitutes abuse and
the individual is unconditionally considered unsuitable. The rationale here is that the military
does not want to risk the possibility of so-called
flashbacks occurring amongst their personnel.

2. Abuse of marijuana or amphetamines: The
determination of abuse here is more flexible and
is left to the judgment of the examining phy-

sician. A general rule of thumb is that use of these drugs on more than six to eight separate occasions or for a period exceeding four to six months qualifies an individual for deferment or discharge for abuse, but this determination is very flexible.

3. Abuse of heroin: This, if reported, requires automatic disqualification of a potential inductee.

II. Reasons for Psychiatric Consultation Prior to Induction

A. Self-referred

1. Individuals seeking to avoid the draft on basis of a legitimate psychiatric illness.

   a. At the time of this writing this is the most frequent motivation of those seeking an evaluation. With the advent of the anticipated all volunteer military and the abolition of the military draft this source may decrease in importance.

2. Individuals who have volunteered for military duty but who, due to emotional problems, do not feel they can meet their obligation. This group will grow larger under the all volunteer military.

3. Individuals who do not want to serve and are seeking an unwarranted diagnosis to get them out.

   a. In the author's experience, these individuals comprise roughly one-third of those falling under the self-referred heading. It goes without saying that it is unwise to write them a sympathetic letter in lieu of a substantiated clinical diagnosis and recommendation. This type of self-referral, of course, should decrease in number when the draft is discontinued.

B. Concerned Parent, Wife or Relative.

1. Seeking help for the potential inductee.
2. Seeking help for themselves.

a. If a wife or dependent of the potential inductee demonstrates significant mental illness such that the inductee's absence from them for basic training would constitute a significant risk to their ultimate health and well-being, that inductee may be recommended for a hardship deferment.

C. Referral from another physician.

III. Considerations for Maximizing the Effectiveness of the Psychiatrist's Recommendations.

A. Always obtain a signed permission from the individual before releasing any information to the military.

B. In the case of a civilian who has not yet been inducted, send recommendations to the nearest armed forces examining station addressed directly to the senior medical officer.

C. In the case of an individual who is already in the military, address your recommendations to his immediate commander and mark them confidential.

D. State clearly at the outset of the letter:
   1. Individual's name and social security number.
   2. The reasons for the psychiatric evaluation.
   3. The date (s) on which the individual was examined.

E. Include pertinent and concise historical information to support the diagnosis and/or recommendation.

F. State the diagnosis clearly and include as much clinical detail as needed to illustrate the symptomatology. (Use standard, approved diagnostic labels. See Chapter I.)

G. Recommendations
   1. The most important thing to keep in mind is that the military cannot concern itself primarily about the individual. (Griffin, 1963) They are primarily concerned with the most effective accomplishment of their mission. Therefore, rec-

ommendations based solely on what is best for the individual will be poorly accepted and may go unheeded. The psychiatrist must key his recommendation to the best interests of the armed forces as well as the individual.

2. State clearly what are likely to be the consequences both to the individual and the military if he were inducted.

   a. Illustrate how this particular individual would present a liability to the service both currently and ultimately (example: currently he is likely to become very dangerous to himself and others around him. Ultimately the experience in the military could very well cause a more serious and longstanding service-connected disability).

   b. In short, the psychiatrist must demonstrate clearly to the military why they would not benefit from having this individual in their ranks (how inducting him would detract from the mission).

3. Always make statements in the form of recommendations, not pronouncements.

4. If treatment has been recommended for the individual, say so in the letter and make some statement to illustrate motivation on his part to follow recommendations for treatment.

5. It cannot be overemphasized that the spirit of the letter should be to provide a service to the military as well as to the individual involved. As such the letter should be closed with an invitation to the military to contact the psychiatrist if they feel he can be of further help in this case.

References

Friedman, H. J.: Military psychiatry. *Arch Gen Psychiatry, 26:* 118, February, 1972.

Griffin, M. D. and Sparks, J. C.: An orientation to military psychiatry. *Milit Med, 128:* 1124, 1963.

EVALUATION OF SEXUAL DYSFUNCTION
JOSEPH R. NOVELLO, M.D.

Psychiatrists are increasingly consulted by patients with sexual disorders. Much of this has followed upon the pioneering work of Masters and Johnson which has led to a new enlightenment among both medical professionals and the general population regarding the nature of human sexual dysfunction.

The identified patient may be an individual or a couple. Although the chief complaint may run the entire medical-psychiatric gamut, the most frequently encountered problems include:

1. Impotence
   a. primary, i.e. the patient has never been able to have an erection
   b. secondary, i.e. the patient has successfully maintained erections in the past, but presently is unable to do so
   c. circumstantial, i.e. the patient is able to maintain an erection only under certain circumstances, such as the male who is potent with a prostitute but impotent with his wife, etc.
2. Premature ejaculation
3. Dyspareunia
4. Vaginismus
5. Orgasmic dysfunction
   a. primary
   b. secondary
   c. circumstantial
6. Diminished libido, lack of interest on part of patient
7. Complaints about the spouse's interest in intercourse, i.e. one partner may complain that the other wants sex too often or too infrequently
8. Repulsion to sex in general or to a particular sexual practice
9. Marital disharmony, i.e. here the problem simply masquerades as a primary sexual problem

Other problems, less frequently encountered, include:

10. Compulsive hypersexuality
11. Compulsive masturbation
12. Problems of conflicted sexual identity or inappropriate choice of sexual object, i.e. homosexuality, transvestism, trans-sexualism, fetishism, exhibitionism, voyeurism, sexual sadism, sexual masochism, etc.

In cases where the psychiatrist is the physician of first contact, he must be prepared to function within the medical model, as a physician, since many of these primary sexual problems may be essentially medical in nature. Therefore, in addition to a competent psychiatric evaluation he must take an adequate medical history. He must be able to recognize a possible medical problem by history and be prepared to make a suitable referral. In fact, until the sexual dysfunction is definitely recognized as being caused primarily by psychological factors, the problem should not be considered psychiatric at all.

Psychiatrists who treat patients with sexual dysfunction will differ in their treatment methods, but common to all must be an accurate collection and assessment of data. The following outline for taking a sexual history is provided for this purpose.

It must be stressed, however, that a sexual history does not exist apart from an overall, skillful professional evaluation that includes all other features of the patient's life. As Masters and Johnson have pointed out, a sex history when taken out of context of the person's total personal history, is about as meaningful as a stomach history or a heart history in general medicine.

Basic Principles:

1. A person's complaint of a sexual dysfunction does not necessarily indicate the presence of psychopathology. Often the cause is nonpsychiatric and the consulting psychiatrist, as a physician, should recognize these cases:
   a. Organic Causes: Many cases of dyspareunia, and primary impotence, for example, may be due to organic

causes. Suspected physical or hormonal abnormalities must be appropriately referred for investigation.

b. Insufficient Knowledge: Many individuals suffer sexual dysfunction simply out of naïveté. Straightforward counseling and/or behavioral modifications are often sufficient in treating these disorders.

c. Poor communication between marital pairs: Married couples may be inhibited in discussing their sexual difficulties with each other. Often communication can be opened in the clinical setting of the physician's office and lead to improvement in sexual functioning without "psychiatric" intervention.

2. The psychiatrist making an initial evaluation of sexual dysfunction should:

a. be comfortable himself with the subject; be able to discuss all aspects of human sexuality openly, without inhibition or embarrassment.

b. be free of prejudice regarding sexual practice and values.

c. be especially alert to countertransference phenomena.

The Sexual History

The following outline is intended as a guide to data collection in the specialized area of the sexual history. It is intended as a reminder to the clinician of the kind of information that is generally required in a sexual history. It is intended to be used with reasonable flexibility. The psychiatrist may choose to collect more or less information according to the requirements of the specific case. The sequence and pace of data collecting should be dictated by the needs of the patient. The outline should not be used as a questionnaire or checkoff list. Such a use would be contrary to sound psychiatric interviewing and may undermine the doctor-patient relationship.

When evaluating a married couple, it is often desirable to interview each spouse separately at an early stage in the evaluation. It is especially important to unearth secrets that may hinder later therapeutic attempts (affairs, clandestine homosexuality, etc.). It is also wise to learn which spouse initiated the professional contact and why, and to learn whether either spouse is present at the interview under duress (threat of divorce, etc.).

The Sexual History (Male)

I. Presenting Problem, Identifying Data
II. Childhood
    A. Which parent was the patient closest to emotionally? Why?
        1. Any special feelings of rivalry or competition to either parent?
    B. Attitude of each parent toward sex.
    C. Which parent did the disciplining? How was it done?
    D. Siblings
        1. Quality of relationships
    E. How did the patient first become aware of physical differences between the sexes?
        1. Did parents discuss it? Which parent? How?
    F. Primal scene experience
        1. Did the patient ever see parents having intercourse? Ever hear something and believe (or fantasize) that it was caused by parents' sexual activities?
    G. Early fantasies re: sex
    H. Recurrent dreams or nightmares in childhood
    I. Earliest memory
        1. Earliest memory of mother
        2. Earliest memory of father
    J. Any sexual contact in childhood?
        1. Seduction, molesting, mutual looking or masturbation, etc.
    K. Childhood masturbation
        1. Extent, how performed, etc.
III. Adolescence
    A. Primary source of sex information
        1. i.e. parent(s), friends, books, etc.

B. First petting experience
   1. Age, describe circumstances
   2. Describe partner and partner's reaction
   3. Did it involve ejaculation? Other episodes of ejaculation without intercourse?
C. Masturbation
   1. Age at which first began
      a. how discovered?
   2. Pattern through adolescence
      a. frequency
      b. how performed, use of artifacts, fetishes, etc.
      c. guilt or shame
      d. masturbatory fantasies, i.e. what did the patient usually think about while masturbating?
      e. was patient usually in hurry to ejaculate or did he purposefully prolong it? Why?
   3. Present pattern of masturbation
      a. same questions as above
D. Nocturnal emissions
   1. Age at which first experienced?
      a. patient's reaction to it
      b. did parent (s) discuss it with him
E. Homosexual contact
   1. Age at which patient had first homosexual contact or opportunity. Describe, i.e. what was done, patient's reaction, description of partner (s) , etc.
      a. was patient active or passive
   2. Frequency of any subsequent homosexual contact
      a. describe
      b. especially: which erogenous zone is most preferred by the patient (genital, oral, anal, etc.)
IV. First Intercourse and Sex Prior to Marriage
   A. Age
   B. Describe circumstances
      1. Prearranged, spontaneous, etc.

C. Describe the sexual partner
   1. Age, relationship (i.e. in love, stranger, etc.)
   2. What was her reaction?
      a. was she orgastic
      b. did she give any message such as it was good, bad, it hurt, etc.
D. Were drinking or drugs involved? Describe
E. Anticipatory feelings
   1. Fear, joy, guilt, etc.
   2. Did patient anticipate difficulty, etc.
F. The act
   1. Describe: foreplay, intercourse, post-coital period
   2. What thoughts did patient have during the act
   3. At what point did the patient ejaculate
   4. Any problems: impotence, premature ejaculation, etc. and patient's reaction to the problem then and now

V. Marital Sex
  A. Brief marital history
     1. Describe wife
     2. What do they usually disagree about
     3. Current status of the marriage (shared values)
  B. Any past divorce
     1. Reasons why. Related to sexual problem? Describe.
  C. If the patient and his spouse engaged in premarital sex together, has the quality or quantity of their sex life changed since they have been married? Describe.
  D. Honeymoon
     1. Describe circumstances, relationship and sexual data
  E. Current pattern of marital sex
     1. Frequency
        a. especially as compared to earlier patterns
     2. Who generally initiates sex?
     3. How is the act performed?

   a. which position is favored by patient? by wife?
   b. have they shared this information? Why not?
  4. Any problems
   a. wife's orgastic frequency, etc.
  5. Are drinking or drugs involved? Describe.
  6. Fantasies during sex act.
  7. What is the patient's concept of normal marital sex? His wife's concept?
 VI. Extramarital Sex
  A. Description of the general pattern
   1. Frequency, circumstances
   2. Type of female generally chosen and patient's relationship to her, i.e. personality type, etc.
   3. Are drinking or drugs involved? Describe
   4. How is the act usually performed?
   5. How does the extramarital sex compare to patient's sexual experiences within the marriage?
  B. Patient's value system re: extramarital affairs
  C. Any problems
   1. With consummation of the act itself
   2. Guilt or shame
  D. Does the patient's spouse know of this activity?
   1. What might be her reaction?
 VII. Sexual Preferences
  A. At what time in his life and under what circumstances has the patient experienced the most pleasure from sex?
  B. At what time in his life and under what circumstances has the patient experienced the least pleasure from sex?
  C. What sexual practice does the patient enjoy most? Least? Why?
   1. Which erogenous zone is involved, i.e. genital, oral, anal, etc.
   2. Is the patient active or passive in these circumstances?
   3. What are his fantasies during these acts?
   4. What is the reaction of his partner or spouse to these practices?

        5. Patient's own attitudes
        6. Use of accouterments such as vibrators, special
           clothing, etc.
        7. History of wife-swapping or group sex. Describe.
    D. What is the content (and frequency) of the pa-
       tient's dreams and daydreams about sex?
    E. What is the quality of the patient's relationships
       (not necessarily sexual in nature) with women in
       general? with men?
        1. Does he most prefer the company of men or
           women? Why?
    F. Has the patient ever had an especially close rela-
       tionship with a woman that did not involve sex at
       all? Describe.
VIII. Decision for Treatment and Motivation
    A. What led the patient to seek help at this time?
    B. History of any past treatment for the same or re-
       lated condition
        1. When? Why? By whom?
        2. Type of treatment
        3. Result
        4. Patient's evaluation of the experience
    C. What are the patient's current treatment goals?
        1. What is his concept of normal sexual function-
           ing? For himself? For his spouse?
    D. What is the nature of the patient's motivation for
       treatment?
        1. Is he willing to follow recommendations ex-
           plicitly?
        2. Does he have some reservations?
        3. Is he under duress?

The Sexual History (Female)

The sexual history of the female follows the general form
and content of the male sexual history with the exception
that additional information is sought in four areas:

1. Menstrual History: Age of menarche. Had menstruation been explained prior to its onset? By whom? In what
way? What was the patient's reaction (joy, disgust, etc.)?

Any history of menstrual abnormalities (dysmenorrhea, oligomenorrhea, etc.)? Describe patient's reactions to menstrual difficulties and summarize past treatment, if any. Is there a particular time in the patient's menstrual cycle that she is most interested in having sexual relations? least interested? What are her attitudes toward intercourse during menstruation?

2. Pregnancy: Summary of past pregnancies. Were they planned? Patient's initial reaction to learning that she was pregnant? At what point in the pregnancy did she discontinue sexual intercourse? Why? Was this with the mutual consent of her spouse? Description of labor and delivery. Any complications? Did she notice any change in the sexual habits of herself or her spouse following the addition of children into the family?

3. Birth Control: History of the types of birth control practiced by patient and spouse. Does she think birth control has affected her sexual life in any way? If patient is taking birth control pills, specify for how long and which type (sequentials, etc.).

4. Orgastic History: There is almost no male counterpart to primary orgastic dysfunction in the female. Even the impotent male is often capable of orgasm via masturbation. Ask specifically if the female patient is capable of reaching orgasm via masturbation. How is it performed? What are her masturbatory fantasies? Be certain what the patient means by orgasm. Is it a type of profound emotional experience or does she describe a true, genital-pelvic muscular discharge?

Reference

Masters, W. H. and Johnson, V. E.: *Human Sexual Inadequacy*. Boston, Little, Brown and Company, 1970.

PSYCHIATRIC EVALUATION FOR COSMETIC SURGERY
RAYMOND F. ZEH, JR., M.D.

Cosmetic surgery can no longer be regarded as a luxury for vain, wealthy individuals. In some cases it may be considered as a social and economic necessity in light of our current sociocultural emphasis of physical attributes and attractiveness, pressures to conform as well as to individualize, devaluation of middle and older age groups with orientation toward a youth culture, and increased recognition of social, economic and psychiatric consequences of disfigurement. Therefore, plastic surgeons have been becoming increasingly aware of the psychosocial aspects of cosmetic surgery. They are increasingly aware of the complexities involved behind a patient's request for cosmetic surgery.

Associated with this increasing complexity is the current trend toward patient's questioning the results of all types of medical procedures and testing them through the legal system. Cosmetic surgical results are especially vulnerable to litigation. For all of these reasons, plastic surgeons frequently request psychiatric consultation for their patients before making a decision to operate.

The psychiatrist who receives such a consultation request must have some knowledge of the possibilities and limitations of cosmetic surgical procedures and, in addition to the routine psychiatric evaluation, he should be aware of certain specific data that will allow him to reach a decision regarding a patient's suitability for cosmetic surgery with more precision.

The following outline is prepared to aid the psychiatrist in this task.

I. How Patients Come to Psychiatry Referral
   A. In the author's experience in a university teaching hospital patients come to the psychiatrist almost exclusively through the plastic surgeons initiating the request.
II. Most Common Reasons a Person Requests Cosmetic Surgery (Patient's Explicit Motivation)
   A. Socio-cultural-economic concerns
   B. Change for aesthetic concerns
      1. Own
      2. Others who may induce patient to initiate request

III. Why a Psychiatric Consultation is Requested (Surgeon's Motivation)

   A. Aid in dealing with the increasing complexity and pitfalls of decision-making associated with the application of dynamic theory to the understanding of:

      1. Motivation: It is of crucial importance to identify the patient's specific motivation in requesting cosmetic surgery. (Jacobson, 1960)

      2. Somatic Delusions (Druss, 1971)

         a. Psychodynamics of Delusion Formation

            1. Denial of reality: insignificant deformity appears conspicuous and attractive features appear ugly.

            2. Projection: of unconscious fears onto body rather than environment.

            3. Concretization: concentration of above onto specific body part rather than various psychosomatic complaints.

            4. Preoccupation: increased intensity and duration of symptom with private and symbolic meaning determining intensity to extent that inappropriate actions taken.

         b. Significance

            1. May represent encapsulation of emotional disorder, even psychosis, and surgery may focus further attention on psychiatric symptom and confirm to patient its importance.

            2. Large number of unhappy patients are in this category who displace their dissatisfaction with both the surgical outcome and their own lifelong grievances to person of surgeon. These patients, particularly if paranoid tendencies exist, are apt to be litigenous.

   B. Therefore the following questions are most likely to be posed in their psychiatric consultations.

      1. Does the patient have a realistic understanding of the procedure, its limitations, complications

and disability? This emphasizes the psychiatrist's need for understanding these aspects and his responsibility to have the surgeon provide him with such.

2. To what extent, if any, is a somatic delusion a component of the aesthetic concern?

3. To what extent, if any, is the aesthetic concern a response, transitory or otherwise, to an external stress?

4. Does this patient have psychopathology of such a nature that he would tend to regress from his current level of adjustment?

5. Is the dynamic structure of the patient such that dissatisfaction would be expressed, and perhaps litigated, regardless of surgical result?

IV. A Suggested Approach to Assessment

The following outline is suggested as an instrument to collect and organize data.

A. Statement from plastic surgeon to psychiatrist re:
  1. Surgical problem, its degree, description of surgical procedure, limitations, complications and durability of results.
  2. Surgeon's reason for requesting psychiatric consultation.

B. Statement from psychiatrist to patient defining his own role.

C. Statement from patient concerning:
  1. His understanding of psychiatric consultation request.
  2. His own description of feature under consideration for surgical alteration.
  3. His expectations for surgery including understanding of procedures, and their limitations, complications and durability.

D. Psychiatrist's own estimation of degree of deformity.

E. Basic data
  1. Age
  2. Sex

3. Heterosexual situation and estimated level of adjustment.
4. Past and present school and/or work experience.
5. Health
   a. General health
      1. Estimation of degree and number of functional and hypochondriacal concerns.
   b. Surgical history (include complications, litigation, etc.)
      1. General
      2. Other plastic surgery experiences
6. Socio-cultural-economic level including past, current or proposed changes.

F. History of patient's cosmetic concern
   1. Earliest recalled onset
      a. Situations surrounding the awareness.
      b. Attempts to deal with these concerns and result.
   2. Later recurrences
      a. Situations surrounding.
      b. Attempts to deal with and result.
   3. Why presenting to plastic surgery at this time with special attention to:
      a. Transient stress vs.
      b. Long standing stress.
   4. Expectations for surgical results to:
      a. Change perception and limitations of self.
      b. Change others perceptions and interactions with self.
      c. Cure-all.

G. Family history and dynamics
   1. Significant members and patient's relationship to, especially parents.
   2. Assessment of patient's identification models.
   3. Any conscious identification of the undesirable cosmetic feature with a family member or other person.

H. Synthesis of motivational structure (external, internal) from the data
   1. Conscious
      a. socio-cultural-economic.
      b. others
   2. Preconscious (Jacobson, 1960)
      a. might give some cognizance that difficulty involves personality and life experience through:
         1. acceptance of responsibility vs. projection and externalization.
         2. manner of perceiving relations with others.
         3. type of expectations regarding surgical result.
         4. concerns about trusting the surgeon.
         5. attempts to do something about himself.
   3. Unconscious
      a. estimate of to what degree the feature of concern, (i.e. the undesirable cosmetic feature) represents a symbolization of unresolved conflictual identification.
      b. defensive structure and estimate of degree of stability.
I. Assessment of presence and degree of psychopathology and prediction of what result cosmetic surgery might have in relation to the existing psychopathology.
V. Psychiatric Profiles of Patient's Seeking Cosmetic Surgery

In evaluating a patient for cosmetic surgery, it is useful for the psychiatric consultant to be able to compare the psychiatric profile of his patient with the typical profile of other individuals who have undergone cosmetic surgery. The following profiles, male and female, have been constructed from the existing literature. Although the entire data has been collected from patients who were seeking one specific type of surgical operation (rhinoplasty), certain translations can be made to other types of surgical procedures and, at any rate, the reader is presented with an example of how the psychiatrist's data can be organized into a clinically useful form.

A. *Profile of Female Rhinoplasty Patients* (Edgerton, 1971; Jacobson, 1971; Meyer, 1960)
1. General
   a. intellectual capacity average or above.
   b. physical health good with history of few surgical procedures.
   c. low incidence of significant psychiatric disorders.
   d. history of few functional or hypochondriacal complaints.
   e. self consciousness of nose dated from adolescence.
   f. majority identify nose with that of their father's.
2. Family history and dynamics
   a. mother: an inadequate model for learning effective and easy functioning in the feminine role.
   b. father amiable and with whom the patient strongly identified in early life.
   c. in later years this identification came to be felt as disconsolate to comfortable femininity.
   d. this conflict, as represented by a sense of nasal deformity, is associated with a wish to resolve by disassociating from this parental identification.
3. Reactivation and/or reinforcement of psychological conflicts by socio-cultural-age variables
   a. Less than 20 years of age.
      1. Most such patients in these series are Jewish with no desire to disassociate themselves from their faith but a wish not to be socially stereotyped.
      2. Want to be regarded as individuals.

        3. Dating worries and social concerns are prominent.

    b. 21 to 30-year group.

        1. Most of Protestant faith.

        2. Difficulty in dealing with current problems in courtship and marriage; often associated with frustrations to success at work.

    c. Patients greater than 30 years of age.

        1. Marked strain in marriage.

        2. Correction of long-standing sense of nasal deformity felt as a necessary preliminary in coping with threat of depression evoked by interpersonal difficulties.

        3. Link established in adolescence between depressed mood and sense of deformity.

  4. Expectations

    a. More likely (than males) to harbor positive psychological expectations.

    b. More likely (than males) to be hoping for psychological changes in self and less in others.

    c. In so far as transference to the surgeon may occur, more likely to be that of a helpful, available, kindly father.

    d. Congenital deformities more likely to have realistic expectations than acquired deformities.

B. *Profile of Male Rhinoplasty Patients* (Edgerton, 1971; Jacobson, 1960; Jacobson, 1971)

  1. General

    a. intellectual capacity average or above.

    b. physical health good with history of few surgical procedures.

    c. incidence of psychopathology higher than females.

    d. history of few functional or hypochondriacal complaints.

    e. self consciousness of nose dated from adolescence.

    f. majority identify nose with that of their father's.

2. Family history and dynamics

    a. father less available than mother as model through absence, emotional distance, rejection of parental role, unsuitability, etc.

    b. in later life patient consciously resentful, reproachful or contemptuous of father while feelings of love, affection and need for him are relatively unconscious.

    c. patient identifies himself strongly with more available mother in attempt to deal with ambivalent relationship with father; describing mother often as dominant and occasionally overprotective.

    d. in later life can consciously compare his personality with mother's but largely is unconscious of feelings of rage toward her.

    e. conflicts symbolically represented in a sense of nasal deformity and conscious wish to disassociate himself from the father's undesirable traits or weaknesses while unconsciously wishing to disassociate himself from feelings of rage toward mother.

    f. therefore as the nasal deformity is a symptomatic alternative to dealing with the conflicts, so is the request for surgery an attempt at resolution without dealing directly with the conflictual feelings.

3. Reactivation and/or reinforcement of psychological conflicts and socio-cultural-age variables.

    a. these are less important for the male, therefore resulting in fewer requests and the increased emphasis which should be given to internal motivation.

    b. reactivated by any challenge to masculine effectiveness.

      1. serious problems in marriage.

      2. if single had marked difficulty with women and characterized as bashful, shy, self-conscious.

      3. often involved in upward mobility struggles concurrent with request for surgery.

    c. high incidence of first generation Americans associated with wish not to be stereotyped as alien; wish to be viewed as an individual rather than with stereotyped class attributes. (In these series the single largest ethnic group was Catholic-Italian ancestry.)

  4. Expectations

    a. surgeon more likely to be working in field of negative psychological expectations (than with females).

    b. less likely to be hoping for psychological changes in self than in others.

    c. in so far as transference important, more likely to be pessimistic because of previous patterns of disappointment and frustration in previous experiences with father.

    d. congenital deformities more likely to have realistic expectations than acquired.

  5. References for other types of surgical procedures:

    a. *Augmentation Mammaplasty* (Knorr, 1968)

    b. *Congenital Deformity: Otoplasty* (Knorr, 1968)

    c. *Acquired Deformity: Dermabrasion, Facial Scars* (Knorr, 1968)

    d. *Transsexual Patients:* (Edgerton, 1970)

    e. *Various Procedures in an Inmate Population* (Kurtzberg, 1967).

VI. Contraindications for Surgery

  A. Major life crises

    1. Concurrent major alterations in socio-cultural-economic spheres.

    2. Severe marital discord.

    3. Other serious, significant situational reactions.

B. Assessment that feature under consideration is strongly associated with a somatic delusion and its defensive dynamics.
   1. Intensity: rationalization that degree of deformity is appropriate to intensity of feeling.
   2. Denial
   3. Projection: to extent that blames all environmental frustrations on the undesirable cosmetic feature.
   4. Concretization.
   5. Preoccupation: especially to extent that other, more serious physical conditions are ignored.
C. Assessment that defensive structure in B would not be altered or that it would disorganize.
D. In the above cases a waiting period prior to surgery and/or a recommendation for psychotherapy (if only to clarify motives) possibly followed by surgery could be advised.

VII. Post operative Results and Conclusion
A. As a dynamic approach to psychiatrically evaluating the preoperative candidate would predict the theory of the emergence of unbound anxiety or impulses seems to have some relevance with the appearance of episodes of anxiety and temporary patterns of regressive behavior in a significant percentage of patients (Jacobson, 1960; Knorr, 1968; Meyer, 1960).
B. But studies (Edgerton, 1971) have shown that even in the presence of psychopathology (neuroses and an occasional psychosis) many receive substantial benefit if attention is paid to the contraindications.
   1. Some neuroses may be realistic responses to external situations.
   2. Correction of appearance could serve to remove a barrier in relations with others and help gain some self-esteem in a person who might otherwise be unable to manage an effective response.

References

1. Druss, R. G., *et al.:* The problem of somatic delusions in patients seeking cosmetic surgery. *Plast Reconstr Surg, 48:* 246–250, September, 1971.
2. Edgerton, M. T. and Knorr, N. J.: Motivational patterns of patients seeking cosmetic (esthetic) surgery. *Plast Reconstr Surg, 48:* 551–7, December, 1971.
3. Edgerton, M. T., *et al.:* The surgical treatment of transsexual patients. *Plast Reconstr Surg, 45:* 38–46, January, 1970.
4. Jacobson, W. E.; Edgerton, M. T.; *et al.:* Psychiatric evaluation of male patients seeking cosmetic surgery. *Plast Reconstr Surg, 26:* 356–72, October, 1960.
5. Jacobson, W. E.; Edgerton, M. T.; *et al.: Screening of rhinoplasty patients from the psychological point of view. Plast Reconstr Surg, 28:* 279–81, September, 1971.
6. Knorr, N. J.; Hoopes, J. E. and Edgerton, M. T.: Psychiatric-surgical approach to adolescent disturbances in self image. *Plast Reconstr Surg, 41:* 248–53, March, 1968.
7. Kurtzberg, R. L., *et al.:* Psychological screening of inmates requesting cosmetic operations. *Plast Reconstr Surg, 39:* 387–96, April, 1967.
8. Macgregor, F. C.: Selection of cosmetic surgery patients, social and psychological considerations. *Surg Clin North Am, 51:* 289–98, April, 1971.
9. Meyer, E., *et al.:* Motivational patterns in patients seeking elective plastic surgery, I. Women who seek rhinoplasty. *Psychosom Med, 22:* 193–203, 1960.

PSYCHIATRIC EVALUATION FOR TRANSGENDER SURGERY

ROBERT L. HATCHER, Ph.D.

AND

M. JOSEPH PEARSON, M.D.

Although not a major clinical problem in terms of number of patients, this article on evaluation for transgender surgery is included because there is scant information on this topic in the existing literature and it is hoped that the authors' experience at the Gender Clinic (University of Michigan, Department of Psychiatry) will be of some benefit to psychiatrists that may encounter the male patient who is requesting a change of sex operation.

I. Reason for Referral

Most gender patients present themselves for the

explicit purpose of gender surgery and do not come seeking psychiatric evaluation. Generally they are referred from the department of surgery as part of a routine workup. The patient will wish to sell himself as a transsexual in need of surgery. His history, present life situation, the description of sexual activity—everything may be slanted to this aim. Therefore careful, probing and open-ended interviewing is required.

II. Basic Considerations

A. The first step of the interview must be a clear, careful and detailed description of what the patient may expect from the Clinic. He needs to know about the purpose of the evaluation, the cost of the evaluation, the step-by-step procedure that is followed and the Gender Clinic's commitment to him must be clear.

B. In particular, the patient must be aware that it is very unlikely that he will be accepted for surgery, and that no promise is implied. He should be told that the purpose of the interview is to determine to the satisfaction of the examiner and his own satisfaction that gender surgery is the best and most appropriate solution to his problem. This should be a mutual effort, because, no matter how convinced he is that surgery is the answer, any decision of this magnitude should be weighed very carefully by the patient.

C. The evaluation procedure is lengthy and expensive. Because of the expense of the evaluation and the surgery, should it be performed, the patient should have financial resources and be capable of managing money. This is also an index of his reliability and motivation. After one or two screening interviews, the patient's case is discussed by the psychiatric team of the Gender Clinic. If he seems likely to be a suitable candidate for gender surgery, he is seen in further interviews and formal psychological tests are administered. A social history is taken from a relative by the social worker. The evaluation cannot proceed unless a family member is available for this purpose. Following this, the Gender Clinic meets again. If the surgery still seems indicated, the medical team, composed of gynecological, urologic and plastic surgeons, examines the patient; the final decision is reached by the entire medical-surgical-psychiatric team.

III. The Interview

Following these introductory comments, the interview should be free-ranging. The transsexual's feminine identity requires that he deny his actual male sexuality. This denial often affects his personality more generally. Transsexuals tend to be vague, uncertain about facts and unreliable in keeping appointments. This makes the evaluation a real test of the evaluator's interviewing techniques. The following points should be covered to allow an early and effective decision to be reached.

A. Appearance: One of the most important features of the transsexual will strike the examiner immediately: the general appearance of the individual. The examiner's initial reaction to this appearance is important. This response is useful in distinguishing between the convincingly feminine transsexual and the passive homosexual who often displays a caricature of femininity.

B. Differential diagnosis: passive homosexual, transvestite, transsexual

  1. A major problem in evaluating patients seeking transgender surgery is to distinguish between patients who unconsciously value their male genital and those who regard it fundamentally as a superfluous appendage. Certain transvestites and passive feminine homosexuals fall into the first category, for whom surgical castration and penectomy are likely to be disastrous.

  2. Passive Homosexual: A male patient, whose un-

derlying sexual orientation is a passive, effeminate homosexuality, may present himself as a transsexual. These are men whose repugnance at the notion of being homosexual leads them to the defensive wish to be a woman. However, the underlying attachment to their sense of maleness and the penis make them unsuited to transgender surgery. These are often very pathetic patients.

3. Transvestite: The transvestite rarely seeks transgender surgery, since the core of his perversion is an attempt to realize the fantasy of the phallic woman. The transvestite enacts this fantasy and experiences sexual excitement by dressing in feminine clothing. Transvestites may work hard to develop a convincingly feminine appearance, but the penis plays a vital role in their perversion.

4. Transsexual: The transsexual, on the other hand, does not value the penis, and does not retain even a covert sense of maleness. There is no fetishistic excitement in cross dressing, which is more often a relieving and prideful experience for them.

5. The chief problem in the differential diagnosis is that these three categories often merge and blur in individual cases. Particularly, the transvestite may have passive effeminate homosexual features leading these patients to seek evaluation for transgender surgery. Transsexual patients often have had sexual intercourse with men who are usually homosexual. The problem then becomes one of determining the nature of their attraction to these men. Table IV-I listing various features of the transsexual, transvestite and passive effeminate homosexual, should help in these differentiations.

TABLE IV-I

DIFFERENTIAL DIAGNOSIS: PASSIVE HOMOSEXUAL, TRANSVESTITE, TRANSSEXUAL

	Passive Homosexual	Transvestite	Transsexual
Appearance	may appear to be a caricature of femininity	may be convincingly feminine	may be convincingly feminine
Cross-Dressing	less frequent	cross-dressing is exciting	frequent and convincing; not done for sexual excitement *per se*
Attitude Towards Own Penis	more or less conscious, attachment, masturbation may be inhibited	likely to consciously value penis, masturbation important	feels penis is superfluous, no masturbation
Masturbation Fantasy and Sexual Daydreams	sex as a woman with a homosexual partner	derivatives of fantasy of phallic woman	sex as a woman with a normal man
Attitude Towards Women	may be catty, contemptuous; often seeks out sisterly women	selects women who aid and/or join in transvestite activities, over whom he triumphs in fantasy	often has regular girl friends
Attitude Towards and Sexual Activity with Men	often an adoring, submissive attachment to homosexual men; no fear of discovery of penis in homosexual activity	often seen as weak, impotent, contemptible; men not used sexually; sense of triumph if able to fool a man by his cross-dressing	may maintain relatively close, affectionate ties to men; yearning for heterosexual man may preclude present sexual activity because of fear of discovery by partner
Sense of Gender	effeminate but basic masculine identity	masculine	feminine

C. Collection of Data

1. Current Adjustment: Careful review of the patient's current adjustment is required. The typical transsexual patient has experimented with cross dressing and cross living, despite the social risks involved. The patient who has not may be expressing uncertainty about his femininity. The transsexual who cross lives and cross dresses successfully is, of course, fooling everyone he meets. A certain degree of sociopathy is required for this, but extensive evidence of sociopathy in the patient's general adjustment makes him a poor risk for gender surgery.

2. Sexual orientation: The patient's sexual orientation and activities are a major area of concern. A careful history of his sexual experiences needs to be taken, including heterosexual, homosexual and transvestite experiences. How does the patient achieve sexual gratification? Inquire into the occurrence of masturbation, its frequency and duration; and especially the fantasies occurring during masturbation. If homosexuality has been experimented with, it is important to know the nature of the experiments and the amount of involvement. Any fantasies occurring during sex are of particular importance. It is important to know if the patient gets pleasure from simply dressing as a woman, as this is diagnostic of transvestism. Any history that can be obtained of a male transsexual using his genitals for sexual gratification is important to uncover since the person who values his genitals for gratification would not be a good candidate for surgery.

3. Selection of Friends: Inquire into the kind of person the transsexual chooses for friends. Are his friends homosexuals? Other transsexuals? *Normal* men? What does the patient do with these people? What does he like about them?

4. Gender Orientation: Sexual activity must be distinguished from gender orientation, although the patient will describe them together. Find out when and how the patient discovered that he feels himself to be a woman. What did he do about it? What are his plans or hopes for himself, if he were to receive surgery?

5. Family History: A family history should be taken, but special attention given to the family members' attitude toward the patient and his problem. Will a family member be willing to give information in the social history with the social worker?

6. Psychopathology: Close attention should be given to any other psychopathology. Factors which rule against transgender surgery for otherwise *bona fide* transsexual individual include:
   a. Sociopathy, especially criminal behavior
   b. Psychosis
   c. Severe infantile character
   d. Severe impulse disorder
   e. Inability to cross live successfully
   f. Inability to work reliably
   g. Inability to save money
   h. Lack of family cooperation

7. Record-keeping: Careful dictation of the evaluation is necessary because extensive follow-up interviews are done with operated transsexuals as a part of ongoing research. Effective comparison between these interviews and the initial interviews is essential. The following is an outline for dictating the evaluation interviews.

Transsexual Interview Outline

I. Current Life Situation
   1. Name
   2. Age
   3. Physical gender
   4. Current claimed gender

5. Impression of sexual presentation. Is it convincing?
6. Living as a transsexual? How long and in what way? Where? How long? History of cross-dressing? Cross-living?
7. Current and past employment
8. Current savings, insurance
9. Criminal record?
10. Describe manner during the interviews; Cooperative? Overcooperative? Reliability as an informant?
11. General impressions of current life adjustment
12. General impressions of patient as a person

II. Sexual Orientation and Activities
   A. Attitude toward genitals
      1. Pleasures in erection, masturbation? How often? What fantasies?
      2. Indifference, disgust with genitals?
   B. Sexual activities
      1. Sexual activity with partners? History of these contacts.
         a. Are these *normal* men
         b. Homosexuals
         c. Women
      2. What does the patient enjoy about these contacts?
      3. Pleasure, sexual excitement associated with cross-dressing?

III. Gender Orientation
   A. How did patient learn about transsexualism?
   B. How does patient date the onset of transsexualism and wish for sex change operation?
   C. How does patient describe the evaluation of transsexualism and wish for sex change?

IV. Family History
   A. Patient's description of and attitude toward mother, father, siblings and relevant others, (e.g. grandmother, uncles), including their attitude toward the patient and his transsexualism, the possibility

of gender surgery and their willingness to partici-
pate in the evaluation procedure.
   B. Record *verbatim* the earliest memory (ask for age,
details) , the earliest memory of mother, father and
the wish to be a woman.
   C. Earliest play activities; other significant experiences
 V. Surgery
   A. What does surgery involve, as patient imagines it?
   B. What does he believe it will do for him?
   C. What plans and fantasies, post-operative?
   D. Is the plan realistic?
   E. Are there perhaps other motives for surgery?
 VI. Other Psychopathology
   A. Describe other psychopathological features, with
particular attention to: sociopathy, pathological nar-
cissism, infantile or inadequate character.
 VII. Object Relations
   A. Does the patient experience people as distinct, sep-
arate individuals? As need satisfiers? As symbiotic
aspect of himself?
VIII. Summary
   A. Interviewer's conclusions re: sex-orientation, gen-
der-orientation, diagnosis, suitability for gender
surgery.

References

Benjamin, H.: *The Transsexual Phenomenon.* New York, Julian Press, 1966.
Money, J. and Green, R. (Eds.) : *Transsexualism and Sex Reassignment.*
   Baltimore, The Johns Hopkins Press, 1969.
Stoller, R.: *Sex and Gender: The Development of Masculinity and
   Femininity.* New York, Science House, 1968.

EVALUATION OF THE ADOLESCENT PATIENT

DAVID W. PEARSON, M.A., M.D.

   The adolescent patient presents unique problems in clinical evaluation. The psychiatrist is faced with a complex set
of psychodynamics and bio-social factors. In addition, there
may be important legal considerations that vary from state
to state. The following outline is designed to aid the psychi-

atrist in evaluating the adolescent patient so that the data necessary for diagnostic formulation and treatment planning may be gathered in a smooth and optimal fashion.

I. Introduction
   A. Definition: Adolescence is that period in psycho-bio-social development extending from the time of early physical changes that herald the onset of puberty (Males: the beginning in sudden growth spurt of the testicles and the penis. Females: the beginning of growth of pubic hair to the time when the individual has defined and begun to adopt his adult social roles).
   B. Discussion: the difficulties faced in evaluating adolescents can be seen from this definition as it starts with a definable physical event and ends with an extremely complex social-psychological end point. This complexity makes evaluating the adolescent psychiatric patient one of the most complex, demanding and challenging problems facing the psychiatrist. Development during the adolescent phase must be viewed along a series of continua: biological, degree of family relatedness to both family of orientation and family of procreation, peer relationships (both male and female), school adjustment, work adjustment, internal psychological development, sexual and self-identity, etc. Each individual patient may be at different points on each continuum.

II. Stages in the Development of the Adolescent:
   It is important to attempt first to conceptualize the stage of adolescence that the particular patient has reached. (Less precise, perhaps, than the stages of childhood libidinal development but clinically useful nevertheless.)
   A. Two useful stage theories are described:
      1. P. Blos (1962)
         a. Preadolescence
         b. Early adolescence

   c. Adolescence
   d. Late adolescence
   e. Post adolescence
  2. D. Miller (in press)
   a. Early adolescence (puberty)
   b. Mid-adolescence (identity and self-realization)
   c. Late adolescence (coping)
 B. J. M. Tanner (1962) describes the biological basis of such stage theories in great detail in his classic text, *Growth at Adolescence*. He states that secular trends push the actual age of puberty and maximum physical size earlier by three months every decade.
 C. Discussion:
  1. Stage theory emphasizes the evolution of social-psychological pressures on an individual who varies in his biological development within certain broad limits. In evaluating an adolescent it is important to note whether he or she is an early developer. It is important in the early adolescent to assess the family of orientation and the patient's interactions with them, much as one does in the evaluation of a latency child.
  2. The peer group becomes more important in the midadolescence and conflicts with parental values in both sexes are often presenting problems.
  3. As the adolescent enters late adolescence, problems of intimacy within heterosexual relationships, establishing a family of procreation, establishing the self and the roles that the self adopts *vis-à-vis* society and peer groups are of central importance.
III. Interviewing the Adolescent Patient
 A. Helpful factual information to know before approaching an adolescent patient:
  1. The state's laws as to when an adolescent reaches his majority

  2. The hospital's policy as to age of child-adolescent and adult-adolescent distinctions

  3. The legal problems involved in permission to see an adolescent patient

  4. The specific state's definition of an emancipated minor

B. The patient and his parents:

  1. The evaluation of the adolescent patient can be especially threatening and challenging for the young psychiatrist. In part, this is because many of the conflicts that a late adolescent has concerning role models and identity are similar to those of the young psychiatrist who is still developing his own professional identity. Any uncertainty is often picked up by an adolescent who is asking for controls, limits and the assurance that someone does care, and that he has not alienated all of society by his actions or his feelings.

  2. In working with adolescents there are traps that the psychiatrist who is inexperienced in dealing with patients of this age group can fall into by trying to appear too ready an ally or too distant an evaluator. The adolescent who has some sensitivity to the types of professional or personal conflicts within the physician often will put his thumb on the interviewer's insecurities.

  3. Playing it straight and open is important with adolescent patients in varying ways depending upon the developmental stage of the patients.

  4. It is often true that those psychiatrists who wish to maintain a more distant and reflective quality with adolescent patients have difficulty in establishing rapport. It is usually necessary to take a more active stance, framing questions more concretely, and going directly after information. An adolescent who looks withdrawn, terrified, and depressed can blossom once common ground is established and interaction is encouraged.

5. As in all interviewing it is important to make emphatic contact early in the interview without sounding sympathetic or pitying and without infantalizing the patient.

6. It is usually wise to interview the parents and the patient separately. In this case, a colleague (other psychiatrist, social worker, etc.) may see the parents. If the evaluator plans to see the parents it is wise to see the patient in the presence of the parents. This may have therapeutic results and can aid in establishing trust between the psychiatrist and the designated adolescent patient.

C. Factors in diagnostic formulation

1. The Patient: from a developmental orientation in terms of his own experiences, his developmental history, his internal conflicts, his defenses, his present life experiences, his sexual adjustment and his strengths (skilled psychological testing by someone who has had experience with adolescent protocols can be helpful).

2. The Patient's Family: their socio-economic status, their education, their own upbringing, the patient's position within the family, the effect of the patient's problems upon the family and vice versa.

3. The Patient's School: the problems that he presents to school (and vice versa), his achievement, the school's willingness and flexibility to adjust to meet the patient's needs.

4. The Patient's Community: the nature of the patient's peer group and how he relates to others, the actual living arrangements both within the family and within the community.

5. Actual on the spot evaluation of any of these areas may be useful. Rapport with schools, community agencies and other community facilities is essential in adequate planning and management of the adolescent patient.

References

Blos, P.: *On Adolescence: A Psychoanalytic Interpretation.* Glencoe, The Free Press, 1962.

Miller, D.: *That the Young Survive: Helping Adolescents in a Disturbed Society.* New York, Science House, In press.

Tanner, J. M.: *Growth at Adolescence.* Springfield, Thomas, 1962.

Other Recommended Reading

Aichorn, A.: *Wayward Youth.* New York, Viking Press, 1935.

Caplan, G. and Lebovici, S. (Eds.): *Adolescence; Psychosocial Perspectives.* New York, Basic Books, Inc., 1969.

Feinstein, S. C.; Giovacchini, P. L.; and Miller, A. A. (Eds.): *Adolescent Psychiatry; v. 1; Developmental and Clinical Studies.* New York, Basic Books, Inc., 1971.

EVALUATION OF THE CHILD PATIENT

The following outline for data collection in the psychiatric evaluation of pediatric-age patients is the general format used at Children's Psychiatric Hospital, The University of Michigan Medical Center. The first part of the history (I through V) is obtained from one or both parents by either a social worker or by the child psychiatrist who will later evaluate the child.

While a discussion of diagnosis in child psychiatry is beyond the purpose and scope of this handbook, the reader may refer to *Psychopathological Disorders in Childhood: Theoretical Considerations and a Proposed Classification* (Group for the Advancement of Psychiatry, 1966); this diagnostic system is the official diagnostic instrument used at C.P.H. Copies may be obtained by writing: GAP, 419 Park Avenue South, New York, New York, 10016 ($3.50 per copy).

Other references that are especially useful in the diagnostic conceptualization, genetic-dynamic formulation and treatment-planning aspects are listed as Suggested Reading.

I. Introduction
    A. Brief description of the child
        1. Include name, age, sex, race, grade, residence, socio-economic status of family, place in family (natural, adopted, foster child, ordinal position).

B. Referral information
   1. By whom, for what reason, service sought.
C. Information obtained from
   1. Those present at evaluation and from what records to date.
   2. Previous agency contacts and responses to therapeutic/remedial intervention (e.g., speech therapy, medication).
D. Examiner's view of problem and service sought
   1. Please note if varying from Intake Statement of problem and service sought.
E. Parents' attitude toward evaluation and their expectation of service.

II. Current Situation and Child Behavior: Present Problem
A. Symptom picture and time of onset, including precipitating events.
B. Behavioral picture: include interaction with family and others. Characteristic handling of hostile and affectionate feelings by child and parents. Discuss fears.
C. Academic picture: grade placement, current levels of achievement, current levels of performance, attitude and management efforts of school personnel.

III. Family Circumstances
A. List family members.
B. Comment on housing, child care and sleeping arrangements, family attitudes toward family size and planning and use of birth controls.
C. Pertinent social and emotional historical data, to include any significant loss of relationship or past traumatic events affecting family life. (Note child's age at the time and his reaction.)
D. Where pertinent, describe child-rearing patterns in families of origin and how this affects current parental attitudes and practice. Discuss special roles of close relatives at present time. Discuss discipline and the child's response to it.

    E. Briefly describe siblings' personalities, relationships with this child and parents' attitude towards siblings.

    F. Describe personalities of each parent and marital relationship. Illustrate with parental interaction in interview, including interaction with examiner.

IV. Developmental History

  A. Birth history

    1. Pregnancy

      a. mother's previous pregnancies, age at time of this pregnancy, length of gestation, course of pregnancy.

      b. attitudes toward pregnancy, expectations for infant, special events during pregnancy, general emotional state of mother and father.

    2. Delivery: length of labor, course, type of delivery, birth weight, complications (Rh factor, transfusions, infant distress, maternal distress).

    3. Neo-Natal Period (0–10d): infant responsiveness, sucking capabilities, activity level, parental reactions to infant's sex and general appearance, mother's emotional state.

  B. Early development

    1. Habit patterns.

      a. Feeding: breast or bottle, schedule, appetite, weaning, introduction of solids, problems (colic, spitting up, pica, food idiosyncracies, thumbsucking). Mother's reactions.

      b. Sleeping: regular or irregular, age when first sleeping through the night, early sleep arrangements, problems (insomnia, wakefulness, nightmares, restlessness).

      c. Elimination: early problems (infant diarrhea, constipation), toilet-training (age, by whom, method, child responses, compare with others in family, quality of parent-child interaction, age completed; bowel and bladder, night and day).

      d. Sexual: present level of development and

identification, autoerotic behavior, curiosity, parent responses, attempts at education, child's level of understanding, traumata.

2. Physical development.
   a. Growth: body size, teething, inordinate growth.
   b. Motor: rolling over, sitting up, crawling, standing up, walking, coordination.
   c. Communication: smile, words, sentences, problems (delay, distortion).
   d. General Health and Physical Condition: illnesses, operations and responses to them.
   e. Specific problems of *organicity,* including hyperkinesis, sensory deficit or perceptual disturbance.

V. School History: Response to Starting School, Grades Repeated, Past Special Placements and Remedial Help, Areas of Subject Difficulty, Moves, Responses to Teachers and Peers, Parental Attitude to School, Parental Expectations.

VI. Interview with the Child
   A. Part I; Descriptive.
      1. Describe child's physical appearance
      2. Describe behavior and interaction with parents and examiner in waiting room.
      3. Describe behavior while in the interview with the examiner; include significant interventions by the examiner.
      4. Discuss rate of activity, flow of ideas, characteristics of thinking, context of thinking, general mood and/or affect, clinical impression of intellectual functioning and capacity, capacity to relate.
      5. What is the child's attitude about coming to see the interviewer?
   B. Part II; Technical interpretation of observed and historical material (support with anecdotal material).
      1. Ego assessment

a. defensive functions; preferred defenses, appropriateness and efficiency.
b. quality of object relations; extent of capacity to relate.
c. relation to reality; capacity to adapt.
d. nature of thinking processes; abstract vs. concrete, utilization of fantasy.
e. drive regulation and control; include development of drive endowment, superego function, assess degree of impulsivity, frustration tolerance, attention span.
f. autonomous functions; intelligence, memory (immediate and remote, lapses or distortions), motor function (coordination, use of body language), perception (distortions; organic or psychologic), language.
g. Synthetic function: assess capacity to integrate and organize experience.
h. Assess ego's general functioning in light of above relative to age and developmental stage.
2. Superego; broadly assess nature and extent of guilt vs. fear of external authority.
3. Results of other examinations.
VII. Genetic-Dynamic Formulation
  A. Discuss major sources of conflict relative to:
    1. Psychosexual phase of development.
    2. External and internalized conflict relative to child.
    3. Major identifications and their contributions to child's adaptations.
    4. Intrafamily relationships.
    5. Community.
VIII. Impression/Diagnosis: Primary diagnosis, with secondary features (*GAP Diagnostic Nomenclature*, 1966).
  IX. Recommendations
    A. Optimal and alternative.
      1. Child; form of intervention and goals.
      2. Parents; form of intervention and goals.

    3. Community; practical suggestions based on available resources.

B. Interpretive Interview with Parents; specific context of interpretations to parents and/or child and their responses. Your prediction of their potential to follow recommendations. (Can be included by an addendum if interview takes place on a later date.)

C. Interpretation to Community Personnel; note whether interview or by mail.

    1. Content of interpretations (if by interview).

    2. Estimate of community's ability to utilize recommendations.

D. Examiner's commitment to plans for follow-up.

Reference

Psychopathological Disorders in Childhood: Theoretical Considerations and A Proposed Classification. Group for the Advancement of Psychiatry, Volume VI, Report No. 62, New York, 1966.

Suggested Reading

Freud, A.: *Normality and Pathology in Childhood: Assessments of Development.* New York, International Universities Press, 1965.

Nagera, H.: *Early Childhood Disturbances, The Infantile Neurosis and the Adulthood Disturbances.* New York, International Universities Press, 1966.

Chapter V

EVALUATION OF PATIENTS FOR PSYCHOTHERAPY

As in general medicine, it is crucial in psychiatry to base treatment-planning upon sound diagnostic evaluation. This can be especially important in psychotherapy.

Although a discussion of the techniques of psychotherapy is beyond the purpose and scope of this handbook, this chapter is designed to aid the psychiatrist in that all-important first step: evaluation, a step that all too often is not given proper attention. To neglect this aspect, however, is to unnecessarily risk treatment failure.

This chapter focuses upon four major forms of psychotherapy: intensive, uncovering psychotherapy; group therapy; marital therapy and family therapy. Its seeks to answer such basic questions as: What are the indications and contraindications for each of these therapeutic modalities? Which patients will benefit most (and least) from each of these treatment methods? What data must the psychiatrist collect in order to match the right patient and the optimum treatment?

EVALUATION FOR INTENSIVE PSYCHOTHERAPY
Dennis Walsh, M.D.

Intensive psychotherapy, for purposes of this outline, refers to psychoanalytically-oriented psychotherapy. It refers to in-depth therapy that proceeds from the surface (conscious) to the unconscious. It implies the use of basic psycho-analytic principles: (1) not to make use of authority and to eliminate, as far as possible, suggestion as an element of treatment; (2) to discard abreaction as a therapeutic tool; (3) to keep manipulation of the patient to a minimum; and (4) to consider the analysis of resistance and transference, and interpretation of unconscious material as the legitimate tools of therapy (A. Freud, 1965).

The outline is divided into three parts: I. The Patient's Qualifications, II. The Therapist's Qualifications, III. The Supervisor's Qualifications.

I. The Patient's Qualifications
   A. Practical Considerations
      A reasonably intact life situation is most desirable. By this is meant that while a patient's psychopathology will sometimes make his life appear chaotic, one would question a patient beginning intensive long-term psychotherapy in the midst of a divorce, a new marriage, a pending move to another city or any realistic life situation which threatens the likelihood of a long-term commitment to therapy. Crisis intervention and short term therapy may well be needed at this point, but a patient's life should be as stable as possible before long-term therapy is begun.
   B. Motivation
      It is preferable if the patient seeks therapy freely of his own volition rather than being referred by an agency or some other person. Sometimes patients who are not self-referred can become genuinely interested in therapy in the course of the pretherapy evaluation. The therapist should be very hesitant, however, about recommending long-term intensive psychotherapy to a patient who, at the end of his evaluation, does not feel that the majority of his problems are internal. If he considers his problems to reside in the environment, intensive psychotherapy is not usually indicated.

C. Degree of Discomfort Caused by the Referring Complaint

The therapist should be able to point out several areas in the patient's life that are causing him acute discomfort. If there is no anxiety or no perceived difficulty in interpersonal relationships, it is unlikely that the patient would be able to generate the necessary motivation to work through unconscious conflicts.

D. Financial Stability

In a clinic setting it is possible to scale down fees to what would be fair and equitable for a person in any financial condition. Nevertheless, it is important to ascertain whether or not there is some stable source from which regular financial support can come to assure that the patient will be able to regularly pay his fee though it may be as low as three or four dollars per session. This is an area where residents especially have difficulty and, by and large, tend to ignore or underevaluate. It is essential that the patient's monthly income and fixed expenses be gone over in some detail so that the fee may be fairly set: not too high, not too low. If the patient can afford to be involved in private psychotherapy he should be so referred so that the number of positions for low cost treatments are not filled by people who could afford to be treated elsewhere.

E. Diagnostic Considerations

1. The optimum treatment case for intensive psychoanalytically-oriented psychotherapy is the patient who has consolidated and integrated his neurotic conflicts into a true neurosis, i.e. although patients may present serious problems in the arenas of narcissism, object relationships and oral and anal fixations, all of these difficulties have been organized into a complex system cluster around a phallic-oedipal core. For a fuller

understanding of this important criterion, the reader is referred to *Early Childhood Disturbances, the Infantile Neuroses, and the Adult Disturbances* (Nagera, 1966).

2. While it is true that patients with more serious disturbances (schizophrenia, borderline syndrome, character disorders, addictions) are sometimes treated in intensive, uncovering psychotherapy these cases should not be attempted by an inexperienced therapist. Even the skillful, experienced therapist encounters great difficulty with such patients.

3. It is obviously imperative that the therapist performs a thorough and careful evaluation of the patient *before* recommending intensive psychotherapy. The evaluation must be performed in depth and must go beyond mere descriptive accounting of behavioral manifestations and defensive mechanisms. Patients who present, on the surface, the same phenomenologic appearance and defensive style may turn out to have significantly different nuclear conflicts upon a skillful evaluation.

II. The Therapist's Qualifications

A. Stage of Training

Residents in psychiatry generally should not undertake an intensive treatment case until they have completed a significant portion of the first year of training. Basic knowledge of dynamic theory and skill in interview technique are minimum prerequisites.

B. Interest

Not all psychiatrists are interested in conducting intensive psychotherapy. Those who are not interested, should not do so, with the one exception, perhaps, of a basic training requirement in a residency program.

C. Personal Therapy

It is generally agreed that the psychiatrist who performs intensive uncovering psychotherapy as a major portion of his clinical practice should himself have undergone intensive psychoanalytically-oriented psychotherapy or formal psychoanalysis. The therapist, obviously, must be aware of his own areas of psychic conflict and be in a position to fully understand countertransference issues as they appear if he is to be of help to the patient in this treatment modality. The therapist will also have a deeper appreciation of the phenomenon of transference, having experienced it himself in a psychotherapeutic setting and his firsthand knowledge of the *process* of therapy (resistance, confrontation, interpretation, working-through) will be invaluable as the treatment proceeds.

III. The Supervisor's Qualifications

Supervisors of intensive psychotherapy in psychiatric training centers should meet the basic requirements of formal psychoanalytic training or personal therapy plus theoretical study. While the resident treats the patient, it is the supervisor that treats the case. Therefore he must be sensitive to the needs of the trainee and skillful in shaping the resident's professional growth and development.

Countertransference issues and psychic blind spots in the resident must be handled with great tact. Supervision takes various forms, varying from frank therapy for the trainee (therapist-oriented) to strict and exclusive attention to the patient (patient-oriented). The supervisor should be skillful and flexible enough to operate at both ends of the spectrum and at several points in between, depending on the needs of the trainee at the moment.

References

Freud, A.: *The Writings of Ann Freud,* Volume VI. New York, International Universities Press, 1965.

Freud, A.; Nagera, H. and Freud, W. E.: Metapsychological Assessment of the Adult Personality: The Adult Profile. *Psychoanalytic Study of the Child XX,* New York, International Universities Press, 1965.

Nagera, H.: *Early Childhood Disturbances, the Infantile Neuroses, and the Adulthood Disturbances.* New York, International Universities Press, 1966.

EVALUATION FOR MARITAL THERAPY

Marital therapy is any therapeutic intervention which has as its major focus the alteration of the marital dyad. Although treatment goals may vary widely from case to case, it is generally agreed that the most fundamental aim in treatment is to assist the couple to better understand their reciprocal marital interaction and to attempt to find ways in which their needs can be mutually satisfied so the growth and development of each partner can be maximized in the relationship. (Olson, 1970)

There are two basic technical approaches to marital therapy: the person-oriented approach and the marriage-oriented approach. In the person-oriented approach the overriding concern is with the individual, regardless whether the therapist is conducting classic 1:1 therapy or he is treating a marital couple in conjoint therapy. The focus is on the growth and development of the individual. Consequently the "marital chips are left to fall where they may." (Olson, 1970)

In the marriage-oriented approach the focus is on the marriage itself. The marriage unit takes precedence over the individual. The goal is to resolve problems that are interfering with each spouse having his or her most important needs fulfilled. (In cases where such a workable solution is not possible, marriage-oriented therapy may be used to ease the path to divorce.) Interactional rather than intrapsychic factors are stressed. Systems theory, communication theory and problem-solving techniques are often employed.

Marital therapy borrows from many theoretical frameworks, but as yet does not rest upon its own theoretical base. The most commonly employed theories include: psychoanalytic, learning theory, behavioral modification, Rogerian systems-communication theory (Haley, 1963; Jackson, 1961;

Satir, 1964), role theory (Hurvitz, 1970), self concepts (Johnsen, 1968) and relationship typology (Bolte, 1970).

Similarly, marital therapists utilize a wide range of techniques that are drawn from the theoretical positions listed above and also including such techniques as transactional analysis, gestalt psychology, sensitivity training laboratories and others.

Part One: Diagnostic Assessment
JOSEPH R. NOVELLO, M.D.

The psychiatrist who is consulted by an individual patient or a married couple because of marital difficulty is faced with several important tasks and questions to be answered:

1. What are the factors to consider in evaluating the marriage? What is the problem?
2. How should the evaluation be conducted?
3. Should treatment be recommended?
4. What type of treatment: Person-oriented or marriage-oriented? What specific form should the treatment take and which techniques should be employed?

The following section on evaluation for marital therapy is designed to aid the psychiatrist in answering these questions.

I. Evaluation of Marital Problems

Hollender (1971) has pointed out that the success or failure of any marriage has little to do with the normality or abnormality of either partner. For example, two reasonably healthy individuals may have an unsteady, unworkable marriage while two relatively sick individuals may have a stable, relatively satisfactory marriage.

In evaluating a marriage, therefore, the psychiatrist must look beyond the assets and liabilities of each spouse and investigate the mutuality of their marital interraction. In marriage one plus one equals three. The psychiatrist must consider not only the two individuals but the marriage itself.

In evaluating the all-important third factor, the

marriage itself, Hollender suggests five criteria that should be examined:

A. Dovetail of Needs

Reciprocal needs of partners foster a good marital fit while clashing needs result in disharmony. For example, a passive-dependent woman married to a man who has a need to dominate and control is likely to have a satisfactory marriage while two dependent types or two controlling types will find it difficult to satisfy their own needs and the marriage will be doomed to repeated friction.

In any marriage there are a number of needs that must be met. The psychiatrist must identify the individual needs of each spouse and then determine if they are being met in the marriage. In what areas do the needs clash? What are the predominate needs of each spouse? What is the relative health or psychic dysfunction of these predominate needs?

B. Attitude Toward Problems

The attitude of the person toward the marital difficulties is often much more crucial than the nature of the problems themselves. Each partner must be prepared to acknowledge his own flaws and to recognize the unfulfilled needs of their spouse. There must be a willingness to change if the marital unit is to achieve a new equilibrium. Marriage-oriented therapy will not work in the marriage that sees one spouse resolutely maintaining that it's all his fault or it's all her fault. If the psychiatrist, on the other hand, comes to agree that the blame resides in one spouse, a course of individual treatment is usually indicated. (Providing, of course, that the person accepts such a recommendation.)

C. Manner In Which The Marital Relationship Is Used Or Exploited

This factor is closely related to attitude toward problems. The person who insists upon utilizing an ego defense of externalization merely converts his own intrapsychic conflict into an interpersonal marital battle. If he lacks sufficient insight and motivation to change, this can be interpreted during the evaluation. If, then, his spouse is willing to live with this arrangement, she too has a problem. The marital fit may then be exposed as unhealthy. If neither spouse opts for change, however, there is little reason to recommend conjoint marital therapy. If, on the other hand, one spouse is interested in self-growth and change, the recommendation for individual therapy may be made.

D. Expectations

What does each spouse actually expect from the marriage? This factor is all important. Are the expectations reasonable or are they in the realm of fantasy? Is there a dovetail of expectations? Often the problem is that one or both partners have unreal, fairy-tale expectations of the marriage.

E. Attitude Toward Marital and Family Stability

The psychiatrist must carefully evaluate this factor in both his assessment of the marital unit and in deciding whether or not to recommend treatment. Some couples, because of individual, cultural and religious reasons, will endure any amount of individual hardship in order to maintain a marriage. They pay a tremendous personal price and are left with a marriage in name only, de facto divorce. Yet under no circumstances are they prepared to accept legal divorce or even to demand change of themselves or their spouse, fearing that to do so might lead to divorce

At the other end of the spectrum are couples who find it easier to separate than to work out even relatively minor differences.

The psychiatrist who utilizes the five criteria listed above will be in a position to perform an accurate marital evaluation.

The method of actually collecting the necessary information from each spouse will vary according to the style of the individual therapist and the dictates of the specific case.

One of the most useful techniques for data gathering is the conjoint marital interview. The following section provides guidelines for the conjoint interview and outlines specific data that the therapist might obtain in order to construct a profile of the marriage. He will then be able to submit the profile to diagnostic scrutiny and answer such questions as: (1) How does the marriage rate on the five criteria listed above? (2) Is treatment indicated? (3) If so, for whom? The marital unit? One spouse? (The question of what kind of treatment should be prescribed is taken up in Part Three.)

Part Two: The Conjoint Marital Interview

ARTHUR R. WILLIAMS, Ed.D.

The following format is designed for use as a diagnostic tool in the conjoint marital interview, and is best suited to the initial or intake interview. The conjoint interview is especially valuable in assessing the dynamics of the interpersonal relationship of the marital partners. This technique may be used alone or in combination with individual interviews of each spouse separately.

This format for the conjoint marital interview is based upon clinical application of research data which indicate (1) specific areas of agreement common to successful marriages, and (2) the sequence through which successful marital relationships proceed to healthy adjustment. The essential keys to adjustment here are (1) an effective and functioning communication system within the marriage dyad, and (2) *agreement* between husband and wife concerning shared feelings and attitudes in each area. To facilitate the use of this format, the outline lists the specific steps to be followed chronologically during the interview. Followed as presented, the format will yield marriage history information and data relevant to present functioning and/or dysfunctioning of the marriage relationship, and help provide the basis for formulating the treatment plan.

I. Preparation of the Couple for Information Giving

Couples are invariably anxious when they come for a psychiatric evaluation. They have little knowledge as to what to expect, and what expectations they do have are often distorted. Many times the therapist is perceived as a judge who will hear their case. The purpose of the substeps here are to erase misperceptions as to the nature of the process and to lower the anxiety states in an effort to solicit more correct information in the next phase of the interview.

A. Explain the role of the therapist as one whose purpose is to help all present gain insight into the problems of the relationship; not one who is there to judge or penalize.

B. Identify the patient. That is, make it clear that the patient in this process is not the husband or wife but rather the marriage. This can be strongly reinforced by overtly asking the partners to help, as cotherapists, as all look at the patient: the marriage. (This tactic has proved immensely valuable as a tension-reducer in the initial stages of therapy.)

C. Introduce the inventory. Best done in an informal way, again stressing the need for their cooperation.

II. Taking the Marital Inventory

The six areas listed below are the common areas of agreement in successful marriages. They are listed in the order in which most couples resolve them, and it should be noted that evidence suggests the longer it takes for a couple to resolve them, the poorer the prognosis for eventual adjustment.

These areas make up the inventory and, when thoroughly explored, will reveal a reasonably complete history and present status of the marriage. The extent to which they can be explored in the initial interview will depend upon time and sensitivity of the therapist and level of cooperation of the couple. *All* should be touched upon to some extent in the initial interview, and the preferred procedure is to elicit the information casually and informally. Critical points and objects for each area are listed under each heading. Throughout the inventory it is essential that the therapist be aware of level of *communication* and *agreement* or *disagreement* of the partners.

A. Religion
1. Family religious background, if any, of each.
2. Present views *of the couple* with regard to religion.
3. Discernment of values, life goals, etc., of each partner and degree of similarity between the two.

Object here is to attempt to find out if the couple presents a *unified* philosophy of life.

B. Friends
1. Ability of the couple to distinguish his friends, her friends, and their friends.
2. Extent of agreement concerning feelings and attitudes towards all three classes of friends.

Object here is to ascertain ability of couple to differentiate the three types of friends in marriage and the degree of shared attitudes concerning the friends.

C. In-Laws
1. Perceived effect of in-law relations upon marriage.
2. Attitudes of each concerning in-law relations.
3. Degree of consensus concerning feelings towards in-laws.

Object here is to determine the extent to which the couple agrees concerning the feelings and attitudes towards the in-laws and whether or not those stated feelings and attitudes are in fact employed by the couple as a unit in dealing with the in-laws.

D. Activities
1. Feelings and attitudes of each toward the vocational activities of themselves and of their partner.
2. Feelings and attitudes of each toward the avoca-

tional activities of themselves and of their partner.

3. General idea of time allotment to separate vocational and avocational activities.
4. General idea of time allotment to shared vocational and avocational activities.
5. Ability to identify positive or negative feelings
   towards any of the above.

Object here is twofold:

   a. Ascertainment of general time allotment for
      activities.
   b. Exploration of feeling level and content for
      each activity.

E. Budget

   1. Attitude toward income level.
   2. Attitude toward spending and/or saving level.
   3. Agreement as to specific allocation of income.
   4. Exploration of the mechanics of decision-making
      and purchasing of major items (e.g. cars, appli-
      ances, etc.)
   5. Money management patterns in each family of
      origin.

   Object here is to determine to what extent the partners agree as a couple on the generation and expenditure of income and to try to elicit subjective
   feelings in this area.

F. Sex

   1. Degree of agreement as to the present adequacy
      of the conjugal relationship *without regard to
      specifics* such as frequency, position, etc. (See
      section on Evaluation of Sexual Dysfunction
      for detailed discussion, Chapter IV.)

   Object here is to determine the *present* level of
   satisfaction for each partner with the marital sexual adjustment.

   NOTE: Information concerning sexual adjustment
   at this stage may lend itself to one or a
   combination of three possible interpreta-

tions and the therapist should be aware of these possibilities:

    a. Reported dissatisfaction with sexual adjustment may indicate a truly sexual adjustment problem in the marriage.

    b. Reported dissatisfaction with sexual adjustment may indicate dysfunction and lack of open communication in one of the other areas which is being presented symptomatically as a sexual adjustment problem.

    c. Where there is reporting of maladjustment in the other areas but no maladjustment as far as sex is concerned, we may be reasonably certain that failure to report sexual maladjustment is indicative of persistent defensiveness to the therapy environment.

III. Recapitulation for the Partners

It is best to close this interview by summarizing the information which has come to light. This should be done by pointing out the apparent strengths of the relationship to the partners as well as indicating to them the areas in which communication of feelings and consensus of attitudes seem to be blocked.

IV. Recommendations

The therapist, at this point, should have a clear concept of the present status of the marital relationship. He has taken the information obtained in the conjoint interview (and also from separate interviews with each spouse if this technique is used) and scrutinized it carefully. Each of the articles in the profile (Religion, Friends, In-Laws, Activities, Budget, Sex) has yielded valuable data that allow him to assess the marriage in terms of how it meets Hollender's five criteria listed in Part One:

1. Dovetail of Needs
2. Attitude Toward Problems

3. Manner In Which The Marital Relationship Is Used or Exploited
4. Expectations
5. Attitude Toward Marital and Family Stability

Based on this assessment, the psychiatrist is ready to make his recommendations. In some cases he may decide that no treatment is indicated. This may be so for many reasons: There may in fact be no problem requiring therapy, the problem may be surfaced and worked-through during the evaluation, the marriage may be beyond repair, one or both partners may resist treatment and a wide-variety of other possibilities.

In other cases the psychiatrist may decide that the problem is basically due to the severe psychopathology of one of the partners. The psychotic husband of a reasonably stable wife obviously needs treatment above and beyond the marital unit. In this case the psychiatrist may recommend individual treatment for the husband or he may combine the husband's individual treatment with conjoint therapy for the couple.

In cases where the psychiatrist identifies the marital unit itself as the patient, he will recommend some form of marital therapy.

Part Three: Selection of Specific Treatment Modality In Marital Therapy

JOSEPH R. NOVELLO, M.D.

The psychiatrist, as a physician, knows that diagnostic skills alone are not enough if he is in the practice of treating patients. The physician who correctly diagnoses a case of pneumonia must then select the proper antibiotic or his diagnostic skill is wasted. Similarly, the psychiatrist who has conducted a thorough evaluation of a marital unit and has developed a specific diagnostic assessment must then recommend the proper and specific treatment course that is best tailored to the needs of the patient, in this case the marital unit.

Too little attention is generally paid to the problem of

selecting a specific psychotherapeutic treatment approach based on specific diagnostic findings. It usually happens that if a couple goes to a therapist who does 1:1 therapy, they will get 1:1 therapy; if they go to a therapist who does group therapy with married couples, they will get group therapy with married couples and so forth.

Fortunately, the psychiatrist who recommends marital therapy has several options from which to choose. There exist several approaches and techniques in marital therapy, each with their own inherent strengths and weaknesses, indications and contraindications. The psychiatrist, by carefully considering the pros and cons of each approach, may fit the treatment to the patient instead of fitting the patient to the treatment. The following outline is an effort to provide the psychiatrist with this information and to permit him to intelligently tailor treatment to diagnosis.

This outline is based upon the findings of Dr. Bernard L. Greene (1970) and Dr. Peter A. Martin (1970).

I. Individual Therapy
    A. Description: classic 1:1 therapy. The person recognizes a marital problem and designates *himself* as the patient. The spouse does not enter treatment. Any changes in the marriage, therefore, will be incidental to changes in the patient's own psychodynamics.
    B. Indications
        1. Secrets, i.e. the therapist has learned about a secret from one spouse (infidelity, etc.). The patient is not prepared to share the information with his partner at this time.
        2. Preference of one or both partners.
        3. An emotional immaturity exists in one spouse which precludes the sharing of a single therapist.
        4. One spouse believes he must work out his own problems regardless of the consequences to his partner.
        5. Where it is evident that the husband and wife

have widely differing goals in terms of their marital problem (s) .

C. Contraindication

    1. When the spouse who is not in treatment has paranoid-like reactions to being *told on* in the therapy or being influenced by the other spouse in collaboration with the therapist. This suspiciousness leads to repeated questioning as to what is going on in the partner's individual treatment and can seriously interfere with therapy. Such a situation is best handled in conjoint treatment.

II. Consecutive Treatment of Marital Partners

  A. Founder: Oberndorf (1938)

  B. Description: One person enters treatment which continues to completion. The spouse then enters treatment with the same therapist.

  C. Indications: This type of approach is of historical interest. It was the first step in the evolution from individual (1:1) therapy to the several other types of approaches now available in marital therapy.

III. Concurrent (Simultaneous) Dyadic Therapy

  A. Founders: Mittelman (1944)

  B. Description: Each spouse is treated simultaneously in 1:1 therapy by the same therapist. (Followed the introduction of consecutive treatment as the second step in the evolution from purely individual treatment to other forms.)

  C. Indications

    1. Where one spouse simply overwhelms the other.

    2. Where each partner must first gain insights into their own disturbed behavior patterns before the marital relationship itself can come into treatment.

    3. Where a trial conjoint therapy has indicated that one or both partners requires a deeper understanding in the intrapersonal, interpersonal and environmental spheres.

D. Contraindications
1. Severe psychosis or severe character disorder.
2. Paranoid reactions, especially suspicious attitudes toward what the other spouse is communicating in therapy.
3. Excessive *sibling-rivalry* attitudes that preclude sharing the same therapist.

IV. Collaborative Dyadic Therapy (Stereoscopic)
A. Founders: Martin and Bird (1953)
B. Description: Each spouse is seen by a different therapist in 1:1 treatment. The therapists, with permission of the patient, confer regularly and share information.
C. Indications:
1. Where one or both partners are too disturbed or lacking in ego strength for conjoint therapy.
2. Opposition of one spouse to being treated by the same therapist as his partner.
3. Initial hostility of one spouse to the therapist.
4. Referral of patient from another therapist because of his own personal reasons: Inexperience with conjoint approach, nonacceptance of the triadic therapy, countertransference difficulties, etc.
5. Referral of one partner from another therapist because this patient has created therapeutic complications and it is evident to the referring therapist that the husband and wife have widely differing treatment goals.
D. Contraindication
1. Same as individual therapy

V. Collaborative Combined Therapy
A. Description: Each spouse is treated individually by separate therapists. The therapists meet regularly as in the stereoscopic technique. In addition, all four participants (each spouse and their respective therapists) meet regularly in combined group sessions.

B. Indications
  1. Where one or both partners will need a continuing relationship for his own maturation and/or help with the mourning process should the couple separate.
  2. Ineffective stereoscopic approach because of continued distortions between partners.
  3. To resolve pressing interactional difficulties that threaten the success of stereoscopic or simultaneous dyadic therapy.
  4. As preparation for shift to conjoint therapy.
C. Contraindications
  1. Secrets.
  2. Severe psychosis or severe character disorder.
  3. Where transference issues may become confused because of the periodic combined sessions.

VI. Conjoint Triadic Therapy
  A. Founders: Watson (1963), Satir (1965), Haley (1963)
  B. Description: One therapist sees both partners together. May be conducted on various models: person-oriented or marriage-oriented. Most common approach is interactional (marriage-oriented).
  C. Indications
    1. Where there is a special need to focus on the current marital relationship.
    2. Where explosiveness in the marital situation demands speed in bringing order to the marriage.
    3. There is a special need to foster communication between the partners.
    4. Couples in which the problems in the marriage are largely acted out.
    5. Couples who perceive relationships between events and their own responses only when directly confronted with them.
    6. To more readily identify and work through distortions.
    7. To minimize transference and countertransference phenomena.

8. Where one spouse reacts with paranoid or suspicious behavior toward the spouse that is in therapy.
9. Economic, i.e. the cost of treatment is usually less.

D. Contraindications
   1. Secrets
   2. Excessive *sibling rivalry* attitudes toward therapist.
   3. Severe psychosis or severe character disorder.

VII. Combined Marital Therapy
   A. Founder: Greene (1965).
   B. Description: Combination of individual, concurrent, and conjoint sessions depending on the needs of treatment at any particular time. Allows for flexible shift of focus at various points in therapy.
   C. Indications
      1. Where conjoint triadic sessions have been used initially to achieve stability and harmony; the shift is then to individual sessions to work on entrenched intrapersonal conflicts.
      2. Therapeutic impasse with other techniques.
      3. Acting out by one or both partners that cannot be dealt with by other techniques.
      4. One spouse's relationship with a single parent is introjected to the degree that he is threatened by a dyadic setting (sexual, hostile or oral dependent needs).
      5. An impasse in concurrent therapy because of transference difficulty: either too intense (libidinal or aggressive) or involving insufficient emotional involvement.
      6. Where a therapeutic impasse occurs in dyadic therapy because the dyadic transference neurosis can be activated and interpreted only in the triadic sessions.
      7. Where one spouse's obsessive-compulsive personality style makes it necessary to enlist the cooperation of the other spouse.

D. Contraindications
1. Secrets
2. Excessive *sibling-rivalry* attitudes toward therapist.
3. Severe psychosis or severe character disorder.

VIII. Family Therapy
A. Founder: Ackerman (1958)
B. Description: The basic form of family therapy is for a single therapist or cotherapists to see all members of the immediate family together in each session. In kin network therapy, the nuclear family is expanded to include members of the extended family, and even friends and neighbors in some cases. In multiple family group therapy, a group made up of several complete families is treated. (See Evaluation for Family Therapy, this chapter.)
C. Indications
1. Where a child is contributing to the marital discord by acting out parental unconscious impulses.
2. Where a child is being used as a pawn in the struggle between spouses.
3. Where a child is being used as a scapegoat in the marital conflict and this is producing increased marital and family friction.
4. Where there are pressing family concerns (such as serious juvenile delinquency, etc.) that must be resolved before the deeper marital conflicts can be explored.
5. All indications listed for conjoint triadic therapy also apply to family therapy.
D. Contraindications
1. Secrets
2. Excessive *sibling rivalry* attitudes toward therapist.
3. Severe psychosis or severe character disorder.
4. Where there is an irreversible trend to breakup of the family.

IX. Coordinated Family Group Therapy (Multiple Impact Therapy)
    A. Founder: Slavson (1965)
    B. Description: A single therapist or team of therapists meets with individual family members and with various subgroups of the family.
    C. Indications
        1. More flexibility than traditional family therapy approach.
        2. Prevents distortions if all therapists meet regularly.
        3. Avoids confusion in transference.
        4. Especially useful if adolescents are involved since they can be seen as a subgroup.
        5. Where secrets or excessive *sibling rivalry* threaten the success of traditional family therapy approach.
    D. Contraindications
        1. Where there exists a pathologic tendency to fragmentation of the family such an approach might subtly reinforce the process.
 X. Treatment of a Couple by a Couple
    A. Founder: Reding (1964)
    B. Description: The married couple is treated by a male-female therapist couple. In some cases the therapists themselves may be married to each other.
    C. Indications:
        1. Include all those indications listed under conjoint triadic therapy with the exception of No. 3, economic, since the addition of another therapist usually increases the fee.
        2. Where educative, *role-modeling* techniques are important to treatment.
        3. Where it is necessary to block seductive acting out by one of the patients toward an individual therapist of the opposite sex as in conjoint triadic therapy.

4. Where one of the partners resists being treated by a therapist of the opposite sex, yet prefers the conjoint approach.
   D. Contraindications
   1. Secrets
   2. Severe psychosis or severe character disorder.
   3. Where unresolved conflicts exist between the two therapists that would interfere with treatment.
XI. Married Couple Group Therapy
   A. Founder: Blinder (1967)
   B. Description: Therapy group is comprised of married couples (usually three or four couples) and therapist or cotherapists. Where cotherapists are employed, it is customary that they are a male-female team. Various theoretical foundations are used; common to all is some element of group process.
   C. Indications:
   1. Where one person or a couple is unable to observe the results of interactions because of poor insight (maladaptive learning) or resistance, this method increases the opportunity to observe behavioral styles in the here and now and provides the patient (couple) opportunities to experiment with alternatives.
   2. Where the therapist team may effectively utilize educative, *role-modeling* techniques.
   D. Contraindications
   1. Where the marriage is so unstable as to be almost beyond repair it can have a destructive effect on the rest of the group.
   2. Where the addition of other persons into the treatment setting may be predicted to increase the destructive acting out of a particular patient.
   3. Secrets
   4. Where unresolved conflicts exist between the cotherapists that would interfere with treatment.
   5. Psychosis or severe character disorder.

References

Ackerman, N. W.: *The Psychodynamics of Family Life.* New York, Basic Books, 1958.

Blinder, M. G. and Kirschenbaum, M.: Married couple group therapy. *Arch Gen Psychiatry, 17:* 44, 1967.

Bolte, G. L.: A communications approach to marital counseling. *The Family Coordinator, 19:* 32–40, 1970.

Greene, B. L.; Broadhurst, B. P. and Lustig, N.: Treatment of marital disharmony. In Greene, Bernard L. (Ed.) *The Psychotherapies of Marital Disharmony.* New York, The Free Press, 1965.

Green, B. L.: *A Clinical Approach to Marital Problems: Evaluation and Management.* Springfield, Thomas, 1970.

Haley, J.: Marriage therapy. *Arch Gen Psychiatry, 8:* 213–224, 1963.

Hollender, M. H.: Selection of therapy of marital problems. In Masserman, J. H. (Ed.) *Current Psychiatric Therapies,* Vol. II, New York, Grune and Stratton, 1971.

Hurvitz, N.: Interaction hypotheses in marriage counseling. *The Family Coordinator, 19:* 64–75, 1970.

Jackson, D. D. and Weakland, J. H.: Conjoint family therapy: some considerations on theory, technique and results. *Psychiatry, 24:* 30–45, 1961.

Johnsen, K. P.: Self-concept validations as a focus of marriage counseling. *The Family Coordinator, 17:* 174–180, 1968.

Martin, P. A. and Bird, H. W.: An approach to the psychotherapy of marriage partners, the stereoscopic technique. *Psychiatry, 25:* 123–127, 1953.

Martin, P. A.: An historical survey of the psychotherapy of marriage partners. In Sipe, A. W. R. (Ed.) *Hope—Psychiatry's Commitment.* Papers presented to Leo H. Bartemeir, M.D. New York, Bruner/Mazel Publishers, 1970.

Mittelman, B.: Complementary neurotic reactions in intimate relationships. *Psychoanal Q, 13:* 479–491, 1944.

Oberndorf, C. P.: Psychoanalysis of married couples. *In J Psychoanal, 25:* 453, 1938.

Olson, D. H.: Marital and family therapy: Integrative review and critique. *J Marriage and the Family,* 501–538, November, 1970.

Reding, G. R. and Ennis, B.: Treatment of the couple by a couple. *Br J Med Psychol, 37:* 325, 1964.

Satir, V.: *Conjoint Family Therapy: A Guide to Theory and Technique.* Palo Alto, Science and Behavior Books, 1964.

Satir, V.: Conjoint marital therapy. In Greene, B. L. (Ed.) *The Psychotherapy of Marital Disharmony.* New York, The Free Press, 1965.

Slavson, S. R.: Coordinated family therapy. *Int J Group Psychother, 17:* 44, 1965.

Thomas, A.: Simultaneous psychotherapy with marital partners. *Am J Psychother, 10:* 716–727, 1956.

Watson, A. S.: The conjoint psychotherapy of married partners. *Am J Orthopsychiatry, 33:* 912–922, 1963.

EVALUATION FOR FAMILY THERAPY
JOSEPH R. NOVELLO, M.D.

Family therapy is not as much a specific treatment method as it is a philosophy. It assumes that the family is the central most crucial factor in the etiology of individual psychopathology. From this it follows that it is the family unit itself that becomes the focus of therapy. Consequently, family therapy has been defined as *any therapeutic intervention which has as its major focus the alteration of the family system.*

Although family therapists share in common the basic philosophical beliefs described above, they differ dramatically in their technical approaches. They differ in the extent to which they deal with such factors as conscious and unconscious, content and process, past and present. They also differ in the degree that they emphasize the intrapsychic, the interpersonal and the environmental.

Haley reinforces this notion when he states that "family therapy is not a method of treatment but a new orientation to the human dilemma. Given that orientation, any number of methods might be used." He goes on to explain that, as a matter of fact, "as family therapists become more experienced, they often tend to avoid a method approach and become problem-oriented."

Family therapists, therefore, tend to subscribe to the systems theory. They believe that change in one person in the family system will necessarily cause change in another and (conversely) "an individual cannot change unless his family system changes." (Haley)

The following outline is designed to aid the psychiatrist in evaluating a family unit for possible family therapy. It is a guide to the collection and organization of data, to indications and contraindications for family therapy, and to customary therapeutic goals for this approach.

I. Indications
    A. There has been little systematic research that an-

swers whether there are particular conditions that respond best to family therapy as compared to alternative approaches. The most fundamental indication for family therapy, therefore, grows out of the therapist's belief in the philosophical tenets of family therapy. The indications for family therapy, among practiced family therapists, tend to be broad since their philosophical outlook is broad-based.

B. Certain therapists have identified specific conditions for which they feel family therapy is especially indicated:

1. Problems of adolescents in separating from the family (Ackerman, Wynne).

2. Marital problems that are tied to larger family concerns, especially where children are being used as pawns or scapegoats in the marital conflict. (See Evaluation for Marital Therapy, this chapter.)

   a. includes preparation for divorce, remarriage, etc.

3. Treatment of schizophrenia (Lidz, Fleck)

4. Failure of other treatment methods

II. Contraindications

A. The most fundamental contraindication to family therapy is any condition that chronically interferes with either the physical presence of vital family members (lack of motivation, hospitalization, justifiable work commitments, etc.) or with psychological accessability (such as acute psychosis, etc.) (Wynne)

B. Other specific contraindications have been noted: (Ackerman)

1. The presence of a malignant, irreversible trend toward the breakup of the family, which may mean that it is too late to reverse the process of fragmentation. (Yet family therapy may be used in this case to control the fragmentation and make it less traumatic.)

2. The dominance within the group of a concentrated focus of malignant, destructive motivation.
3. One parent who is afflicted with an organized, progressive paranoid condition, or with incorrigible psychopathic destructiveness or who is a confirmed criminal or sexual deviate.
4. Parents, one or both, who are unable to be sufficiently honest; lying and deceitfulness that are deeply rooted in the group negate the potential usefulness of family therapy.
5. The existence of a certain kind of family secret.
6. The existence of an unyielding cultural, religious or economic prejudice against this form of intervention.

III. Goals
    A. Therapeutic goals in family therapy may differ as widely as those in any other type of psychotherapy. Yet there appear to be a relatively constant set of primary therapeutic goals that are generally sought by present-day family therapists. A survey of family therapists conducted by the Group for the Advancement of Psychiatry in 1970 revealed the following primary goals:
        1. Improved communication (90 percent)
        2. Improved autonomy and individuation (87 percent)
        3. Improved empathy (71 percent)
        4. More flexible leadership (66 percent)
        5. Improved role agreement (64 percent)
        6. Reduced conflict (60 percent)
        7. Individual symptomatic improvement (56 percent)
        8. Improved indvidual task performance (50 percent)

IV. Theoretical Frameworks in Family Therapy
    A. In addition to practical application of the general systems theory, the following theoretical frameworks

are utilized in family therapy, sometimes exclusively but more often in various combinations.

1. Psychoanalytic
2. Small group theory
3. Communication theory
4. Behavioral theory
5. Learning theory
6. Existential theory
7. Transactional analysis
8. Gestalt psychology

V. Techniques in Family Therapy
  A. Conjoint
    1. A single therapist or cotherapists see all members of the family in all sessions.
  B. Multiple impact therapy
    1. A team of therapists work with individual family members and with various subgroups of the family. The therapists meet regularly, and, in training centers, have a single common supervisor.
  C. Kin network therapy
    1. The nuclear family is expanded to include members of the extended family, and even friends and neighbors in some cases.
  D. Multiple family group therapy
    1. A group of several complete families are seen together.

VI. Family Evaluation
The first step in successful family treatment is an accurate collection of data in order to formulate reasonably accurate diagnostic impressions and make intelligent treatment plans. This is especially difficult since the family as a group has a long and multifaceted history (unlike the usual therapy group that does not exist as a group until it is brought together for therapeutic intention). The family is composed of separate individuals and subgroups each with their own dynamic(s). Each unit relates within the family and

within the community in a particular way that must be carefully evaluated. The following outline of a family evaluation is presented as a tool for collecting and organizing data. (Parts of the outline have been adapted from Ackerman, 1958.)

A. Presenting problem
   1. How initial referral or contact was made
   2. Which family member is identifying a *problem?*
      a. how do other family members view the *problem?*
B. The individual family members
   Each family member is evaluated separately as though for individual psychotherapy. This evaluation must, of course, be skillfully tailored according to the age of each family member. With younger children, for example, it will take the form of play. (An outline of special techniques in family evaluation is included later in this outline.) This information should lead to a concise metapsychological profile for each individual. Basic information should include:
   1. Name
   2. Age
   3. Sex
   4. Appearance
   5. Family role
   6. Significant past medical, psychiatric, social history
   7. Relationship to other family members
   8. Subgroup preferences within the family
   9. Attitude toward possible family therapy
   10. Early memories, recent and recurrent dreams
   11. Metapsychological assessment
       a. dynamic (including characteristic ego defenses employed)
       b. economic
       c. topographic
       d. genetic
       e. adaptive

C. Parents' natal families

In addition, each parent should be interviewed re: their *own* natal family.

1. Description of natal family
2. Place in sibship
3. Quality of relationship to other family members
4. Any family problems

D. Marital history

A developmental history of the marriage should be obtained. The amount of information required will vary considerably from case to case but should contain, as a minimum, the following data:

1. Brief history of courtship and marriage
2. Were each of the pregnancies planned? Attitudes and special problems surrounding pregnancies.
3. Shared values and goals
4. A brief assessment of Hollender's five criteria should be attempted. (See Evaluation for Marital Therapy, this chapter, for more detailed description.)
   a. dovetail of needs
   b. attitude toward problems
   c. expectations of each partner
   d. manner in which the marital relationship is used or exploited
   e. attitude toward marital and family stability

E. The Family

1. Chronological family history
   a. chronological family history i.e. births, deaths, geographical moves, major events, etc.
   b. social and financial status at various periods
   c. significant past *family crises*
      1. especially tragedies, family deaths, etc.
   d. situations surrounding births of children in immediate family
2. Internal organization
   a. emotional climate
   b. style of communication

      c. method of crisis and problem resolution
      d. division of labor
      e. lines of authority, how maintained
      f. family values, goals, means of attaining
      g. activities, pleasures
      h. subgroups
      i. stability
        1. continuity in time
        2. conflicts
        3. present status
    3. External organization
      a. socioeconomic status
      b. how the family and its members relate to the community
      c. conflict and/or complementarity in the requirements of intrafamilial and extrafamilial roles
F. Special techniques in family evaluation
    1. Home visit
      The home visit is an invaluable tool in family evaluation. The task is for the evaluator (s) to informally observe the family in action. The visit should, therefore, be arranged for a time when all family members are present. The family is told that the evaluator (s) wants to see them in as natural a setting as possible. There will be no formal questioning, etc.; the evaluator (s) simply watches the family unobtrusively and interacts only if invited. The most common criticism of this technique is that the family will not act natural under such circumstances. It can be answered that psychotherapists, as trained observers, should have little difficulty in extracting truths.
      a. focus of observations
        1. family interactional patterns
        2. family role adaptations
        3. emotional climate of the home

        4. cultural and psychosocial identity of the family

   b. organization of data

     The observations required above can be described within the following organizational schema:

        1. chronology of the visit, i.e. what happened, when, etc.

        2. interactions of the family as a group

        3. brief description of each individual

        4. description of the home, neighborhood

        5. miscellaneous

2. Other techniques

   a. As part of the evaluation of the individual family members the evaluator may choose to employ any of the standard psychological tests. (See Psychological Testing In Clinical Psychiatry, Chapter III.) Such tests are designed, of course, to reveal information in the individual dimension rather than the group or family dimension and, as such, have limited usefulness in evaluation of the family as a unit.

   b. Other tests have been designed by family therapists to elicit responses more appropriate to the assessment of *family* relationships. It is not possible to fully describe each of these tests here; the reader may refer to the references for original source material.

     1. Family Relations Indicator (Howells and Lickorish)

        a. thirty-three pictures showing basic family groups and interactions. The subject is asked to say what he thinks the people are saying or doing in the pictures.

     2. Test of Family Attitudes (Jackson)

        a. eight pictures; standard questions may be asked concerning each picture.
3. Two Houses Technique (Szyrynski)
        a. names of all family members are recorded. Two houses are drawn on a sheet of paper. The subject is asked to divide the family between the two houses and explain his decision.
4. Family Relations Test (Anthony and Bene)
        a. subject chooses statements printed on cards and sorts them out according to which family member he believes each statement most closely applies.
5. Fels Rating Scale (Baldwin, Kalhorn, Breese)
        a. thirty rating scales of family and individual variables
6. Revealed Differences (Strodtbeck)
        a. each family member independently answers a 15-item questionnaire on family life. The family then meets as a group to discuss their responses.
7. Draw-a-Family Test (Novello)
        a. each member of the family is asked to draw a picture of the family. Analysis is similar to draw-a-person test with added family dimension. Followup drawings at various points in treatment course may be useful in assessing change.
G. Diagnostic formulation and treatment plans
  1. Diagnosis
      a. how does the therapist conceptualize the case? How does he view the *problem?*
  2. Family liabilities
      a. what family factors are contributing to the problem?
  3. Family assets

      a. what are the family's assets that could allow them to grow and change, i.e. to *solve the problem?*

4. Motivation and availability for treatment

      a. identify the motivation of each family member for treatment.

         1. is there any interfamilial threat or duress such as wife threatening husband with divorce unless he enters treatment, parents threatening children, etc.?

      b. will the entire family be consistently available for a suitable length of time if family treatment is recommended?

         1. special considerations re: appointment times, transportation, etc.

      c. Any financial difficulties

5. Treatment goals

      a. given the diagnostic formulation, what are the therapist's treatment goals?

      b. how do these goals compare to the explicit and implicit goals of the family?

6. Treatment plan

      a. what stress will be placed on intrapersonal techniques? interactional? behavioral modification? environmental manipulation?

      b. what specific techniques will be used? in what sequence?

      c. list specific criteria for success.

      d. proposed length of treatment, duration of each session, number of sessions per week, fee.

      e. is the therapist sufficiently flexible to deviate from the initial treatment plan if the needs of the family change during the course of therapy?

References

1. Ackerman, N. W.: *The Psychodynamics of Family Life.* New York, Basic Books, 1958.

2. Anthony, E. J. and Bene, E.: A technique for the objective assessment of the child's family relationships. *J Ment Sci, 103:* 541–555, 1957.
3. Baldwin, A. L.; Kalhorn, J. and Breese, F. H.: The appraisal of parent behavior. *Psychol Monogr, 63:* 4, 1949.
4. Group for the Advancement of Psychiatry: *The Field of Family Therapy,* New York, 1970.
5. Haley, J.: An editor's farewell. *Family Process, 8:* 149–158, 1969.
6. Hollender, M. H.: Selection of therapy for marital problems. In Masserman, Jules H., M.D. (Ed.) *Current Psychiatric Therapies,* II. New York, Grune & Stratton, 1971.
7. Howells, J. G. and Lickorish, J. R.: *The Family Relations Indicator.* Edinburgh, Oliver & Boyd, Ltd., 1967.
8. Jackson, L.: *A Test of Family Attitudes.* London, Methven, 1952.
9. Lidz, T,; Fleck, S. and Cornelison, A. R.: *Schizophrenia and the Family.* New York, International Universities Press, Inc., 1965.
10. Novello, J. R.: (unpublished)
11. Strodtbeck, F. L.: Husband-wife interaction over revealed differences. *Am Sociol Rev, 16:* 468–473, 1951.
12. Szyrynski, V.: The 'two-houses' technique. *Can Psychiatr Assoc J,* April, 1963.
13. Wynne, L. C.: Some indications and contra-indications for exploratory family therapy. In Boszormenyi-Nagi, I. and Framo, J. L. (Ed.): *Intensive Family Therapy: Theoretical and Practical Aspects.* New York, Harper and Row, 1965.

EVALUATION OF PATIENTS FOR GROUP THERAPY

NAOMI E. LOHR, Ph.D.

The term *group therapy* is nearly as varied in its referent as is the term *miscellaneous.* Group therapy refers to everything from lectures with large audiences to psychoanalysis with an audience; from fifty members to four; from ego supportive to uncovering unconscious conflicts; from psychopathology suppression and neglect to invitations to act out; from a limited number of sessions to open-ended, years-long treatment; from leaderlessness to multiple leaders plus observers and recorders; from marathon sessions to infrequent get togethers; from exclusive focus upon action in the group process itself to exclusive focus upon early childhood; from homogeneous to heterogeneous patient populations, etc.

In the context of such diversity there cannot be one single *right* way to evaluate or select patients for group therapy.

The therapist must adjust his evaluation procedures to the type of *group therapy* that he intends to perform. The following outline is provided to aid the therapist in such evaluations.

I. Basic Considerations
    A. Selection of patients for group therapy
        1. General considerations
            a. Patients who might benefit from group therapy are not so basically different from other patients, i.e. most patients who come to an agency or a private practitioner for psychotherapeutic help can best be given a general evaluation in which possible treatment recommendations would always include: no treatment, supportive or uncovering treatment, crisis intervention or long-term treatment, and individual or group therapy. Taking into consideration available treatment opportunities, the patient's needs, motivations and socioeconomic circumstances, the evaluator would recommend what he felt most advantageous.
            b. Other factors set aside, the most efficacious treatment modality for analyzing intrapsychic conflict is generally individual, one-to-one, therapy. The *other factors* set aside, of course, include such things as availability of a competent therapist, motivation and ego resources of the patient, etc.
            c. Combined individual and group therapy is a viable option, and indeed, the treatment of choice for certain patients.
            d. Any group will lose some patients via their *dropping out*. These patients may have been poorly prepared, for group or for therapy more generally. It is useful for the group leader (s) to explore with a prospective patient (on a one-to-one basis before he actually

enters the group) his fantasies about therapy and about group therapy, his expectations, his fears, his past experiences with groups, etc. Sufficient time should be allowed for this exploration, to educate the new patient regarding group therapy, to allay anxiety and begin analyzing the patient's unconscious motives for and against entering group therapy. The extent of preparation will vary with the needs of the patient and the type of group.

2. Selection by diagnosis

   While the selection of a therapeutic modality for a particular patient cannot be made solely on the basis of his diagnostic label, certain generalizations are possible.

   a. Basically, *normal* people may benefit from a *sensitivity training group experience, consciousness raising,* or other special interest kinds of groups, i.e. a woman's group, Weight Watchers, etc.

   b. Patients who have neuroses, character problems, some borderline conditions and some who have symptoms significantly affecting their social interactions and relationships can often profit from either uncovering group therapy or uncovering combined therapy.

   c. Patients who have significant ego deficits, i.e. borderline or psychotic conditions, usually benefit most from supportive group therapy.

3. Selection by *special problems*

   A category of supportive or anxiety-allaying groups should be mentioned. Often relatively healthy people or patients who complain of a fairly circumscribed problem can be treated very usefully in a homogeneous special interest group (e.g. Weight Watchers, AA, primapara mothers, people who have had heart attacks, Parents without Partners, undergraduates about to practice teach, men with congenital sterility problems, drug addiction, recent psychiatric hospital admissions, black children being bussed to a predominantly white school, applicants for vasectomies, etc.). Such groups provide specific psychological benefits: dispelling the person's sense of being alone with his *problems,* exploring fantasies, supporting anxiety reduction, and others. In simple economic terms, this group approach can provide help to more people at less cost in time, money, trained personnel, etc.

4. Selection by role choice

Any group, therapeutic or otherwise, can be described in terms of interpersonal roles played by various members. The term *played* does not mean faked or put on, but rather, that when any collection of people gather, certain relationships emerge characteristic of the interactions of those people. Some will lead, some follow, some facilitate, some instigate, some obstruct, some question, some nurture, some compete, some exploit, some emote, some reflect, some aggress, some advise, some sacrifice, some punish, etc. The recognition of such roles in group process and information about the preferred roles a person assumes, permit the selection of people for a treatment group who combine to meet basic *group needs,* facilitating the group's capacity to jell and get to work. All groups need some balance in preferred roles (which do, of course, shift with changes within the patients or the additions of new members.) Helpful roles to have include an *instigator,* an *emoter,* a *reflecter* and a *nurturer.*

5. Random selection of members

There is so much controversy concerning selection of patients for group therapy, an argument could be made for no selection. This may not be the best method but can, at times, produce well functioning groups.

B. Size of the Group

Because dropouts are bound to occur, a useful size to keep the group is between eight to ten members. This keeps the group size from ever shrinking below six, which appears to be a crucial number, i.e. less than six people have a difficult time cohering into a therapy group, often remaining individuals taking turns working individually in front of an audience.

II. Basic Types of Psychotherapy Groups

A. Supportive Group Psychotherapy

1. Definition of supportive group psychotherapy

Supportive group therapy denotes a group, open-ended or time-limited, of six to ten patients who are sharing personal communications for the purpose of receiving support of reality testing, defenses against anxiety, cathexis of external reality, appropriate social behavior. Such a group may also have goals of learning new social skills or of providing socialization opportunity and gratification.

2. Indications for supportive group therapy

The indications for this sort of treatment group would be similar to the indications for supportive therapy on an individual basis: a patient with ego deficits who requires minimization of his defects and support of his ego strengths, who has neither the ego structure nor the motivation for participation in this basic type of ego reconstructive treatment. If a supportive group is available and such a patient is motivated for a group and if he would fit in with the other patients in the group, supportive group therapy is indicated.

B. Uncovering group psychotherapy

1. Definition of uncovering group psychotherapy

Refers to a heterogeneous, open-ended group of six to ten patients who are analyzing both their interactions with one another and their fantasies (dreams, etc.) to uncover unconscious conflicts, work through the conflicts and experience increased access to personality options. (The valid question of whether or not working through is possible in a group setting lies beyond the scope of these comments. The assumption is that working through unconscious contents is done most efficiently in individual therapy, but is possible in group therapy.) The patients in an uncovering group may or may not be simultaneously in individual therapy. The two together are generally called combined therapy. The individual therapist may be the same person or different from the group therapist. Groups may function with a heterogeneous mix of exclusively group patients, combined therapy patients, same therapist, individual therapist different from the group therapist, etc. All the combinations have both succeeded and failed with different patients at different times.

2. Indications for uncovering group psychotherapy
   a. Indications include: the patient who is oblivious to the aspects of himself that other people consider his symptom (e.g. chronic disdain and sarcasm); the patient who is especially naive about psychological issues, unaccustomed to introspection and intellectually bewildered by the process of psychotherapy; the patient who is paralyzed in a one-to-one situation by either the need to produce a session's worth of material or by the potential intimacy; the patient who is motivated to work on interpersonal symptoms but is unable to see the value of exploring intrapsychic concomitants; the patient who needs dilution of the emotional charge of an intimate relationship (e.g. a person

who fears losing control of murderous rage while alone with an individual therapist often feels safer in a group) ; the patient who needs reality feedback to maintain his capacity to discern real reactions from transferential projections; the patient who needs reality feedback because significant figures from his past were emotionally unresponsive to him; the patient who for any reason would benefit from splitting the transference relationship and slowing down, diluting or preventing the development of a transference neurosis.

b. Thus, patients suffering from characterological problems, some borderline conditions, or neuroses characterized by social inhibition and constriction or extreme naïveté make likely candidates for uncovering groups. In addition, regardless of the nature of the psychopathology, patients whose motivation centers on interpersonal conflict or who have progressed in therapy to a point where trying out new behaviors is possible and desirable might well either begin in a group or add group therapy somewhat later in their treatment. Combined therapy is often the treatment of choice for many borderline and/or schizoid personalities, especially to facilitate an anticipated change in therapists, to provide extra support while doing uncovering work, to dilute overly emotional relationships, to dilute dependency, to broaden the range of cathexes to external objects, etc.

c. A frequent erroneous referral is of a basically psychotic patient to group therapy rather than individual therapy. The more correct decision would be to refer the patient to supportive therapy, whether it be individual or group. Such a patient will decompensate every bit as quickly in an uncovering group as in uncovering individual treatment. Another frequent erroneous judgment is to refer a basically unmotivated patient to group therapy; such a patient is just as likely to drop out of group as individual treatment.

3. Contraindications for uncovering group therapy
   a. Patients with a mild developmental crisis, trauma reaction or uncomplicated neurosis; patients whose problems include no particular indication for group (or combined) therapy and for whom it is practical, should be referred to a competent individual therapist.
   b. Patients who are in some important way, out of step with the other group members; who unbalance the group roles, e.g. more aggressive women than the passive men in the group can work with; patients who make more withdrawn silence than the emoter and instigator can stir up; patients who make more nagging bosses than the masochists can hold their own against, etc.
   c. Patients who have a symptom better treated in a homogeneous group (homosexuality, addiction).
   d. Some contraindications have to do with group therapy in general, and some with a particular group.
   e. Further contraindications for uncovering group, at least at a particular point in time for a given patient, have more to do with the patient's symptoms and unconscious motives. For example, a patient with very strong inhibition of, or conflicts about, unconscious exhibitionistic impulses tends to become a group dropout. One girl indicated these conflicts by wearing her sunglasses a good half hour into the diagnostic interview. Others gave

little indication other than evident shyness, but later, in individual treatment confessed shamefacedly to voyeuristic or exhibitionistic behavior. Patients who are extremely masochistic or passive may too readily accept a referral to group therapy; soon, however, they may be faced with intolerable ambivalence or anxiety and will have to drop out. Patients with extreme social phobias may need a fairly long preparation before being able to work in a group. Generally, if the person's anxiety will be increased by group process to an unmanageable degree, group process is contraindicated.

f. In selecting a patient for group the therapist must also attend to the patient's own unconscious motives for desiring group therapy. He may be able to talk convincingly about conscious motives for group, yet undermine his own progress; to attempt to gratify his own need for support, help, attention, being done for; masochistic wishes for condemnation, etc.; or to display himself rather than understand himself. The nature of group interactions can facilitate a contagion of acting out; an emotional catharsis the patient can perceive as not being him, but rather in response to the needs of other members; and can allow, in a similar way, the patient to leave the instigation of affects and behaviors to other members of group, thus evading ownership and consequent guilt. For some patients entering group therapy means unconsciously supporting denials and maintaining, *I don't really need treatment,* (i.e. individual) so the therapeutic work accomplished has a subtle *as if I were in therapy* quality.

g. Contraindications for combined uncovering

therapy include inability of the individual therapist and group therapists to communicate frankly, helpfully, and noncompetitively; the patient who has a motivation toward one therapy setting as resistance against the other; a past history of inconsistent parental figures that suggest the patient only becomes frightened and confused by the splitting of transference reaction, i.e. that the transference projections become fragmented more than split.

III. The Process of Evaluation for Group Psychotherapy

In addition to a routine diagnostic evaluation of presenting complaints, precipitating events, personality structure, symptoms, dynamics, attitudes, moods, ego strengths, motivation for treatment, history, life circumstances, etc., the therapist should collect other data specifically relevant to the patient's suitability for group therapy.

A. Assessment of the patient's motivation for group therapy

Explore with the patient his expectations and fantasies regarding group treatment. If he expresses no reservations at all, suspect he indeed has some that he is unaware of at the time. In such cases, it is wise to extend the evaluation.

1. Manifest motives: Patients usually articulate motives in terms of needing to learn to get along with people better. They may, however, speak of wanting to know about how others solve their problems.

2. Latent motives: Latent motives often include evasion of *real* therapy; unconscious wishes for gratification of exhibitionistic, voyeuristic, dependency or power needs; the avoidance of intimacy or reestablishment of a family. Obviously the variety of such latent motives is infinite.

B. Assessment of the character of the patient's past and present interpersonal relationships, especially in regard to capacity for intimacy and quality of social interaction style
1. Preschool socializing (with playmates, nursery school, availability of parents, quality of play).
2. Relationships with siblings.
3. Relationships with parents and other significant adults.
4. School-age socializing (chums, friendships groups, best friends, ages of playmates, roles taken with others).
5. Dating history (age, variety, steadies, quality of interaction, ease of intimacy, marriage, divorce circumstances).
6. Nature and variety of current friendships (nature of relationships with parents, employers, teachers, nature of relationships with people at work, servants, service and store personnel).
C. Assessment of how the patient believes other people see him
1. It is often useful to ask how the patient imagines other people characterize him in various settings.
D. Assessment of past group participation
1. Has the patient previously participated in group therapy?
2. Similar information should be gathered about family, classroom, play, activity groups.
E. Exploration of the patient's questions, expectations and fantasies re: group therapy
F. Describing group therapy to the prospective patient
1. If an appropriate group therapy placement is available, recommendation for group therapy is then made to the patient. This usually includes describing group therapy, giving a thumbnail sketch of the group in mind (e.g. there are seven current members; four men and three women;

half are married; ages range between 20 and 30; kinds of problems vary, but what you describe is a problem also to several members. . . .) , and clarifying the advantages and disadvantages of group treatment for that particular patient. The evaluator would also clarify with the patient the nature of the therapeutic task and point out that in a group he would have the responsibility of trying to help others, as well as the responsibility of helping himself.

G. Common concerns patients express about group psychotherapy

1. Patients wonder if other patients can be trusted to keep material confidential. The evaluator may simply reassure the patient directly, regarding the mores of the particular group in question, or may investigate with him the source of the concern.

2. Another question is, How can *sick* people help others? Uusually this is best answered once the patient is participating in group. *Sick* people may draw upon their own experience to understand, share problem-solving attempts, and, most of all, have *healthy* grasp of areas outside their own blindspots. The group therapist is there to ensure patients can be objective and helpful with each other.

3. Other concerns include trusting strangers, being attacked by other patients, not having enough time if the others talk too. The patient needs to be told that he can be actively involved in his own treatment while listening or understanding similar problems in others or his reactions to others.

4. Other frequent questions concern whether or not personal matters can be discussed in group therapy (they can) ; what to do about shame,

guilt, embarrassment (discuss it with the group and understand it) ; what about frightening irrational thoughts; (others have come to terms with similar things) ; what if you meet a group member in a social situation? (Group customs differ on this.)

Suggestive Reading

Bach, G.: *Intensive Group Therapy.* New York, Ronald Press, 1954.

Slavson, S. R.: *A Textbook in Analytic Group Psychotherapy.* New York, International Universities Press, 1964.

Yalom, I. D.: *The Theory and Practice of Group Psychotherapy.* New York, Basic Books, 1970.

Chapter VI

HOSPITAL
PSYCHIATRY

ALTHOUGH THERE EXISTS a rich and voluminous literature devoted to all aspects of hospital psychiatry, there are some gaps in that literature that this chapter on hospital psychiatry is designed to fill. While not a text on the practice of treating psychiatric inpatients, this chapter aims to provide the psychiatrist with some practical, clinically-oriented guidelines that are not elsewhere available in this form.

The first article, Criteria for Admission to a Psychiatric Hospital, starts right at the beginning. When should a person be admitted as an inpatient on a psychiatric unit? Indications and contraindications are listed.

Treatment Planning for Psychiatric Inpatients reviews all phases of inpatient treatment and provides the psychiatrist with a handy checklist for quick reference when he must write orders and formulate his overall therapeutic approach.

The third article, Planning for Discharge from a Psychiatric Hospital, addresses a topic that has been largely ignored in the past. It focuses upon criteria for discharge. A checklist of items to consider before discharge and factors to consider in planning for after care is provided.

The last article, The Problem-Oriented Record-Keeping System in Hospital Psychiatry, details a new method of clinical record-keeping that is adapted from the problem-oriented systems being used in general medicine. It can be a particularly valuable adjunct in the practice of hospital psychiatry.

The reader is instructed in its use in an easy step-by-step manner.

CRITERIA FOR ADMISSION TO A PSYCHIATRIC HOSPITAL

GAIL BARTON, M.D., M.P.H.

The decision to admit a patient to a hospital psychiatric unit must not be taken lightly. There are several important factors to consider. The following outline is designed to aid the psychiatrist in reaching this decision.

I. Criteria for Admission of Patient to Hospital Psychiatric Unit
   A. For admission
      1. Patient is a danger to himself or others
         a. usually hospitalization is the treatment of choice
         b. occasionally there is sufficient community support, i.e. relatives, a therapist who can see him through crisis as an outpatient, etc.
      2. Patient is a nuisance to the community
         a. usually has to do with bizarre, inappropriate behavior
         b. may include antisocial behavior which deserves evaluation
      3. Alcohol or drug habituation
         a. patient motivated for withdrawal
         b. patient motivated for psychotherapy
      4. Confusion or memory disturbance
      5. Request from another unit of hospital
         a. patient unmanageable there, even with psychiatric consultation to medical-surgical staff. (See Psychiatric Consultation to Medical-Surgical Units, Chapter VII.)
         b. patient would be potentially helped by treatment on new ward
      6. Political pressure

  a. not valid reason without evidence of mental illness

  b. facility should be potentially helpful, not custodial

7. Private therapist feels that he cannot manage patient through a crisis as an outpatient

8. Court requests an inpatient evaluation

9. Patient desires treatment and requests time away from present living environment

10. Transportation to an outpatient facility extremely difficult or impossible for patient

11. No other facility more appropriate has beds available (i.e. V.A., state hospital, nursing home, etc.)

12. Diagnostic problem that requires hospitalization for more intensive evaluation

13. Research interest (with full consent of patient)

B. Against admission

1. Patient needs to work through transference problems with current therapist

2. Patient would be evading responsibilities; such is the case with many chronic alcoholics or sociopaths

3. Patient already being followed by another agency and when they are notified about contact, they wish to see patient themselves rather than have him admitted

4. Patient or relatives requesting admission but evidence by evaluation of patient and situation does not warrant inpatient care

5. Patient would lose more than he would gain from admission such as being forced to lose his job, place in school, etc.

6. Patient not motivated for therapy

7. Patient really only needs lodging, not psychiatric treatment

8. Patient better suited to another type of facility

such as nursing home, medical ward, school for retarded, etc.

The psychiatrist must not only be mindful of the general type of patient that best meets criteria for hospitalization but he must also know the strengths and weaknesses of his own unit. This factor can be decisive in deciding whether or not to admit a patient.

 II. A list of factors that the usual inpatient service can be expected to provide

  A. Distancing from environmental stress

  B. 24-hour crisis intervention short-term treatment (few weeks) or long term residential treatment (many months or longer)

  C. Specialized therapy (O.T., R.T., group, milieu, supportive, etc.)

  D. Distance from objects of paranoia

  E. Identification models

  F. Opportunity to learn and practice new modes of venting feelings with opportunity for immediate feedback

  G. Place to monitor drugs as to safety, efficacy especially with drugs such as Lithium Carbonate® or Prolixin® (Fluphenazine Hydrochloride)

  H. Place to combine physical diagnosis and treatment with emotional illness diagnosis and treatment

  I. Relief of burden on relatives

  J. The unit's ability to handle the violent, aggressive patient should be established as a matter of policy. If there are not such facilities, the patient should be transferred elsewhere.

 III. Additional factors that may weigh against admission:

  A. Increases burden on family

   1. Time, i.e. visits to hospital

   2. Stress, i.e. burden on all family members with hospitalization of one

   3. Financial burden

    a. Especially if no insurance or other financial aid available

      b. If have to hire homemaker, child care, transportation, etc.

      c. If relatives will need time off from work to visit hospital

      d. If a spouse or other relative must quit work to care for the patient's family (children)

    4. Social: stigma, decreased time for other activities

  B. Increases difficulties for patient

    1. May increase the strain upon patient-family relationships

      a. i.e. he is separated physically from them

      b. i.e. his hospitalization changes the roles of each family member

    2. Strain upon patient-employer relationships or patient-employee relationships

    3. Stigma of mental illness to carry in the community greater after being an inpatient

    4. Patient may have more time on his hands at hospital than usual, so he has increased time to brood

References

Hartlage, L. C.; Freeman, W. and Horine, L.: Expediting admissions procedures. *Ment Hyg, 53:* 71–77, January, 1969.

Rock, Ronald: *Hospitalization and Discharge of the Mentally Ill.* Chicago, University of Chicago Press, 1968.

Smith, Kathleen; Pumphrey, M. W. and Hall, J. C.: The "last straw": The decisive incident resulting in the request for hospitalization in 100 schizophrenic patients. *Am J Psychiatry, 120:* 228–233, September, 1963.

Spitzer, S. and Denzin, M.: *The Mental Patient: Studies in the Sociology of Deviance.* New York, McGraw Hill, 1968.

TREATMENT PLANNING FOR PSYCHIATRIC INPATIENTS

GAIL BARTON, M.D., M.P.H.

Once the decision to admit a patient to the psychiatric unit has been made, the psychiatrist must give careful attention to constructing an effective treatment plan. It is complex task with a great many factors to be considered.

I. Items to Consider in a Treatment Plan
  A. Which ward milieu is most suitable: Not all patients can be expected to fit into the same kind of ward milieu. If feasible, it is important to choose the most appropriate milieu, according to the needs of the patient.
    1. *Therapeutic community* setting is usually geared for a patient who can be up and about, is capable of verbalizing, has sufficient strength to withstand a certain amount of responsibility and who has a capacity to care about others. There are usually more real-life kinds of activities during the day and evening in which the patient is expected to participate. The therapeutic emphasis is on group dynamics and may feature some form of *patient government*.
    2. *Hierarchical milieu*. This is more of a medical model than the former milieu. The lines of authority are clearly drawn, with the patient at the bottom of the hierarchy. This kind of milieu is especially suited for patients who are in intensive psychotherapy. The highlight of the patient's week is his psychotherapy; the rest of the time is filled with busy activities or times for thought, which act as lulls between the important therapy sessions.
    3. *Custodial milieu*. This is a much more low key environment where the basics of room, board, medications, and perhaps bodily nursing care is given. It may approximate a routine medical ward or a nursing home environment.
  B. Diet
    1. In most cases the routine house diet is in order, but if the patient has medical problems such as diabetes, hypertension, etc., a special diet should be prescribed.
  C. Medications
    1. Type of medication

a. Consider first the best drug for the target symptoms. (See Psychopharmacology, Chapter IX.)

2. Number of medications
   a. Keeping the number of different medications to a minimum keeps it simple for the nursing staff and the patient, as well as decreasing the likelihood of synergism or incompatibility effects.

3. Route
   a. Fast action requires I.V. or I.M. route and is especially wise with an obstreperous patient.
   b. Liquid medication may be better orally than pill form if the patient is suicidal. These latter patients seem to almost play a grizzly game of seeing how many pills they can tongue and then collect for taking all at once at some later time.

4. PRN Medication
   a. Sometimes time saving for both nurse and doctor, but it is a practice that is to be discouraged routinely. It creates ambiguity from a doctor-nurse standpoint since it essentially leaves up to the nurse when a medication should be given should the situation change, but requires no awareness on the doctor's part on what is new in the patient's behavior.
   b. It is better to leave open communication possibilities between the doctor and the nurse as to new developments in behavior with joint decision-making resulting. Re: the prescribing of medication.
   c. PRN medication also makes the patient-nurse-doctor relationship strained since the patient is thrust into the role of deciding when he needs medication. Then he must convince the nurse. If she refuses to give the medication, the patient may angrily report the in-

cident to the doctor in an attempt to malign the nurse, and the potential set-up for division within the treatment team exists.

    d. Even the seemingly more innocuous medications, such as aspirin and milk of magnesia should be prescribed only when they are truly needed so that a change in the patient's physical health can be a part of the therapist's awareness.

  5. Sedation

    a. There are occasions, such as the first few nights that a patient is hospitalized, that night sedation might be indicated.

    b. The abuse of this group of drugs is so well-known, however, so that the therapist should be extremely loathe to perpetuate poor medical practice by prescribing it regularly.

    c. It would also be important to use the less addicting, less abused medications. This not only diminishes the likelihood of dependence but also guards against a serious suicide attempt should the patient deceitfully save the pills for himself or another suicidal patient.

    d. Benadryl®, Valium®, chloral hydrate, and more recently, Dalmane® appear to be less dangerous than other sedatives.

    e. Often the staff's simply giving the patient more attention at bedtime can be more successful than using a sedative.

 D. Phone restrictions

  1. Most of the time, to encourage self-reliance, no phone restrictions are necessary. If there is a particularly paranoid patient who as part of his delusional system wants to call the President, the FBI, etc., it is best to withhold his privileges for a time until he is better able to control himself and will not be bothering the community.

  2. If a patient is particularly despondent, it is often

best to temporarily suspend phoning since these calls tend to be prolonged, tear-gathering and stressful. As the patient improves, they might be only time-limited, person-limited or monitored by a staff nearby to act as a brake if the patient loses control.

E. Visiting restrictions
   1. Ordinarily, visiting is to be encouraged since it keeps the patient linked more realistically to his family and the community.
   2. Visitors might well be restricted in the case of patients being withdrawn from drugs or alcohol, since those ordinarily acquainted with the patient are often involved in the habituation either overtly or covertly.
   3. Visitors might also be restricted if it seems that they are coming to see the hospital or the patient out of curiosity and have no real meaning in the life of the patient.

F. Selection of roommate
   1. The patient who is suicidal would do better to have a roommate than to be assigned a single room. The roommate acts not only as a diversion from morbid thoughts, but can also act as an interested, concerned, watchful person. It is far better to have someone like a roommate acting as a deterrent to self-harmful actions than an impersonal sitter who is hired to watch a suicidal patient.
   2. Often a patient in homosexual panic would be better without a roommate until his discomfort is lessened by getting accustomed to the hospital routine, the other patients and the personnel.
   3. It is preferable to allow the patients already in the hospital to be instrumental in inviting the new patients to be their roommates, if possible, rather than have arbitrary incompatible assignments made by the staff. It is courteous for the

staff to notify an *old* patient ahead of time that he is getting a new roommate if he is unable to be involved in the decision.

G. Belonging search

1. If the person is a potential danger to himself or others or is to be treated for an addiction, the patient's belongings should be searched upon admission. It is best to inform the patient at the outset that this will be done and that he may assist in the search and should be present while it is done. An explanation as to the need for search is a courteous and honest approach on the part of the staff.

H. Therapy

1. Crisis Intervention: Emphasis placed on defining as clearly as possible what the circumstances were that created the crisis at this point in time for the patient. Efforts are made to solve the crisis from a practical standpoint as well as an intrapsychic standpoint. Attempts at achieving better anticipatory problem-solving and overall crisis-coping is the goal. Attempts are not directed at uncovering or at major personality reconstruction.

2. Supportive: Day to day activities and socializing skills are emphasized. Delusional and other symptoms of pathology are discouraged, healthy topics are encouraged.

3. Intensive Psychotherapy: Varying degrees of personality reconstruction are attempted in order to make the patient more aware of the predisposing ideas, causes and interrelationships. Directiveness depends on the degree of depth in therapy and the length of time available for therapy. (See Evaluation for Intensive Psychotherapy, Chapter V.)

4. Group Therapy: Use of uncovering and/or supportive techniques as well as peer pressure to

assist a person in changing some of his personality characteristics. The patient's strengths are drawn upon by the group through his efforts to help the others. (See Evaluation of Patients for Group Therapy, Chapter V.)

5. Behavior Therapy: Use of conditioning and deconditioning techniques upon particular symptomology which has been clearly defined in the evaluation phase of treatment.

I. Assistance with aspects of daily living
   1. Some patients will need help with such basic concerns as keeping clean, eating, dressing or social situations.
   2. If this is so, it is helpful to direct the staff's attention to this from the outset and perhaps work out the details as part of a team effort.

J. Potentially suicidal patient
   1. If a patient is likely to be harmful to himself, either because of depressive thought or delusional ideas, then he should be under constant surveillance by another person who is willing to take on that responsibility (a staff member, a relative or another patient).
   2. It is best if this helping person knows the patient and has an accepting, helping relationship with him; not an antagonizing or estranged one.
   3. This watchfulness should include accompanying the patient to shower and bath until the acute phase has passed.
   4. Sudden mood change to optimism or peace of mind on the part of the patient should be viewed with alarm, since it is often an indication that the patient has accepted the inevitability of his suicide and has decided on a plan.
   5. Staff members should be alerted to the underlying dynamics of the depression and the cues the patient may have previously given in order to signal for help, so that they can be aware of

even the most subtle communications from these patients, and can respond appropriately.

6. (See also comments under Medication, Phone Restrictions, Visiting Restrictions, Selection of a Roommate and Belonging Search.)

K. Potentially violent or homocidal patients

1. If there is the potential for violence in the patient, it is best to plan ahead so that the staff and the other patients are protected.

2. Words or situations that might trigger violence in the patient should be ascertained from the outset so that action can be taken to protect others immediately and so that efforts can be made to divert or short circuit an outburst.

3. Often simply having a large number of people immediately available is quite calming to a patient. He will often feel that even if he gets out of control, there are enough people around him to help him maintain or regain control.

4. The use of adequate doses of tranquilizing medication not only at the outset of hospitalization, but also routinely, will usually prevent outbursts of violence entirely. If an outburst should occur early in hospitalization, swift and heavy medication will often give the patient a secure feeling that adequate help is available.

5. The use of heavy sedation, restraints, and seclusion-type rooms are a last resort and only a stop-gap in most instances. The more creative, cohesive staff will rarely, if ever, need to use these techniques.

6. One other preventive measure which is useful is a staff trained in self-defense. The attitude of assuredness and absence of fear of the patient may have a calming effect on the potentially violent patient.

L. Potential nuisance to other patients

1. It is important to ascertain if the new patient

has disturbing medical problems (noctural epileptic attacks), compulsions (taking 20 baths a day), steals, wanders (confusion) or has sexual difficulties (rapist, exhibitionist). Planning here is also helpful, informing the staff and other patients about the nature of the problem and individualizing a method of dealing with the problem leads to therapeutic benefits.

M. Negative feelings toward hospitalization
   1. Supportive techniques can be supplied by staff if alerted to these feelings by the admitting physician. Often the other patients themselves can be quite supportive in stilling not only the overt negative feelings, but also in reducing the covert fearful and anxious feelings in the newly admitted patient.

N. Escape
   1. Once the staff and patients are told that a patient is an escape potential, they can be alert to any cues or overt attempts. Most of the time, firm direction and statement of expectations on the part of the staff will interrupt a patient's flight.
   2. Supportive patients may also firmly discourage the action. Medication promptly and supportively administered is also helpful.
   3. A locked section of the ward, or an entire locked ward, may be necessary.
   4. The best preventive is a firm verbal contract prior to admission that specifies the responsibilities and expectations of both the hospital and the patient.

O. Activity program
   1. There are often many alternatives and modalities in selecting an activity program for the patient. This is usually worked out as part of the individual treatment prescription with the prerequisite that it will be updated depending on the progress of the patient.

2. Portions of the activity program to be considered include:
   a. Ward activities: Such things as ward meetings, meals in the dining room, card games, watching TV, ward clean-up, discussions with patients and/or staff.
   b. Outside activities: Such things as shopping trips, walks, movie or play going, picnics with other patients and staff.
   c. Occupational therapy: Such things as activities of daily living, socializing while involved in a task-oriented group, learning leisure skills such as ceramics or woodworking.
   d. Recreational therapy: Such things as active participation in a sport to learn coordination, cooperation or leisure time skill. Could include being spectator at sporting event to enhance interest in leisure activity or in personal improvement of existing skills.
   e. Community activities: Actually becoming a member of a community sponsored group activity to prepare for socializing and participation in the community.
   f. Passes: Actually attending activities outside the hospital on own. Passes should be judiciously used for therapeutic purposes.
P. Social work with relatives
   1. The treatment plan should include some efforts to assist the important people in the patient's life in a number of different areas, depending on the needs of the individual case:
      a. Advice for financial assistance if required, i.e. referral to agencies, etc.
      b. Family or marital counseling.
      c. Therapy geared toward helping the family accept the patient better upon his discharge.
      d. Advice re: legal assistance if required.
      e. Guidance concerning patient's future living arrangements after discharge.

        f. Assistance in finding another treatment disposition following discharge (state hospital, nursing home, private psychiatrist).

Q. Work or occupational intervention

    1. Quite often an entering patient leaves a job behind which rightfully should receive some attention, not only to keep the job secure but to provide thoughtful community relations.

    2. Efforts might include:

        a. Contact with the employer about holding the job open.

        b. Arrange an extended sick leave.

        c. Arrange for the patient to work part-time or even stay on full-time while hospitalized.

        d. Counseling about more appropriate job.

        e. Job training.

R. School intervention

    1. A patient's hospitalization may come at a time when the person is still attending school. Attention might be given to help the student in several different ways:

        a. Arrange to allow the student to continue full-time or half-time.

        b. Arrange to have the patient take a leave of absence.

        c. Arrange with dormitory or landlord to either hold the room or rent to another.

        d. Arrange to have classmates visit.

        e. Arrange tutoring if attending classes would be counter-therapeutic.

        f. Counsel (if appropriate) a change of major, school or living situation.

S. Medical problems

    1. Appropriate treatment of existing medical problems must be arranged immediately and proper follow-up provided.

T. Predictions about the patient's hospitalization

    1. These should be an integral part of the initial treatment plan since they assist those concerned

with the patient's treatment in goal-setting and pacing the program.

2. Things to predict include:
   a. Length of time of inpatient care
   b. Clinical course
   c. Criteria for discharge
   d. Type of after-care (See the Problem-Oriented Record-Keeping System in Hospital Psychiatry, this chapter.)

U. The patient's expectations
   1. It is important to ascertain what goals the patient himself has concerning the hospitalization. The therapist can then negotiate a meaningful treatment contract and therapy receives an immediate impetus.

V. Staff participation in treatment planning
   1. Inviting the staff to join in the planning of the patient's treatment not only results in a more comprehensive plan, but also gives the staff the feeling of participating in the therapy. They are more likely to work with enthusiasm and creativity in caring for the patient if they have helped plan his care than if they have been passive recipients of orders to be followed.

References

Freeman, H. L.: *Psychiatric Hospital Care: A symposium.* London, Bailliere, Tindall and Cassell, 1965.

Margolis, P. M.; Meyer, G. G. and Louw, J. C.: Suicidal precautions: A dilemma in the therapeutic community. *Arch Gen Psychiatry, 13:* 224–231, September, 1965.

Samorajczyk, J. F.: Crisis intervention in the mental hospital. *Ment Hyg, 53:* 477–9, July, 1969.

PLANNING FOR DISCHARGE FROM A PSYCHIATRIC HOSPITAL

GAIL BARTON, M.D., M.P.H.

While it is imperative for the psychiatrist to carefully establish criteria for admission to the hospital and then to thoughtfully construct a treatment program that is tailored to the needs of the individual patient, it is also important to establish, in advance, the criteria that will be used to determine when the patient has achieved maximum benefits from his hospitalization and is ready for discharge.

Such criteria will be the standards against which the progress of the patient is measured. Without such standards the psychiatrist cannot intelligently evaluate the efficacy of his treatment.

The problem-oriented record allows the psychiatrist to maximally individualize treatment goals and discharge criteria. (See The Problem-Oriented Record-Keeping System in Hospital Psychiatry in this chapter.) Where such a record-keeping system is not employed, the psychiatrist should, nevertheless, carefully formulate treatment goals and discharge criteria at an early stage of the patient's hospitalization.

It is best if the decision for discharge is a consensus decision involving doctor, patient, staff, family and other interested parties (such as courts, etc.). All should agree that the patient:

1. has received maximum or satisfactory benefits of treatment.
2. is not a danger to himself or others.
3. is in control of his emotions and actions.
4. will not be a nuisance to the family or the community.
5. has sufficient family and/or community support or (in the absence of these factors) is able to care for himself.

In addition to determining the patient's suitability for discharge from the hospital, the psychiatrist faces one more crucial task: arranging for follow-up care in the posthospitalization period.

Close attention to *after care* is an important part of the psychiatrist's responsibilities to the patient. In fact, the ultimate success or failure of treatment can hinge on this factor. Intelligent consideration of *after care* should be an integral part of the psychiatrist's overall treatment plan and must be completed prior to the patient's discharge from the hospital.

The following check list is provided to aid the psychiatrist in planning for effective *after care*:

1. Is the patient being referred back to his own physician or to an agency which provides his psychiatric care?
   a. It is important to send a summary to this source.
   b. To provide continuity of care this summary should include a brief synopsis of the patient's hospital course, present medications and any other important information.
2. If there is no referral source: Is there a clinic affiliated with the hospital that would be appropriate to follow the patient?
   a. Often the hospital clinics are useful in maintaining continuity of care for the patient.
3. Is there a therapy group that would be suitable for the patient?
   a. This is particularly useful for character disorders, drug abusers, etc.
4. For heroin addicts consider:
   a. Methadone Maintenance Clinic.
   b. Synanon, a national organization of exaddicts who provide group support for withdrawal and changing lifestyles.
5. For alcoholic patients consider:
   a. Alcoholics Anonymous. AA has the advantage of availability 24 hours/day, relatives groups and the understanding support of former alcoholics.
6. Recovery, Incorporated; if the patient is likely to need long term support.
   a. This is a group which is sponsored by expsychiatric patients who hold group discussions and readings geared toward helping people adjust to their chronic illness or past history of illness.
7. Public health nurse
   a. In the community, the public health nurse, is able to observe whether the patient is able to care for himself and is taking his medications as prescribed.
8. A homemaker service

a. This Red Feather Agency service will often help the returning patient who needs assistance in organizing everyday tasks, especially helpful for women who require assistance in meeting household responsibilities.

b. The homemaker services may be contacted prior to the patient's discharge from the hospital and assume a role in the household prior to the patient's returning home.

9. Community agency
   a. Agencies such as Catholic Social Services or Family Service are useful resources especially in coordination of family involvement in the posthospitalization period.
   b. It helps to arrange this service before discharge so that there is continuity of care.

10. Day care or night hospitalization
    a. These offer a more gradual transition back to the home environment.

11. Half-way house or boarding home
    a. If the patient will need some degree of supervision for his care within the community these are very useful.

12. Community activities
    a. useful to insure sufficient social outlets
    b. YMCA, YWCA
    c. adult education programs
    d. senior citizen groups
    e. special interest clubs
    f. church activities

13. Will the patient require transportation to activities or therapy?
    a. Quite often there are community groups which provide this to those who need it.

14. Is the patient's job secure?
    a. Contact with the patient's employer is often desirable both to secure his job and to arrange for adjustments in the work environment if necessary.

15. Vocational rehabilitation
    a. Assist the patient in counseling job interviewing and placement.
    b. Often have access to more sheltered work situations if the patient should require it.
    c. Can often arrange a sheltered workshop type of job for the more severely incapacitated.
16. Financial assistance
    a. This could provide him with a feeling of security and independence he needs rather than a feeling of oppression caused by financial burdens.
    b. The patient may be eligible for such assistance as Food Stamp Program, Social Security Benefits, Medicaid, Medicare, Aid to the Handicapped, etc.
17. Counseling, medication or other assistance for family planning
    a. Planned Parenthood or referral to a hospital gynecology clinic are possibilities.
18. Discuss the *after care* plans with a family member or concerned individual?
    a. They can often offer support so that the patient can more easily follow through on treatment recommendations.
    b. They can assist patient getting to therapy, taking his medications, remembering what to do if a psychiatric emergency occurs.
19. Routine follow-up contact by therapist
    a. This is often a key to help the patient follow through on recommendations.
    b. Reassures patient to know that someone will be calling to find out how he is doing, will be supporting him in taking him medications if prescribed and offers the therapist an opportunity to gauge the effectiveness of his treatment.
20. Ward staff should be briefed re: what to do if the patient contacts them directly after he is discharged from the hospital
    a. The patient will often see the ward staff as a re-

source in time of crisis, and they can be helpful in steering him toward appropriate helping agencies if this possibility is anticipated.

References

Drieman, J. M. and Minard, C. C.: Preleave planning: Effect upon rehospitalization. *Arch Gen Psychiatry, 24:* 87–90, January, 1971.

Freeman, H. E. and Simmons, O. G.: Consensus and coalition in the release of mental patients—A research note. *Human Organization, 20:* 89–90, Summer, 1961.

Freeman, H. E. and Simmons, O. G.: *The Mental Patient Comes Home.* New York, John Wiley and Sons, Inc., 1963.

Gunn, R. L.; Pearman, H. E.; Groth, C.; et al.: Fractors influencing release decisions. *Hospital and Community Psychiatry, 21:* 290–3, September, 1970.

Lorei, T. W.: A systematic approach to disposition decisions. *Am J Psychiatry, 128:* 281–285, September, 1971.

Mendel, W. and Green, G.: *The Therapeutic Management of Psychological Illness.* New York, Basic Books, Inc., 1967.

Purvis, S. A. and Miskimins, R. W.: Effects of community follow-up on posthospital adjustment of psychiatric patients. *Community Ment Health J, 6:* 374–382, October, 1970.

Safirastein, S. L.: Psychiatric aftercare services: Their place in the continuum of patient care. *J Mount Sinai Hospital, 32:* 578–587, 1965.

Weinstein, L.: Real and ideal discharge criteria. *Mental Hospitals, 15:* 680–683, December, 1964.

THE PROBLEM-ORIENTED RECORD-KEEPING SYSTEM IN HOSPITAL PSYCHIATRY

Joseph R. Novello, M.D.

Accurate record-keeping, important in all aspects of psychiatric practice, is especially critical in hospital psychiatry. Here the psychiatrist may be faced with responsibilities not only for psychiatric management of the patient but also for his medical and social problems. In addition, the psychiatrist may have to direct a ward milieu, consisting of nurses, social workers, psychologists, occupational therapists, recreational therapists and others.

Precise record-keeping is necessary to help make this complex system workable. In addition, good record-keeping can lead to improved patient care and to enriched professional learning.

The problem-oriented approach is especially useful in such a clinical situation. This system of record-keeping is gaining much popularity in general medicine but psychiatry, thus far, has been slow to adopt it. (Weed, 1969)

The psychiatric problem-oriented record system that is described below has been successfully used on a 28-patient adult unit. This system has been found to: meet major criteria for excellence in medical record-keeping (Grant, 1970) ; be adaptable for use in any type of psychiatric treatment setting; allow for more precise determination of treatment goals and patient response; offer more precise guidance to ward staff, while at the same time increasing their learning and their participation in the therapeutic task; be more adaptable for research use than other systems; provide the clinician with a practical and workable instrument that can enhance both his patient's care and his own continued profession growth.

The New System

This new system of psychiatric record-keeping is composed of eight elements: (1) Intake History (2) Planning Conference (3) Problem List (4) Progress Notes (5) Progress Chart (6) Flow Sheet (7) Progress Conference (8) Discharge Conference.

Each of the eight elements of the system will be described around the following case:

A 28-year-old male is admitted to the adult psychiatric unit in an acutely psychotic condition. He has had three previous hospitalizations elsewhere and has been diagnosed as chronic schizophrenia, paranoid type. It is learned that he discontinued medication six weeks prior to admission and that his father passed away one week ago. The patient had recently obtained a job as a stock-boy but the job may be in jeopardy because his employer does not know he is in the hospital. The patient's medical history is unremarkable except for a history of mild (asymptomatic) rheumatic heart disease and a Grade I murmur on physical exam.

1. Intake History

    The initial intake history follows the form of the conventional psychiatric history with the exception that the interviewer is specifically charged to elicit, from the beginning, a sense of the patient's current *problems*, (psychiatric, social, medical and otherwise) ; how they got to be problems; what, if anything, has been done about them; what the patient would like to do about them; and what the therapist and staff can offer toward solving them. Each problem is named according to the level of understanding available at the time of admission. In this case, the primary diagnosis (schizophrenia, chronic, paranoid type) is fairly certain on admission because of the patient's past history but in another case a patient's loss of reality testing and loose associations might be called simply psychosis until further data allowed for a more refined diagnosis, just as fever as an initial medical problem might yield to a diagnosis of pneumonia after a chest x-ray is performed.

2. Planning Conference

    As soon as possible after admission, the patient's therapist meets with the ward staff to formally define a list of problems. Therapist and staff collaborate on formulating the list. The therapist may be most interested in the intrapsychic problems while staff may be more cognizant of ward management problems that they observe in the patient. Treatment planning, therefore, is a team effort. The patient, himself, may be invited to participate if the therapist thinks it appropriate.

3. Problem List

    A list of the patient's problems is generated at the planning conference and each problem is identified by number, (Table VI-I: Problem List) . All further references to a specific problem in the written record contain its identifying number. Although the descriptive term may change (for example, chronic schizophrenia, paranoid type to organic psychosis if it is learned that the patient is, in fact, suffering such a disorder) the identifying number remains the same. This makes it possible for staff or any later outside observer to follow a particular problem in the written records all the way through the course of the patient's hospitalization without having to wade through other data that is not specifically related to the problem under investigation.

The problem list is posted as a permanent face sheet on the first page of the patient's chart. Staff, therefore, get an instant glimpse of the *big picture* every time they

TABLE VI-I

PROBLEM LIST

Problem	Interpretation(s)	Goals	Treatment Plans
1. Schizophrenia			
a. Auditory hallucinations	a. Patient has documented hx of chronic schizophrenia	a. Restore ego functioning	a. Phenothiazine meds
b. Agitation	b. Stopped taking medication six weeks ago		b. Level 1 activities for first week
	c. Father died one week ago		c. 1:1 with staff
			d. Contact previous hospital for records
2. Job in Danger			
	a. Patient's employer does not know he is in hospital	a. We will attempt to hold patient's job until he can return to community	a. Social worker to contact employer
3. Rheumatic Heart Disease			
	a. By history	a. Evaluation	a. Cardiology referral
	b. Has Grade I murmur		
	c. No symptoms		

pick up the patient's chart. The problem list consists of four parts: (1) Each problem by number, (2) dynamic interpretation (s) of each problem when appropriate, (3) the treatment goals, focusing on what criteria will be established to denote maximum hospital benefits for this particular patient and what criteria will be used to determine suitability for discharge from the hospital, and (4) the treatment plans.

The problem list is an ever-changing, dynamic part of the patient's record. In this problem list presented in Table VI-I, for example, Problem 2 might be easily resolved by a phone call from the social worker to the patient's employer. It would then be marked *resolved* and deleted. (The number 2, however, is not assigned to a new problem. If the patient's job status should ever become a problem again, it would re-enter the record as Problem 2. Therapist and staff could then easily trace it back to its origins in the record.)

Similarly, new problems that arise are given new numbers and are entered on the face sheet. Dynamic interpretations are updated as new information becomes available. Goals may be readjusted. Treatment may be revised.

4. Progress Notes

Daily progress notes by staff and therapists are linked specifically to each problem by number (Table VI-II: Progress Note). Each staff person having information to be added into the record, therefore, must carefully conceptualize the material in terms of how it relates to the overall plan and to systematically divide all entries into specific problem areas.

The progress notes are composed of six elements: (1) the problem number, (2) subjective, i.e. what the patient says, (3) observation, i.e. what the staff observes, (4) response, i.e. what staff says or does in reply, (5) result, i.e. what resulted from the interaction and (6) other comments.

Provision is also made for any material that does

TABLE VI-II: *Progress Note*

12/18/72   Problem # 1:   Schizophrenia

    Subj: Patient told me that "voices"
             said he was evil.

    Obj: Agitated, pacing floor all day.

    Resp: Reassurance, maintained 1:1 contact.

    Result: Continues to be agitated.

    Other: Should we increase Medication?

             (signed)_____Jane Doe, R. N._____

not seem to fit into any of the existing problem categories. Such information is simply marked with an asterisk (*). These entries are later reviewed at the progress conference. Often they can be placed within existing problem headings; at other times they serve to identify an emerging problem not previously recognized.

5. Progress Chart

Prior to the weekly progress conference, all staff that are working with the patient, (therapist, nurses, O.T., R.T., social worker, attendants, etc.) are asked to rate the patient's progress in each problem area. The compendium of ratings that results is called the Progress Chart (Table VI-III: Progress Chart). The scoring is done on a basis of —2, —1, 0, +1, +2 with +2 indicating significant improvement, 0 indicating no discernible change, and —2 indicating significant regression. Each staff person enters his score by marking his own initials in the appropriate column so that the information is retrievable on a personal basis. In this way staff can be questioned about scores that seem to deviate significantly from the mean.

TABLE VI-III: *Progress Chart*

Problem	-2	-1	0	+1	+2	Comments
# 1	J.D.	A.B. J.R.N.				?Increase meds −J.D.
# 2				J.D. C.D.	A.B. J.R.N.	Have social worker attend Conference −A.B.
# 3			J.D. J.R.N. C.D. A.B.			Cardiology has not yet answered referral −J.R.N.

The patient may be invited to score his own progress and enter his initials on the chart. This may be the most enlightening and meaningful input into the system and gives the patient a unique sense of participation.

6. Flow Sheet

The flow sheet (Figure VI-1: Flow Sheet) is simply a graphical record of the week-to-week progress in each problem area. It is constructed by taking the average weekly score from the progress chart for each problem. Where the progress chart is static, the flow sheet provides a continuous overview of the patient's ever-changing hospital course.

The sample flow sheet for problem 1 (Figure VI-1) documents that the patient has made steady progress over five weeks of hospitalization. Similar flow sheets are constructed for each identified problem. The flow sheet becomes a part of the permanent record and is continually updated on a week-to-week basis. It provides an instantaneous glimpse of the patient's clinical course, is a ready indicator of treatment response and serves to identify those lesser problems that need further attention and that might, otherwise, go overlooked.

7. Progress Conference

Figure VI-1: Flow Sheet

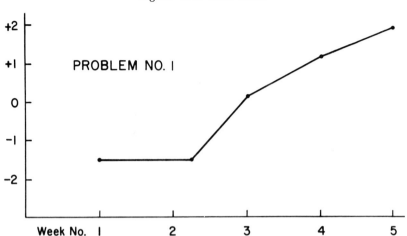

The patient's progress is reviewed formally at a weekly staff conference. The progress chart and flow sheet are constructed *prior* to this meeting and are posted prominently in the meeting room while the patient is being discussed.

Discrepancies between raters, if significant, are investigated. At times, such discrepancies are the result of a particular staff person's inexperience or uncertainty regarding the previously established criteria (*goals* on the problem list). At other times, a staff person may have important information that has not been available to other staff. This information might lead him to make a discrepant, but valid entry.

This open sharing of information among staff members at the progress conference results in enhanced learning and participation.

The final step at the progress conference is to update the problem list. The current status of each problem is carefully reviewed. Goals and treatment plans are similarly examined. Adjustments are made, if indicated.

8. Discharge Conference

Prior to the patient's discharge, the staff participates in a discharge conference. At this time the entire case is again reviewed. The focus is divided equally between judging the patient's suitability for discharge and evaluating staff performance vis-a-vis this particular patient and the problems that he presented for solution.

Suitability for discharge is determined on the basis of the previously determined treatment goals. Does the patient meet the criteria? If so, what type of after-care will he require? If the patient meets the previously established goals of treatment and if necessary follow up and other arrangements have been made, he may be discharged from the hospital.

Staff performance is evaluated on a problem by problem basis. It is often useful to compare the patient's flow sheet to flow sheets of other patients with similar problems. In this case, for example, it is seen that problem 1 was resolved in five weeks. How does this compare with other cases of acute schizophrenia that the staff has treated? Such comparison to similar cases can serve to identify both weaknesses and strengths in the therapeutic milieu. Staff members may also be evaluated individually since their entries into the patient's record are all retrievable individually and on a problem by problem basis.

References

Grant, R. L., Maletzky, B. M.: *A Scientific Approach to Psychiatric Record-Keeping.* San Francisco, Presented at American Psychiatric Association Meeting, May 15, 1970.

Weed, L. L.: *Medical Records, Medical Education and Patient Care.* Cleveland, Press of Case Western Reserve University, 1969.

Chapter VII

PSYCHIATRY
IN MEDICINE

THE ROLE OF PSYCHIATRY in medicine is evolving from a narrow search for psychologic factors in the etiology, onset, and course of physical illness (*classic* psychosomatic theories) to a broadly based psycho-medico-socio concept that includes such factors as patient interviewing, doctor-patient relationship, the physician's own psychological role, characteristic reactions to physical illness, the dying patient, the role of the family, the hospital milieu and many other considerations. In these cases the psychiatrist stands at the crossroads. Because of his unique training and skills in both medicine and psychiatry, he is in the best position to facilitate communication, understanding and change in these areas.

This chapter is devoted to the many interfaces that exist between psychiatry and medicine. While the first article, Psychiatric Consultation to Medical-Surgical Units, outlines some of the more classic disease-oriented approaches, i.e. Table VII-I (Psychiatric Manifestations of Commonly-Used Drugs in Medicine and Surgery) and Table VII-II (Medical Syndromes with Major Psychiatric Manifestations), it also stresses that the psychiatrist must consider the entire milieu as his patient when consulting to medical-surgical units. The psychiatrist is uniquely-equipped for this broad, systems approach. Table VII-III (Common Consultation Requests) outlines the most frequent type of psychiatric referrals and suggests a treatment approach for each.

Normal laboratory values in clinical medicine outlines normal values for the most common diagnostic procedures in general medicine. It is included as a handy reference for the psychiatrist who may have need of such information from time to time.

PSYCHIATRIC CONSULTATION TO MEDICAL-SURGICAL UNITS

Jesse H. Wright, M.D.

Psychiatric consultation to medical-surgical units within a general hospital setting can be an important stimulus for improving comprehensive patient care. The consultation process can go beyond handling problems of individual patients to have an impact on the entire hospital system. The following section gives guidelines for working effectively within the general hospital setting.

I. General Principles: The main functions of psychiatric consultation in a general hospital are diagnosis, advising on patient management, therapy, resolving conflicts within the patient and clinical team, and teaching (Lipowski, 1967). The psychiatric consultant serves as a specialist in dealing with the total milieu of an illness. His knowledge of psychiatric principles coupled with his training as a physician make him especially well equipped to work with the complex interrelationships between psychosocial factors and organic processes. In his consultations, the psychiatrist can demonstrate to members of the medical team the value of his broad medical-psychiatric background and thus have an important influence on the nature of patient care.

II. Liaison Development: Establishing a successful consulting relationship calls for considerable sensitivity and perseverance on the part of the psychiatrist. The understandable distrust which greets a new psychiatric consultant must be patiently overcome. Initial overzealousness on the part of the psychiatrist can lead to alienation which will prevent the growth of a mutually beneficial relationship. The following principles are important in facilitating the development of a working liaison:

A. Availability: Be accessible to staff by regularly attending rounds and being present when help is needed. The consultant's interest and dependability are then in evidence. Personal relationships can begin to develop which will bridge the general uneasiness most medical staff feel in encountering a psychiatrist. Stereotypic prejudices and fears usually give way when the psychiatrist is known as an individual.

B. Preparation:

1. Be knowledgeable about the psychiatric manifestations of toxic and organic illness. In this area especially, the psychiatrist and his medical colleague can speak the same language. Proving one's status as a physician by making correct observations in these cases is often the first step toward winning the acceptance necessary for the beginning of an effective consultation relationship.

2. Table VII-I (Psychiatric Manifestations of Commonly Used Drugs in Medicine and Surgery) lists the most frequent psychiatric side-effects that are observed with commonly-employed therapeutic drugs. The psychiatrist who is called to a medical-surgical unit to consult on a patient who has suddenly exhibited unusual or bizarre behavior, should have a high index of suspicion for an idiosyncratic drug reaction.

3. Table VII-II (Medical Syndromes with Major Psychiatric Manifestations) lists several important medical illnesses that are often associated with a characteristic psychiatric component. In fact, these basically medical illnesses may first present themselves as a psychiatric problem. The psychiatrist who consults to medical-surgical

TABLE VII-I

PSYCHIATRIC MANIFESTATIONS OF COMMONLY-USED DRUGS IN MEDICINE AND SURGERY

Drug	Psychiatric Side Effects
Amphetamines	excitement, sleep disturbance, psychosis with paranoia
Barbiturates	dullness, slow speech, memory loss, disturbed judgment
Belladona Alkaloids (atropine, scopalamine)	delirium, disorientation, visual hallucinations
Bromide (in some over-the-counter sedatives)	lethargy, emotional lability, disorientation, memory loss, psychosis
Corticosteroids	anxiety, emotional lability, psychosis, premorbid personality important in reaction to drug
Digitalis	confusion, disorientation, delirium, hallucinations
Epinephrine	restlessness, tremor, anxiety
Ethacrynic Acid (Edecrin®)	psychosis can follow development of hearing loss
L-dopa (Larodopa®)	euphoria, increased sexual interest, anxiety, depression, psychosis with auditory and visual hallucinations
Methyldopa (Aldomet®)	sedation, depression
Morphine	drowsiness, difficulty in concentration, euphoria
Pentazocine (Talwin®)	sedation, anxiety, bizarre ideation, hallucinations, drug dependence
Progesterone	easy fatigability, depression
Propranalol (Inderal®)	depression
Reserpine	sedation, depression
Sodium Diphenylhydantoin (Dilantin®)	bizarre behavior, psychosis

units is in a unique position to identify these psychic manifestations of medical illnesses. His own medical training will be invaluable in documenting the final diagnosis on the basis of symptoms, physical findings and laboratory tests.

4. Get to know the milieu. What is it like to be a patient in this hospital? How do members of the medical team work together and what are the unique pressures that bear on them? A thorough knowledge of the psychosocial

TABLE VII-II

MEDICAL SYNDROMES WITH MAJOR PSYCHIATRIC MANIFESTATIONS

Syndrome	Psychological Manifestations	Other Important Features
A. *Endocrine and Metabolic:*		
Alcoholic Encephalopathy	irritability, combativeness, visual hallucinations, confabulation	ophthalmoplegia, delirium tremens, poor nutrition and general health
Addisons' Disease (Deficiency of Adrenocortical Hormones)	depression, anxiety, may lead to delirium or psychosis	pigmentation of skin, weakness, weight loss, hypotension
Cushings' Disease (Elevated Adrenocortical Hormones)	depression, irritability, euphoria, distortions of body image and sexuality, often progresses to psychosis	truncal obesity, osteoporosis, muscle wasting, atrophy of skin, striae, easy bruisability
Hepatic Failure	restlessness, visual hallucinations, delirium, coma	jaundice, varices, ascites, tremor
Hyperthyroidism	anxiety, irritability, emotional lability, may progress to psychosis	goiter, exophthalmos, tremor, increased perspiration, hyperactive reflexes
Hypoglycemia	anxiety, syncope, nausea, headache, may progress to confusion and hallucinations	related to food intake, abnormal glucose tolerance test
Hypothyroidism	dullness, apathy, may progress to psychosis, i.e. Myxedema madness	dry skin, brittle hair, bradycardia, myxedema
Pancreatitis	visual and auditory hallucinations, agitation, disorientation, confabulation	upper abdominal pain, nausea and vomiting
Porphyrias	great variety of psychological symptoms including excitement, catatonia, mood disorder, hallucinations	abdominal pain, seizures, brownish-red urine, skin pigmentation, sensitivity to drugs (e.g. barbiturates, sulfa, ergot)
Uremia	apathy, irritability, difficulty concentrating, memory loss, delirium, coma	pale and dry skin, uriniferous breath, nausea, weakness
B. *Cerebrovascular Disorders and Dementias:*		
Cerebral Arteriosclerosis	impaired memory (recent more than past), decreased awareness, emotional lability, sleep disturbance	evidence of arteriosclerosis elsewhere in body, symptoms fluctuate in intensity

TABLE VII-II Continued

Syndrome	Psychological Manifestations	Other Important Features
Hypertensive Encephalopathy	restlessness and confusion which can progress to stupor and coma	elevated blood pressure, retinal hemorrhages, seizures, C.V.A.
Presenile Dementia (Picks' and Alzheimers' Diseases)	slowly evolving dementia, depression, anxiety, behavioral changes	shuffling gait, occasional apraxia or aphasia, onset usually at age 50 to 60
Senile Dementia	impaired memory (recent more than past) poor judgment, emotional lability, personality traits are exaggerated, paranoia	signs of generalized aging, steady downhill course
C. *Brain Tumor, Injury, Sepsis, and other Neuropathological States:* (See also: Chapter VIII, Neurology for Psychiatrists)	may mimic any psychiatric syndrome with varied symptoms such as depression, emotional lability, psychosis	neurological signs, papilledema, headache, seizures
D. *Vitamin Deficiencies:*		
Beri Beri (Thiamine Deficiency)	fatigability, irritability, sleep disturbance, memory loss, may progress to delirium	neuropathies, ophthalmoplegia
Pellagra (Niacin Deficiency)	initially depression, then psychosis with paranoia or catatonia	diarrhea, dermatitis, tremor, seizures, primitive reflexes
Pernicious Anemia (Vitamin B_{12} Deficiency)	irritability, depression, memory loss, disorientation, hallucinations	glossitis, weakness, abdominal pain, evidence of posterior column degeneration
Scurvy (Vitamin C Deficiency)	weakness, irritability, depression	hemorrhagic and bone abnormalities

fabric of the hospital is essential because each problem has ramifications at many levels of interaction. For example: A psychiatrist is called to see an elderly gentleman who has suffered a C.V.A. and is now said to be depressed because of his paralyzed left side. In discussing this situation with a neurosurgical resident making the referral, the psychiatrist learns that the paralysis occurred during a carotid arteriogram suggested by a staff physician. The resident and other house staff members had argued against this procedure because of the patient's advanced age. In this case, the psychiatrist must deal not only with the patient's grief but also with the resident's feelings about the circumstances and the implications they have for the functioning of the entire neurosurgical team.

5. Be aware of common consultation problems. In addition to the hypothetical problem outlined above, there are other types of cases that are regularly referred to the psychiatrist by in-patient medical-surgical units. Table VII-III (Common Consultation Requests) lists six of the most common requests made of psychiatrists by medical-surgical units. A separate clinical approach is suggested for each consultation request.

6. Be knowledgeable about the characteristic reactions to physical disease. A person's psychological reaction to his own illness will, of course, be determined by his own particular intrapsychic blend of conscious and unconscious forces. Yet there are some reactions such as anxiety, depression and grief that many hospitalized patients share in common. There is a growing fund of knowledge about these phenomena in the medical and psychiatric literature. The psychiatrist who will be called to consult on these problems should be familiar with this information. (See Psychiatric Evaluation of the Dying Patient, Chapter IV.)

7. Review the literature concerning the classic psychosomatic illnesses such as tension headache, peptic ulcer, asthma, etc. Valuable references include: Alexander (1950), Kimball (1970), Weiss and English (1949).

Recent thinking about psychosomatic illness tends to reject the search for direct causal links between distinct personality types and specific

TABLE VII-III

COMMON CONSULTATION REQUESTS

Problem	Approach
1. Differential Diagnosis	1. Thorough medical history and physical exam, psychiatric evaluation including mental status exam and laboratory studies as indicated. Keep multiple possibilities in mind.
2. Disruptive Behavior	2. Analyze behavior within context of social situation. Therapeutic intervention at level of disturbance (e.g. patient-staff communication problems, intrapsychic conflict within patient, etc.) with supportive psychotherapy, group process, psychotropic drugs or other modalities. Use of a psychiatric nurse as a co-consultant can be very helpful in advising staff on management of difficult patients.
3. Suicidal Threats	3. Same as number 2 but institute necessary precautions or transfer to psychiatric ward if suicidal risk is high. (See Evaluation of the Suicidal Patient, Chapter IV.)
4. Severe Psychological Reactions To Organic Disease	4. Psychiatric evaluation aimed at assessing need for social or individual therapeutic interventions. Provide environment conducive to ventilation of feelings.
5. Patient With Known Psychiatric Disorder	5. Evaluation of relationship of psychiatric history to present illness. Usually patients with prior psychiatric diagnoses do quite well as medical patients and the primary task is to reassure the medical staff. On other occasions, help in management or recommendations for psychiatric care become necessary.
6. Refusal To Give Consent For Operative Procedure	6. Same as number 2. Advise on legal procedures if indicated.

disease states. Instead, illness is viewed as the final common pathway resulting from the interworkings of social, intrapsychic and physiological factors.

References

Alexander, F.: *Psychosomatic Medicine.* New York, W. W. Norton, 1950.

Kimball, C. P.: Conceptual developments in psychosomatic medicine: 1939–1969. *Ann Intern Med, 73:* 307–316, 1970.

Lipowski, Z. J.: Review of consultation psychiatry and psychosomatic medicine I. general principles. *Psychosom Med, 29:* 153–171, 1967.

Weiss, E. and English, O. S.: *Psychosomatic Medicine.* Philadelphia, W. B. Sanders, 1949.

Other Recommended Reading

Kubler-Ross, E.: *On Death and Dying.* New York, Macmillan, 1969.

Lipowski, Z. J.: Review of consultation psychiatry and psychosomatic medicine II. clinical aspects. *Psychosomatic Medicine, 29:* 201–224, 1967.

Meyer, E. and Mendelson, M.: Psychiatric consultations with patients on medical and surgical wards: patterns and processes. *Psychiatry, 24:* 199–222, 1961.

Schwab, J. J.: *Handbook of Psychiatric Consultation.* New York, Appleton, Century, Crofts, 1968.

NORMAL LABORATORY VALUES IN CLINICAL MEDICINE

Reprinted with permission R. B. Conn, "Normal Laboratory Values of Clinical Importance," In *Current Therapy,* Philadelphia, W. B. Saunders, 1972.

Hematology

Test	Normal Value
Acid hemolysis test (Ham)	No hemolysis
Alkaline phosphatase, leukocyte	Total score 14–100
Bleeding time	
Ivy	Less than 5 min
Duke	1–5 min
Carboxyhemoglobin	Up to 5% of total
Cell counts	
Erythrocytes: Males	4.6–6.2 million/cu mm
Females	4.2–5.4 million/cu mm
Children	4.5–5.1 million/cu mm
(children: varies with age)	
Leukocytes	
Total	5000–10,000/cu mm
Differential	Percentage
Myelocytes	0
Juvenile neutrophils	3–5
Segmented neutrophils	54–62
Lymphocytes	25–33
Monocytes	3–7
Eosinophils	1–3

Test	Normal Value
Basophils (Infants and children have greater relative numbers of lympho-cytes and monocytes)	0–0.75
Platelets	150,000–350,000/cu. mm
Reticulocytes	25,000– 75,000/cu mm 0.5–1.5% of erythrocytes
Clot retraction, qualitative	Begins in 30–60 min Complete in 24 hrs.
Coagulation time (Lee-White)	5–15 min (glass tubes) 19–60 min (siliconized tubes)
Cold hemolysin test (Donath-Landsteiner)	No hemolysis
Corpuscular values of erythrocytes (Values are for adults; in children values vary with age) M.C.H. (mean corpuscular hemoglobin) M.C.V. (Mean corpuscular volume) M.C.H.C. (mean corpus-cular hemoglobin concentration)	27–31 picogm 82–92 cu micra 32–36%
Fibrinogen	200–400 mg/100 ml
Fibrinolysins	0
Hematocrit Males Females Newborn Children (varies with age)	40–54 ml/100 ml 37–47 ml/100 ml 49–54 ml/100 ml 35–49 ml/100 ml

Test	Normal Values
Hemoglobin	
Males	14.0–18.0 grams/100 ml
Females	12.0–16.0 grams/100 ml
Newborn	16.5–19.5 grams/100 ml
Children (varies with age)	11.2–16.5 grams/100 ml
Hemoglobin, fetal	Less than 1% of total
Hemoglobin A	1.5–3.0% of total
Hemoglobin, plasma	0–5.0 mg/100 ml
Methemoglobin	0.03–0.13 grams/100 ml
Osmotic fragility of	
erythrocytes	Begins in 0.45–0.39% NaCl
	Complete in 0.33–0.30% NaCl
Partial thromboplastin time	60–70 sec
Kaolin activated	35–45 sec
Prothrombin consumption	Over 80% consumed in 1 hr
Prothrombin content	100% (calculated from
	prothrombin time)
Prothrombin time (one stage)	12.0–14.0 sec
Sedimentation rate	
Wintrobe: Males	0– 5 mm in 1 hr
Females	0–15 mm in 1 hr
Westergren: Males	0–15 mm in 1 hr
Females	0–20 mm in 1 hr
(May be slightly higher	
in children and during	
pregnancy.)	

Test	Normal Value
Carbon dioxide, content, serum	24–30 mEq/liter Infants: 20–28 mEq/liter
Carbon dioxide tension (Pco$_2$), blood	35– 45 mm Hg
Carotene, serum	50–300 mcg/100 ml
Ceruloplasmin, serum	23– 44 mg/100 ml
Chloride, serum	96–106 mEq/liter
Cholesterol, serum Total Esters	 150–250 mg/100 ml 68–76% of total cholesterol
Cholinesterase, serum RBC	0.5–1.3 pH units 0.5–1.0 pH units
Copper, serum Male Female	 70–140 mcg/100 ml 85–155 mcg/100 ml
Cortisol, plasma	6– 16 mcg/100 ml
Creatine, serum	0.2–0.8 mg/100 ml
Creatin phosphokinase, serum Male Female	 0–50 ml U/ml (30°) (Oliver-Rosalki) 0–30 ml U/ml (30°) (Oliver-Rosalki)
Creatinine, serum	0.7–1.5 mg/100 ml
Cryoglobulins, serum	0
Fatty acids, total, serum	190–420 mg/100 ml

Test	Normal Values
Thromboplastin generation test	Compared to normal control
Tourniquet test	Ten or fewer petechiae in a 2.5 cm circle after 5 min with cuff at 100 mm Hg

Bone marrow, differential cell count	Average
Myeloblasts	2.0%
Promyelocytes	5.0%
Myelocytes: Neutrophilic	12.0%
Eosinophilic	1.5%
Basophilic	0.3%
Metamyelocytes (juvenile forms)	22.0%
Polymorphonuclear neutrophils	20.0%
Polymorphonuclear eosinophils	2.0%
Polymorphonuclear basophils	0.2%
Lymphocytes	10.0%
Plasma cells	0.4%
Monocytes	2.0%
Reticulum cells	0.2%
Megakaryocytes	0.4%
Pronormoblasts	4.0%
Normoblasts	18.0%

Biochemistry (blood, plasma, serum)

For some procedures the normal values may vary depending upon the methods used.

Test	Normal Values
Acetone, serum	
Qualitative	Negative
Quantitative	0.3–2.0 mg/100 ml
Aldolase, serum	0.8–3.0 ml U/ml (30°) (Sibley-Lehninger)
Alpha amino nitrogen, serum	4–6 mg/100 ml
Ammonia nitrogen, blood	75–196 mcg/100 ml
plasma	56–122 mcg/100 ml
Amylase, serum	80–160 Somogyi units/100 ml
Ascorbic acid	See Vitamin C
Base, total, serum	145–160 mEq/liter
Bilirubin, serum	
Direct	0.1–0.4 mg/100 ml
Indirect	0.2–0.7 mg/100 ml (Total minus direct)
Total	0.3–1.1 mg/100 ml
Calcium, serum	4.5–5.5 mEq/liter (9.0–11.0 mg/100 ml) (Slightly higher in children) (Varies with protein concentration)
Calcium, serum, ionized	2.1–2.6 mEq/liter (4.25–5.25 mg/100 ml)

Test	Normal Value
Fibrinogen, plasma	200–400 mg/100 ml
Folic acid, serum	7–16 nanogm/ml
Glucose (fasting)	
blood, true	60–100 mg/100 ml
Folin	80–120 mg/100 ml
plasma or serum, true	70–115 mg/100 ml
Haptoglobin, serum	40–170 mg/100 ml
Hydroxybutyric	
dehydrogenase, serum	0–180 ml U/ml (30°) (Rosalki-Wilkinson) 114–290 units/ml (Wroblewski)
17-Hydroxycorticosteroids, plasma	8–18 mcg/100 ml
Icterus index, serum	4–7
Immunoglobulins, serum	
IgG	800–1500 mg/100 ml
IgA	50– 200 mg/100 ml
IgM	40– 120 mg/100 ml
Iodine, butanol extractable, serum	3.2–6.4 mcg/100 ml
Iodine, protein bound, serum	3.5–8.0 mcg/100 ml (May be slightly higher in infants)
Iron, serum	75–175 mcg/100 ml

Test	Normal Value

Iron binding capacity, total,
  serum
  percent saturation
	250–410 mcg/100 ml
	20–55%

17-Ketosteroids, plasma	25–125 mcg/100 ml
Lactic acid, blood	6–16 mg/100 ml

Lactic dehydrogenase, serum	0–300 ml U/ml (30°)
	  (Wroblewski modified)
	150–450 units/ml
	  (Wroblewski)
	80–120 units/ml (Wacher)

Lipase, serum	0–1.5 units (Cherry- Crandall)
Lipids, total, serum	450–850 mg/100 ml
Magnesium, serum	1.5–2.5 mEq/liter (1.8–3.0 mg/100 ml)
Nitrogen, nonprotein, serum	15–35 mg/100 ml
Osmolality, serum	285–295 mOsm/liter

Oxygen, blood
  Capacity
 	
  Content: Arterial
            Venous
  Saturation: Arterial
            Venous
  Tension: Po_2 Arterial
	
	16–24 vol %
	  (varies with Hb)
	15–23 vol %
	10–16 vol %
	94–100% of capacity
	60–85% of capacity
	75–100 mm Hg

pH, arterial, blood	7.35–7.45
Phenylalanine, serum	Less than 3 mg/100 ml

Test	Normal Value
Phosphatase, acid, serum	1.0–5.0 units (King Armstrong) 0.5–2.0 units (Bodansky) 0.5–2.0 units (Gutman) 0.0–1.1 units (Shinowara) 0.1–0.63 units (Bassey-Lowry)
Phosphatase, alkaline, serum	5.0–13.0 units (King-Armstrong) 2.0– 4.5 units (Bodansky) 3.0–10.0 units (Gutman) 2.2– 8.6 units (Shinowara) 0.8– 2.3 units (Bassey-Lowry) 30–85 milliunits/ml (I.U.) (Values are higher in children)
Phosphate, inorganic, serum	3.0–4.5 mg/100 ml (Children 4.0–7.0 mg/ 100 ml)
Phospholipids, serum	6–12 mg/100 ml as lipid phosphorus
Potassium, serum	3.5–5.0 mEq/liter

Proteins, serum
  Total
    Albumin
    Globulin
	
	6.0–8.0 grams/100 ml
	3.5–5.5 grams/100 ml
	2.5–3.5 grams/100 ml

Electrophoresis Albumin	 3.5–5.5 grams/100 ml 52–68% of total

Test	Normal Value
Globulin	
Alpha$_1$	0.2–0.4 gram/100 ml
	2–5% of total
Alpha$_2$	0.5–0.9 gram/100 ml
	7–14% of total
Beta	0.6–1.1 grams/100 ml
	9–15% of total
Gamma	0.7–1.7 grams/100 ml
	11–21% of total
Pyruvic acid, plasma	1.0–2.0 mg/100 ml
Serotonin, platelet suspension	0.1–0.3 mcg/ml blood
serum	0.10–0.32 mcg/ml
Sodium, serum	136–145 mEq/liter
Sulfates, inorganic, serum	0.8–1.2 mg/100 ml (as S)
Thyroxine, free, serum	1.0–2.1 nanogm/100 ml
Thyroxine binding globulin (TBG), serum	10–26 mcg/100 ml
Thyroxine iodine (T$_1$), serum	2.9–6.4 mcg/100 ml
Transaminase, serum: SGOT	0.19 ml U/ml (30°) (Karmen modified)
	15–40 units/ml (Karmen)
	18–40 units/ml (Reitman-Frankel)
SGPT	0.17 ml U/ml (30°) (Karmen modified)
	6–35 units/ml (Karmen)
	5–35 units/ml (Reitman-Frankel)

Test	Normal Value
Triglycerides, serum	0–150 mg/100 ml
Urea, blood plasma or serum	21–43 mg/100 ml 24–49 mg/100 ml

Urea nitrogen,
    blood (BUN)
    plasma or serum
	10–20 mg/100 ml
	11–23 mg/100 ml

Uric acid, serum
    Male
    Female
	2.5–8.0 mg/100 ml
	1.5–6.0 mg/100 ml

Vitamin A, serum	20–80 mcg/100 ml
Vitamin B_{12}, serum	200–800 picogm/ml
Vitamin C, blood	0.4–1.5 mg/100 ml

Urine

Test	Normal Value
Acetone and acetoacetate	0

Addis count
    Erythrocytes
    Leukocytes
    Casts (hyaline)
	0–130,000/24 hrs
	0–650,000/24 hrs
	0–2000/24 hrs

Alcapton bodies	Negative
Aldosterone	3–20 mcg/24 hrs
Alpha amino nitrogen	50–200 mg/24 hrs (Not over 1.5% of total nitrogen)
Ammonia nitrogen	20–70 mEq/24 hrs
Amylase	35–260 Somogyi units/hr

Test	Normal Value
Bence Jones protein	Negative
Bilirubin (bile)	Negative
Calcium	
Low Ca diet (Bauer-Aub)	Less than 150 mg/24 hrs
Usual diet	Less than 250 mg/24 hrs
Catecholamines	
Epinephrine	Less than 10 mcg/24 hrs
Norepinephrine	Less than 100 mcg/24 hrs
Chloride	110–250 mEq/24 hrs (Varies with intake)
Chorionic gonadotrophin	0
Copper	0–30 mcg/24 hrs
Creatine	
Male	0– 40 mg/24 hrs
Female	0–100 mg/24 hrs (Higher in children and during pregnancy)
Creatinine	15–25 mg/kg of body weight/24 hrs
Cystine or cysteine, qualitative	Negative
Delta aminolevulinic acid	1.3–7.0 mg/24 hrs

Test	Normal Value	
Estrogens	Male	Female
Estrone	3– 8	4– 31
Estradiol	0– 6	0– 14
Estriol	1–11	0– 72
Total	4–25	5–100
	(Units above are mcg/24 hrs) (Markedly increased during pregnancy)	
Glucose (reducing substances)	Less than 250 mg/24 hrs	
Gonadotrophins, pituitary	5–10 rat units/24 hrs 10–50 mouse units/24 hrs (Increased after menopause)	
Hemoglobin and myoglobin	Negative	
Homogentisic acid, qualitative	Negative	
17-Hydroxycorticosteroids Male Female	3–9 mg/24 hrs 2–8 mg/24 hrs (Varies with method used)	
5-Hydroxyindole-acetic acid (5-HIAA) Qualitative Quantitative	Negative Less than 16 mg/24 hrs	
17-Ketosteroids Male Female	6–18 mg/24 hrs 4–13 mg/24 hrs	
Osmolality	38–1400 mOsm/kg water	

Test	Normal Value
pH	4.6–8.0, average 6.0 (Depends on diet)
Phenylpyruvic acid, qualitative	Negative
Phosphorus	0.9–1.3 gm/24 hrs (Varies with intake)
Porphobilinogen Qualitative Quantitative	Negative 0–0.2 mg/100 ml Less than 2.0 mg/24 hrs
Porphyrins Coproporphyrin Uroporphyrin	50–250 mcg/24 hrs 10– 30 mcg/24 hrs
Potassium	25–100 mEq/24 hrs (Varies with intake)
Pregnanetriol	Less than 2.5 mg/24 hrs in adults
Protein Qualitative Quantitative	0 10–150 mg/24 hrs
Sodium	130–260 mEq/24 hrs (Varies with intake)
Solids, total	30–70 grams/liter, average 50 grams/liter (To estimate total solids per liter, multiply last two figures of specific gravity by 2.66; Long's coefficient)

Test	Normal Value
Specific gravity	1.003–1.030
Sugar	0
Titratable acidity	20–40 mEq/24 hrs
Urobilinogen	Up to 1.0 Ehrlich unit/2 hrs (1–3 P.M.) 0–4.0 mg/24 hrs
Vanillylmandelic acid (VMA)	1–8 mg/24 hrs

Gastric Analysis

Test	Normal Value	
Basal gastric secretion (one hour)	Concentration Mean ± 1 S.D.	Output Mean ± 1 S.D.
Male	25.8 ± 1.8 mEq/liter	2.57 ± 0.16 mEq/hr
Female	20.3 ± 3.0 mEq/liter	1.61 ± 0.18 mEq/hr

After histamine stimulation
   Normal
   Duodenal ulcer
	
	 Mean output = 11.8 mEq/hr
	 Mean output = 15.2 mEq/hr	

After maximal histamine stimulation
   Normal
   Duodenal ulcer
	
	 Mean output = 22.6 mEq/hr
	 Mean output = 44.6 mEq/hr	

Diagnex® blue (Squibb)	Anacidity 0–0.3 mg in 2 hrs Doubtful 0.3–0.6 mg in 2 hrs Normal Greater than 0.6 mg in 2 hrs	
Volume, fasting stomach content	50–100 ml	

Test	Normal Value
Emptying time	3–6 hrs
Color	Opalescent or colorless
Specific gravity	1.006–1.009
pH (adults)	0.9–1.5

Cerebrospinal Fluid

Test	Normal Value
Cells	Fewer than 5 cu mm
	all mononuclear
Chloride	120–130 mEq/liter
	(20 mEq/liter higher than serum)
Colloidal gold test	Not more than 1 in any tube
Glucose	50–75 mg/100 ml
	(20 mg/100 ml less than blood)
Pressure	70–180 mm water
Protein, total	15–45 mg/100 ml
Albumin	52%
Alpha, globulin	5%
Alpha, globulin	14%
Beta globulin	10%
Gamma globulin	19%

Semen

Test	Normal Value
Volume	2–5 ml, usually 3–4 ml
Liquefaction	Complete in 15 min

Test	Normal Value
pH	7.2–8.0; average 7.8
Leukocytes	Occasional or absent
Count	60–150 million/ml
	Below 60 million/ml is abnormal
Motility	80% or more motile
Morphology	80–90% normal forms

Feces

Test	Normal Value
Bulk	100–200 grams/24 hrs
Dry matter	23– 32 grams/24 hrs
Fat, total	Less than 6.0 grams/24 hrs
Nitrogen total	Less than 8.0 grams/24 hrs
Urobilinogen	40–280 mg/24 hrs
Water	Approximately 65%

Serologic Procedures

Test	Normal Value
Antihyaluronidase	Less than 1:200. Significant if rising titer can be demonstrated at weekly intervals.
Antistreptolysin O titer	Normal up to 1:128. Single test usually has little significance. Rise in titer or persistently elevated titer is significant.

Test	Normal Value		
Bacterial agglutinins	Significant only if rise in titer is demonstrated or if antibodies are absent.		
Complement fixation tests	Titers of 1.8 or less are usually not significant. Paired sera showing rise in titer of more than two tubes are usually considered significant.		
C reactive protein (CRP)	Negative		
Heterophile titer			
	Unabsorbed	Absorbed With G.P.	Absorbed With Beef
Normal	1:160	1:10	1:160
Inf. mono.	1:160	1:320	1:10
Serum sickness	1:160	1:5	1:10
Proteus OX-19 agglutinins	1:80 Negative 1:160 Doubtful 1:320 Positive		
R.A. test (latex)	1:40 Negative 1:80 –1:160 Doubtful 1:320 Positive		
Rose test	1:10 Negative 1:20 –1:40 Doubtful 1:80 Positive		
Tularemia agglutinins	1:80 Negative 1:160 Doubtful 1:320 Positive		

Toxicology

Test	Normal Value
Arsenic, blood	3.5–7.2 mcg/100 ml
Arsenic, urine	Less than 100 mcg/24 hrs
Barbiturates, serum	0 Coma level: Phenobarbital approximately 11 mg/100 ml; most other barbiturates 1.5 mg/100 ml
Bromides, serum	0 Toxic levels above 17 mEq/liter
Carbon monoxide, blood	Up to 5% saturation Symptoms occur with 20% saturation
Dilantin, blood or serum	Therapeutic levels 1–11 mcg/ml

Ethanol, blood
  Marked intoxication
  Alcoholic stupor
  Coma
	Less than 0.005%
	0.3–0.4%
	0.4–0.5%
	Above 0.5%

Lead, blood	0–40 mcg/100 ml
Lead, urine	Less than 100 mcg/24 hrs
Lithium, serum	0 Therapeutic levels 0.5–1.5 mEq/liter Toxic levels above 2mEq/liter
Mercury, urine	Less than 10 mcg/24 hrs

Test	Normal Value
Salicylate, plasma	0
Therapeutic range	20–25 mg/100 ml
Toxic range	Over 30 mg/100 ml
Death	45–75 mg/100 ml

Liver Function Tests

Test	Normal Value
Bromsulphalein (B.S.P.)	Less than 5% remaining in serum 45 minutes after injection of 5 mg/kg of body weight
Cephalin cholesterol flocculation	0–1 in 24 hours
Galactose tolerance	Excretion of not more than 3.0 grams galactose in the urine 5 hours after ingestion of 40 grams of galactose.
Glycogen storage	Increase of blood glucose 45 mg/100 ml over fasting level 45 minutes after subcutaneous injection of 0.01 mg/kg body weight of epinephrine.
Hippuric Acid	Excretion of 3.0–3.5 grams hippuric acid in urine within 4 hours after ingestion of 6.0 grams sodium benzoate

OR

Test	Normal Value
Hippuric Acid (cont.)	Excretion of 0.7 grams hippuric acid in urine within 1 hour after intravenous injection of 1.77 grams sodium benzoate
Thymol turbidity	0– 5 units
Zinc turbidity	2–12 units

Pancreatic (islet) Function Tests

Test	Normal Value
Glucose tolerance tests	
Oral	Patient should be on a diet containing 300 grams of carbohydrate per day for 3 days prior to test. After ingestion of 100 grams of glucose or 1.75 grams glucose/kg body weight, blood glucose is not more than 160 mg/100 ml after 60 minutes, 140 mg/100 ml after 90 minutes, and 120 mg/100 ml after 120 minutes. Values are for blood; serum measurements are approx. 15% higher.
Intravenous	Blood glucose does not exceed 200 mg/100 ml after infusion of 0.5 gram of glucose/kg body weight over 30 minutes. Glucose concentration falls below initial level at 2 hours and returns to preinfusion levels in 3 hours or 1 hour. Values are for blood; serum measurements are approximately 15% higher.

Test	Normal Value
Cortisone glucose tolerance test	The patient should be on a diet containing 300 grams of carbohydrates per day for 3 days prior to test. At 8½ and again 2 hours prior to glucose load patient is given cortisone acetate by mouth (50 mg if patient's ideal weight is less than 160 lb). An oral dose of glucose 1.75 grams/kg body weight, is given and blood samples are taken at 0, 30, 60, 90 and 120 minutes. Test is considered positive if true blood glucose exceeds 160 mg/100 ml at 60 minutes, 140 mg/100 ml at 90 minutes and 120 mg/100 ml at 120 minutes. Values are for blood; serum measurements are approx. 15% higher.

Renal Function Tests

Test	Normal Value
Clearance tests (corrected to 1.73 sq. meters body surface area)	
Glomerular filtration rate (G.F.R.) Inulin clearance Mannitol clearance, or Endogeneous creatinine clearance	Males 110–150 ml/min Females 105–133 ml/min

Renal plasma flow (R.P.F.) p-Aminohippurate (P.A.H.), or Diodrast	Males 560–830 ml/min Females 490–700 ml/min
Filtration fraction (F.F.) $$FF = \dfrac{G.F.R.}{R.P.F.}$$	Males 17–21% Females 17–23%
Urea clearance (C_u)	Standard 40–65 ml/min Maximal 60–100 ml/min
Concentration and dilution	Specific gravity > 1.025 on dry day Specific gravity < 1.003 on water day
Maximal Diodrast excretory capacity T_{Mp}	Males 43–59 mg/min Females 33–51 mg/min
Maximal glucose reabsorptive capacity T_{MG}	Males 300–450 mg/min Females 250–350 mg/min
Maximal PAH excretory capacity T_{MPAH}	80–90 mg/min
Phenolsulfonphthalein excretion (P.S.P.)	25% or more in 15 min 40% or more in 30 min 55% or more in 2 hrs After injection of 1 ml P.S.P. intravenously

Thyroid Function Tests

Test	Normal Value
Protein bound iodine, serum (P.B.I.)	3.5–8.0 mcg/100 ml
Butanol extractable iodine, serum (B.E.I.)	3.2–6.4 mcg/100 ml
Thyroxine iodine, serum (T_1)	2.9–6.4 mcg/100 ml
Free Thyroxine, serum	1.4–2.5 nanogram/100 ml
T_3 (index of unsaturated T.B.G.)	10.0–14.6%
Thyroxine-binding globulin, serum (T.B.G.)	10–26 mcg T_1/100 ml
Thyroid-stimulating hormone, serum (T.S.H.)	0 up to 0.2 milliunits/ml
Radioactive iodine (I^{131}) uptake (R.A.I.)	20–50% of administered dose in 24 hours
Radioactive iodine (I^{131}) excretion	30–70% of administered dose in 24 hrs
Radioactive iodine (I^{131}), protein bound	Less than 0.3% of administered dose per liter of plasma at 72 hours
Basal metabolic rate	Minus 10% to plus 10% of mean standard

Gastrointestinal Absorption Tests

Test	Normal Value
d-Xylose absorption test	After an 8-hour fast 10 ml/kg body weight of a 5% solution of d-xylose is given by mouth. Nothing further by mouth is given until the test has been completed. All urine voided during the following 5 hours is pooled, and blood samples are taken at 0, 10 and 120 minutes. Normally 26% (range 16–33%) of ingested xylose is excreted within 5 hours, and the serum xylose reaches a level between 25 and 40 mg/100 ml after 1 hour and is maintained at this level for another 60 minutes.
Vitamin A absorption test	A fasting blood specimen is obtained and 200,000 units of vitamin A in oil is given by mouth. Serum vitamin A level should rise to twice fasting level in 3 to 5 hours.

References

Castleman, B. and McNeely, B. U.: *N Engl J Med, 283:* 1276, 1970.

Davidshon, I. and Henry, J. B.: *Clinical Diagnosis by Laboratory Methods,* 14th ed. Philadelphia, W. B. Saunders Co., 1969.

Department of Laboratory Medicine: *The Johns Hopkins Hospital: Clinical Laboratory Handbook,* Baltimore, 1971.

Henry, R. J.: *Clinical Chemistry—Principles and Techniques.* New York, Harper & Row, 1964.

Long, C.: *Biochemists' Handbook.* Princeton, D. Van Nostrand Co., 1961.

Miale, J. B.: *Laboratory Medicine—Hematology*, 3rd ed. St. Louis, C. V. Mosby Co., 1967.

Miller, S. E. and Weller, J. M.: *Textbook of Clinical Pathology*, 8th ed. Baltimore, Williams and Wilkins Co., 1971.

Stewart, C. P. and Stolman, A.: *Toxicology, Mechanisms, and Analytic Methods*. New York, Academic Press, 1960.

Sunderman, F. W. and Boerner, F.: *Normal Values in Clinical Medicine*. Philadelphia, W. B. Saunders Co., 1949.

Tietz, N. W.: *Fundamentals of Clinical Chemistry*. Philadelphia, W. B. Saunders Co., 1970.

Wintrobe, M. M.: *Clinical Hematology*, 6th ed. Philadelphia, Lea & Febiger, 1967.

Chapter VIII

NEUROLOGY FOR PSYCHIATRISTS

I T APPEARS APPROPRIATE to include a chapter devoted to neurology in this handbook for several reasons. Psychiatry and neurology share common historical roots. The psychiatrist and neurologist are both devoted to an understanding of the mind although from different perspectives. Because organic disease of the central nervous system often produces psychiatric symptoms, the psychiatrist must have a fundamental knowledge of neurology and must be prepared to apply it in the day to day clinical setting. Finally, board certification in psychiatry acknowledges the continuing importance of neurological training by requiring candidates to be examined in basic and clinical neurology.

This chapter is designed as a brief guide to the recognition of neurological disorders as they are apt to be encountered in the practice of psychiatry. Special emphasis is placed on the differential diagnosis of certain psychiatric and neurologic entities. Although quite complete, this chapter is not intended as a substitute for comprehensive textbooks in neurology; several are listed as references for the interested reader.

The Neurological Examination is a concise review of the basic clinical examination in neurology. Diagnostic Workup in Neurology reviews the ancillary diagnostic laboratory procedures and offers guidelines for the psychiatrist to follow in requesting these tests; in addition, the procedure for lumbar puncture is reviewed step-by-step since psychiatrists may frequently have to perform this procedure. Differential Diagnosis of Symptoms: Neurological vs. Psychiatric reviews the most common neurological symptoms that the psychiatrist encounters in clinical practice and presents useful information for differential diagnosis, particularly from psychiatric disorders.

THE NEUROLOGICAL EXAMINATION
A. KEITH W. BROWNELL, M.D.

This article outlines the neurological examination. The individual tests of cranial nerves, motor and sensory function, etc. are listed in a step-by-step fashion to aid the psychiatrist in organizing the sequence of the examination and in recalling diagnositic possibilities. For readers interested in a more encyclopedic source of information, the major reference is DeJong's *The Neurological Examination* (DeJong, 1967).

Mental status testing in the neurological examination is very similar to a psychiatric evaluation of mental status. It investigates orientation, cooperativeness, memory, recall, ability for abstract thought, judgment, fund of knowledge, etc. See The Psychiatric History and Mental Status Examination, Chapter II.

I. Cranial Nerves
    A. Olfactory nerve (I.)
        1. Function: Smell
        2. Tests: Ability to distinguish odors presented individually to each nostril
        3. Common causes of abnormalities: Nasal allergy, upper respiratory infection, post-traumatic, tumor affecting olfactory nerve.
    B. Optic nerve (II.)
        1. Function: Vision
        2. Tests:
            a. Acuity by Jaeger cards, newsprint
            b. Visual fields by confrontation and perimetry
            c. Pupillary size at rest
            d. Direct and consensual pupillary reaction

      e. Ophthalmoscopic examination (Funduscopic)
3. Common causes of abnormalities:
      a. Decreased acuity secondary to refractive errors, lens opacity, retinal disease, optic neuitis and optic atrophy.
      b. 1. total loss of vision in one eye = optic nerve disease, retinal vein thrombosis, retinal detachment, glaucoma, other retinopathy.
         2. bitemporal or binasal hemianopsia = chiasmal lesion
         3. homonymous hemianopsia = optic tract, lateral geniculate body, optic radiation or calcarine cortex lesion.
         4. quadrantic defect one eye = retinal disease or chiasmatic lesion.
      c. 1. unilateral dilated pupil = trauma, Adie's syndrome, oculomotor nerve lesion, mydriatic drugs, acute glaucoma, transtentorial herniation.
         2. unilateral constricted pupil = Horner's syndrome, Argyll-Robertson pupil, miotic drugs.
      d. 1. absent direct light reflex = blind eye, eye dilated with mydriactic.
         2. normal direct light reflex but absent consensual response; lesion in midbrain or contralateral oculomotor nerve.
      e. Absence of venous pulsations, venous engorgement, elevation of disc margin and hemorrhages is papilledema of any etiology.
C. Oculomotor (III.); D. Trochlear (IV.); and E. Abducens (VI.)
    1. Function:
      a. motor control of eye
      b. pupillary reaction (along with optic).
    2. Tests:

       a. position of eyes at rest and complete range of eye movements.

       b. pupillary reaction (see optic nerve).

       c. look for nystagmus.

  3. Common causes of abnormalities:

       a. congenital strabismus, isolated lesions of any of the nerves, myasthenia gravis, ocular myopathies and brainstem lesions.

       b. see optic nerves.

       c. disease of eye, vestibular system, cerebellar system or brainstem, anticonvulsant and tranquilizing drugs.

F. Trigeminal (V.)

  1. Function:

       a. Motor to muscles of mastication

       b. Sensory to face

  2. Tests:

       a. Motor: open and close mouth, strength of bite, protrude and retract jaw.

       b. Sensory: all sensory modalities (see sensory examination), corneal reflex.

  3. Common causes of abnormalities:

       a. Motor abnormalities are usually bilateral and secondary to disease in brainstem nuclei, such as motor neuron disease. Entities as myasthenia gravis, primary myopathies and bilateral strokes may be implicated.

       b. See under sensory examination. Decreased corneal reflex seen in contact lens users and abnormalities affecting first division of trigeminal. In many cases cause of isolated trigeminal disturbance is not found. May be present in cerebellopontine angle tumors.

G. Facial (VII.)

  1. Function:

       a. motor to muscles of facial expression.

       b. taste from anterior two-thirds of tongue.

2. Tests:
   a. motor: wrinkle brow, close eyes tightly, retract the angles of mouth and contract platysma.
   b. taste: anterior two-thirds of tongue
3. Common causes of abnormalities:
   a. peripheral paralysis: Bell's palsy, tumor, trauma or infection affecting nerve, myasthenia gravis, motor neuron disease.
   b. central paralysis (brow not affected), cerebral hemisphere lesion, such as stroke or tumor.
   c. unilateral loss of taste: Bell's palsy.
H. Statoacoustic (VIII.)
   1. Function:
      a. hearing.
      b. equilibrium.
   2. Tests:
      a. hearing: whispered voice, watch.
      b. equilibrium: posture, nystagmus, caloric tests.
   3. Common causes of abnormalities:
      a. hearing defect: otologic disease, such as chronic infection, presbycusis, otosclerosis and tumor of nerve.
      b. equilibrium defect: vestibular disease, such as acute infection, trauma, Meniere's and brainstem disease of variable etiology.
I. Glossopharyngeal (IX.) and J. Vagus (X.)
   1. Function:
      a. motor: soft palate, pharynx and larynx.
      b. sensory: all modalities for soft palate and pharynx and taste to posterior one-third of tongue.
   2. Tests:
      a. motor: movement of soft palate and pharynx plus voice assessment.
      b. sensory: taste is rarely tested. Routine sen-

sory testing is confined to touch stimuli to elicit gag reflex.

   3. Common causes of abnormalities:

     a. motor: rarely do isolated lesions occur. Abnormalities usually secondary to brainstem tumor, vascular or degenerative disease or basal meningitis.

     b. sensory: isolated sensory defects rarely occur.

K. Spinal accessory (XI.)

   1. function: motor

   2. tests: strength of sternomastoid and trapezius

   3. common causes of abnormalities: trauma, high cervical cord lesions and basal meningitis.

L. Hypoglossal (XII.)

   1. Function: Motor to tongue

   2. Tests:

     a. observe for atrophy and fasciculation

     b. strength testing

   3. Common causes of abnormalities: Trauma, upper motor neuron disease such as stroke and motor neuron disease.

II. Cerebellar System

A. Function: Coordination of motor activities

B. Tests:

   1. Patient's finger to patient's nose to examiner's finger.

   2. Patient's great toe to examiner's thumb.

   3. Rapid repetitive tapping of hand on a table.

   4. Rapid repetitive tapping of foot on the floor.

   5. Rapid alternating pronation and supination of forearm.

   6. Rapid alternating protrusion and retraction of tongue.

   7. Tremor: postural and intention.

   8. Gait.

C. Common causes of abnormalities:

   1. Drugs: anticonvulsants and tranquilizers

    2. Alcohol: acute and chronic
    3. Tumor
    4. Vascular disease
    5. Hereditary degenerative disease of cerebellum
    6. Multiple sclerosis

III. Motor System
    A. Function: Movement
    B. Tests:
        1. Observation of muscle mass looking for atrophy, hypertrophy or abnormal movements.
        2. Assess tone and check for clonus
        3. Strength testing
        4. Gait
        5. Muscle stretch reflexes (deep tendon reflexes)
        6. Cutaneous reflexes
    C. Common causes of abnormalities:
        1. Tone: clasp knife in upper motor neuron disease, lead pipe in extrapyramidal disease and decreased in lower motor neuron disease.
        2. Muscle atrophy seen in lower motor neuron disease, myopathies and peripheral neuropathies. Hypertrophy is seen in some dystrophies. Abnormal movements include fasciculations (anterior horn cell disease); chorea, tremor and athetosis (basal ganglia disease); myoclonic jerks (pathologic substrate unclear).
        3. Weakness can be generalized as in myasthenia gravis, proximal as in myopathies and distal as in neuropathies. Weakness may be focal as in stroke, root disease or spinal cord disease.
        4. Gait: a spastic gait is seen in hemiplegia, foot drop gait seen in peripheral neuropathy, festinating gait in Parkinsonism and the dancing gait in Huntington's Disease.
        5. Muscle stretch reflexes are decreased in neuropathies, myopathies and anterior horn cell disease and are increased in upper motor neuron disease.

6. Cutaneous reflexes: the Babinski sign is present in upper motor neuron disease, snout and suck reflexes are present in frontal lobe disease.

IV. Sensory System
   A. Function: All sensations
   B. Tests:
      1. Peripheral modalities
         a. touch
         b. vibration
         c. joint position sense
         d. pinprick
         e. temperature
         f. deep pain
      2. Cortical modalities
         a. two-point discrimination
         b. graphesthesia
         c. double-simultaneous stimulation
         d. point localization
   C. Common causes of abnormalities:
      1. Distal involvement of all sensory modalities seen in peripheral neuropathies
      2. In peripheral nerve or dorsal root disorders, the area of sensory abnormality is limited to a localized cutaneous area or a dermatome.
      3. Loss of vibration sense and joint position sense suggests posterior column disease
      4. Dissociated sensory loss suggests spinal cord or brainstem disease
      5. Hemisensory defect suggests lemniscal, thalamic or cortical damage.
      6. Cortical sensory abnormality suggests parietal lobe disease.

DIAGNOSTIC WORKUP IN NEUROLOGY

A. KEITH W. BROWNELL, M.D.

If, after performing a routine neurological examination, the psychiatrist suspects the presence of neurological disease, the customary next step is to request a neurological consultation. There may be instances, however, when it is more expedient for the psychiatrist to proceed to the next diagnostic steps before the neurologist is consulted.

The following outline reviews the basic diagnostic techniques available in neurology and offers the psychiatrist some basic guidelines in how to employ them.

I. Skull x-ray
   A. Indication: Any patient with suspected neurologic disease.
II. Electroencephalogram
   A. Indication: Any patient with suspected neurologic disease.
   B. Preparation:
      1. Ideally, the patient should be off all drugs for one week before the EEG is taken
      2. *Exception:* Never stop anticonvulsant drugs
      3. The hair should be thoroughly washed the night before the EEG
      4. If a sleep record is desired and natural sleep is not obtained, the patient may be given chloral hydrate in the EEG laboratory
      5. Hyperventilation and photic stimulation are routine activating techniques that should be explained to the patient.
      6. Sleep deprivation and drugs can be used as special activating techniques.
III. Echoencephalogram
   A. Indication: Any patient with suspected neurologic disease, especially space-occupying lesions. This is a relatively simple test and requires approximately the same level of patient cooperation as a skull x-ray.
   B. Preparation: None
IV. Brain Scan
   A. Indication:
      1. Focal neurologic abnormality by history
      2. Focal neurologic abnormality on examination
      3. Focal findings on EEF

4. Focal findings on plain skull x-ray.
  B. Preparation: Potassium perchlorate is given prior to brain scanning to block the choroid plexus uptake of isotope. Dosage and timing of dosage varies in different institutions.
  V. Psychometrics: (See Psychological Testing in Clinical Psychiatry, Chapter III.)
 VI. Special studies such as cerebral angiography, pneumoencephalography, myelography and RISA scans.
  A. Indication: Should only be considered after discussion with a neurologic consultant.
VII. Cerebrospinal fluid analysis
  A. Indication:
    1. Suspicion of infection
    2. All other indications are relative
  B. Technique:
    1. Patient is in right or left lateral position
    2. A vertical line drawn from highest point of iliac crest passes through L4-5 interspace
    3. Insert a number 20 or 22 spinal needle into the spinal subarachnoid space at this level, aseptically.
    4. Measure the opening pressure.
    5. Collect cerebrospinal fluid samples
    6. Remove spinal needle. The patient may get up immediately. Rest in bed following a lumbar puncture does not prevent development of a post-lumbar puncture headache.
  C. Procedure for blood tap: If the cerebrospinal fluid is bloody, collect five tubes of fluid and label appropriately. Tube number one is first tube collected, tube number two is second tube collected, etc. Send tubes one, three and five for total red cell counts and have each specimen checked for xanthochromia. If the blood is from a traumatic tap, the total red cell count will fall from tube one to tube three to tube five. If the blood is from a subarachnoid hemorrhage, the total red cell count

will remain the same and xanthochromia likely will be present.

D. Table VIII-I. (Cerebrospinal Fluid, Normal Values) lists the normal values in routine examination of the CSF.

E. Precautions before performing LP:
1. Signed consent
2. Complete neurological exam
3. Rule out papilledema
4. Skull x-ray
   a. rule out pineal shift
   b. rule out erosion of sella turcica

TABLE VIII-I

CEREBROSPINAL FLUID, NORMAL VALUES

Test	Normal Value
Protein	Under 45 mg. percent
-globulin	Under 13 percent of total CSF protein
Colloidal gold	0000000000
Sugar	½ to ⅔ of simultaneously taken blood sugar
Cells	Under 3
Pressure	Under 180 mm. CSF

DIFFERENTIAL DIAGNOSIS OF SYMPTOMS: NEUROLOGICAL VS. PSYCHIATRIC

A. KEITH W. BROWNELL, M.D.

The following is a list of the most common neurological symptoms likely to be encountered by the psychiatrist. Cardinal features of differential diagnosis are outlined to aid the psychiatrist in distinguishing pure neurological illness from neurological manifestations of psychiatric illness. It should be especially useful in psychiatric consultation to medical-surgical units or in the emergency room setting.

I. Headache. Table VIII-II (Headache: Differential Diagnosis) lists differential features that distinguish tension headache, conversion headache and vascular headache.

II. Amnesia. Table VIII-III (Amnesia: Differential Di-

TABLE VIII-II

HEADACHE: DIFFERENTIAL DIAGNOSIS

	Situational Stress, Tension	Conversion Reaction	Vascular
A. Family history	+ or −	+ or −	+
B. Precipating factors	tension	underlying psychiatric disability	tension, alcohol, foods, endocrine
C. Pain location	bifrontal, bitemporal, bioccipital	any location	frequently unilateral
D. Quality of pain	aching, pressure, bandlike	variable	throbbing
E. Duration of pain	as long as tension lasts	days to years	several to 48 hours
F. Associated features	pain in neck, blurred vision, tearing	usually absent	scotomas, sensory and motor deficits, tearing
G. Relief produced by	relaxation	suggestion (in some cases)	rest and sleep
H. Attitude of patient	Distress	Usually some element of belle indifference and secondary gain.	Distress
I. Drug treatment	ASA, muscle relaxants	Psychotropic drugs and/ or psychotherapy	Ergot derivatives

agnosis) distinguishes between organically-determined amnesia and hysterical amnesia.

III. Syncope. Table VIII-IV (Syncope: Differential Diagnosis) distinguishes four causes of syncope: cardiac, vasovagal, orthostatic, and hysterical.

IV. Paralysis
    A. Generalized
        1. Neurologic etiology
            a. periodic paralysis
            b. narcolepsy syndrome
            c. Guillain-Barre syndrome

TABLE VIII-III

AMNESIA: DIFFERENTIAL DIAGNOSIS

	Organic amnesia	Hysterical amnesia
A. Precipitating features	Head trauma, stroke, tumor, subarachnoid hemorrhage, infection, toxins, drugs, electroshock therapy	Psychological stress
B. Onset	gradual or sudden	sudden
C. Associated features	Patient may not complain of defective memory	patient usually complains of inability to remember
	personal identity usually preserved	personal identity usually lost
	frequently there are associated neurologic signs	no associated neurological signs
	patient's amnesia is noted by others	patient frequently appears normal but announces his amnesia to others
D. Recovery	variable but usually some degree of permanent loss even if only for short time	recovery is the rule and amnesic period is usually completely recalled

    2. Hysterical conversion reaction

  B. Focal

    1. Neurologic etiology

      a. cerebrovascular disease

      b. tumors

      c. demyelinating disease

      d. nerve root, plexus or peripheral nerve disease

      e. postictal

    2. Hysterical conversion reaction

  C. Table VIII-V (Paralysis: Differential Diagnosis) distinguishes between neurologic causes of paralysis and hysterical paralysis

  V. Hypersomnia:

    A. Neurologic

      1. Narcolepsy syndrome

      2. Viral encephalitis

      3. Post head trauma

      4. Cerebrovascular disease

      5. Tumors of third ventricle and hypothalamus

TABLE VIII-IV
SYNCOPE: DIFFERENTIAL DIAGNOSIS

	Cardiac	*Vasovagal*	*Orthostatic*	*Hysterical*
A. Precipitating factors	may be none	tight collar, severe pain, sight of blood, other sudden, unexpected psychic trauma	postural change	is person's characteristic style of reacting to stress by histrionic faint
B. Premonitory symptoms	usually none	nausea, blurred vision, weakness, dizziness	usually none	may be of any type; often bizarre
C. Usual circumstances	anywhere, anytime	anywhere, anytime	anywhere, anytime	always in presence of observers
D. Onset	sudden	slow	sudden	slow, dramatic
E. Pulse	absent too slow too rapid	slow and weak	rapid and weak	normal
F. Blood Pressure	unrecordable	low	low	normal
G. Convulsion	may occur	unlikely	unlikely	no
H. Appearance	ashen	cyanotic, sweating, cold	pale, cold	normal
I. Recovery	usually rapid	few minutes but may continue to feel faint for 30 to 45 min.	quick once recumbent posture is attained. May recur on standing.	slow, dramatic

6. Drug intoxication; acute or chronic
B. Psychiatric
1. Depression
2. Schizoid withdrawal phenomenon
3. Catatonic stupor
4. Involutional melochlolia
5. Manic-depressive illness, depressive type
VI. Insomnia:
A. Physiologic in older people
B. Post head-trauma
C. Post encephalitic

TABLE VIII-V

PARALYSIS: DIFFERENTIAL DIAGNOSIS

	Neurologic paralysis	Hysterical paralysis
A. Past History	may be positive	may be positive
B. Patient Type	no particular type	low level of psychological and medical sophistication; frequently female.
C. Precipitating features	infection, heart disease, high carbohydrate intake, vigorous exercise, sleep, trauma, none	emotional stress
D. Onset	slow to rapid	slow to rapid, often dramatic
E. Attitude of patient	very concerned	unconcerned, i.e. belle indifference
F. Secondary Gain	Not present or, if so is incidental to the clinical picture	often a prominent feature and reason for the symptom in the first place
G. Neurologic exam	always abnormal	always normal except for paralysis and sensory deficits which usually do not make sense anatomically
H. Response to reassurance, suggestion, or environmental manipulation	none	may be dramatic cure

D. Post anoxic, hypoglycemia encephalopathy

E. Drug intoxication; acute or chronic

F. Depression

G. Other psychiatric illnesses such as agitated psychosis, manic phase of manic-depressive illness, etc.

VII. Fatigue and Weakness:

    A. Neurologic

        1. Myasthenia gravis

        2. Eaton-Lambert syndrome

        3. Congenital myopathies

        4. Dystrophies and other acquired myopathies

        5. Generalized neuropathies

        6. Drugs

    B. Psychiatric

        1. Depression

2. Neurasthenic, inadequate personality pattern
3. Other

VIII. Sensory Disturbances:

    A. Neurologic
        1. Epilepsy
        2. Migraine
        3. Cerebrovascular disease
        4. Multiple sclerosis
        5. Peripheral neuropathies
        6. Radiculopathies
        7. Delirium tremens

    B. Psychiatric
        1. Hysterical conversion reaction
        2. Hyperventilation syndrome (a form of conversion reaction)
        3. Tactile hallucinations, schizophrenia (diagnosed by presence of other cardinal features of schizophrenia. See Diagnosis of Schizophrenia, Chapter I).

    C. Table VIII-VI (Sensory Disturbance: Differential Diagnosis) distinguishes between neurologic sensory disturbance and hysterical sensory disturbance.

IX. Hallucinations. Table VIII-VII (Hallucination: Differential Diagnosis) distinguishes between hallucinatory phenomena due to neurologic conditions and psychogenic hallucinations.

X. Language Disturbance

    A. Dysarthria; faulty production of speech due to defects in the motor speech apparatus.
        1. Etiology:
            a. upper motor neuron disease, e.g. bilateral cerebral infarcts, motor neuron disease.
            b. lower motor neuron disease affecting cranial nerve nuclei V, VII, IX, X and XII, e.g. brainstem infarction, progressive bulbar palsy, brainstem tumor.
            c. peripheral cranial nerve disease, e.g. trauma, tumors and metabolic disease.

TABLE VIII-VI

SENSORY DISTURBANCE: DIFFERENTIAL DIAGNOSIS

	Neurologic Sensory Disturbance	Hysterical Sensory Disturbance
A. Precipitating Features	variable	emotional stress
B. Onset	gradual to rapid	gradual to rapid, often dramatic
C. Neurologic Exam	may or may not be abnormal	normal except for sensory disturbance which usually does not make sense neurologically
D. Patient Type	no particular type	frequently female, low level of psychological and medical sophistication
E. Attitude of patient	concerned	unconcerned; i.e. belle indifference
F. Secondary Gain	Not present or, if so, usually incidental to the clinical picture	often prominent feature
G. Sensory abnormality	follows anatomical pattern	does not follow anatomical pattern
H. Associated features	headache, altered level of consciousness, pain	none
I. Response to reassurance, suggestion or environmental manipulation	none	good, may be dramatic cure

d. neuromuscular apparatus and muscle disease, e.g. myasthenia gravis and muscular dystrophy.

e. cerebellar disease, e.g. tumor, vascular disease, alcoholic cerebellar degenerations.

f. drugs, e.g. Dilantin, tranquilizers, sedatives

B. Aphasia; Faulty production of meaningful language in spite of an intact motor speech apparatus

1. Types:

a. expressive: lesion in Broca's area

b. receptive: lesion in parieto-temporal area

c. global: site of lesion is variable but usually an extensive cortical or subcortical lesion in the dominant hemisphere.

2. Examination of a patient with aphasia:

TABLE VIII-VII

HALLUCINATION: DIFFERENTIAL DIAGNOSIS

	Neurologic (organic)	Psychiatric
A. Type	Usually visual (formed and unformed)	auditory most common; visual and tactile hallucinations are, by comparison, rare.
B. Associated Features	decreased level of consciousness, as part of a seizure, temporal lobe tumor, decreased visual or auditory perception, narcolepsy syndrome; drug abuse especially hallucinogens, amphetamines	schizophrenia, other functional psychoses
C. Neurologic Exam	frequently abnormal	normal
D. EEG	frequently abnormal	usually normal

a. Determine if the patient can understand verbal communication. This can be done by instructing the patient to do simple tasks, e.g. close your eyes, lift up your right arm, etc.

b. Determine if the patient can understand written communications. This can be done by observing the patient's response to simple written commands, e.g. close your eyes, lift up your right arm, etc.

c. If the patient is unable to respond to verbal communication, further evaluation is restricted to observation of the patient's speech and recording its form and content.

d. An aphasic patient is unable to respond by written word. If a patient appears aphasic but can respond in writing, then the patient is aphonic, not aphasic.

e. Determine the patient's ability to name a group of objects of increasing complexity; e.g. thumb, wristwatch, stem of watch, crystal, etc.

f. If patient is unable to name objects, determine

his ability to identify objects when presented with a list of names of increasing complexity.

    g. Instruct the patient to repeat a sentence the examiner provides.

    h. Instruct the patient to read aloud from a simple passage.

    i. Instruct the patient to write a simple passage dictated by the examiner.

    j. Instruct the patient to copy a simple passage provided by the examiner.

  3. Special features of expressive aphasia:

    a. Little spontaneous speech, poor articulation

    b. Speech comes out in telegram style

    c. Unable to repeat a sentence.

    d. Can carry out commands that do not involve a verbal response.

    e. Great difficulty naming objects.

    f. If given name, can identify the object.

    g. Usually associated with a hemiplegia.

  4. Special features of receptive aphasia:

    a. Spontaneous speech is present, well articulated, normal grammatical skeleton, normal rhythm and melody.

    b. Speech often meaningless because of use of incorrect words and nonsense words.

    c. Usually able to repeat a sentence.

    d. Usually not associated with a hemiplegia.

  5. Etiology of aphasia:

    a. cerebrovascular disease

    b. tumor.

    c. trauma.

    d. metabolic disorder.

    e. postictal.

XI. Seizures:

  A. Major clinical types

    1. Grand mal

    2. *Petit mal*

3. Focal motor or sensory
4. Temporal lobe
5. Myoclonic
6. Akinetic
7. Mixed

B. General characteristics of seizures:
 1. Frequent presence of an aura.
 2. Sudden alteration in state of consciousness.
 3. Presence of motor activity.
 4. Short duration.
 5. Postictal confusion and drowsiness.

C. Etiology:
 1. Idiopathic
 2. Tumors
 3. Drug withdrawal
 4. Post-traumatic
 5. Metabolic
 6. Psychiatric
    a. grand mal seizure on basis of hysterical conversion reaction is relatively rare.
    b. generally more bizarre and dramatic than organic types.
    c. patient rarely gives history of actually hurting himself in a fall to the floor or biting his tongue, etc.
    d. other characteristics listed above do not fit well either.
    e. belle indifference, secondary gain.

D. Special comments on temporal lobe seizures:
 1. Most often confused as being due to psychiatric disease.
 2. Auras frequently consist of altered emotional state, hallucinations and visceral disturbances.
 3. To a casual observer, there may be little evidence of a change in state of consciousness.
 4. Bizarre or stereotyped motor activity may be carried out during the seizure.

TABLE VIII-VIII

TEMPORAL LOBE SEIZURE VS. DISSOCIATIVE STATE

	Temporal lobe seizures	Dissociative states
Precipitating factors	sleep deprivation, hyper-ventilation, failure to take anticonvulsants	terror, guilt, fear, shame; i.e. emotional factors
Aura	frequently present	none
Level of consciousness	may appear nearly normal, show delerium or stupor	may appear nearly normal, show delerium or stupor
Motor activity during attack	very variable, may be bizarre, stereotyped, posturing	very variable, frequently bizarre
Length of an attack	Usually a matter of minutes	may go on for hours, days or weeks
EEG during an attack	abnormal because of spikes, sharp waves or other paroxysmal activity	normal. If abnormal, does not show paroxysmal activity
Appearance after an attack	drowsy, confused	normal
Response to anticonvul-sants	attacks decrease in frequency or stop	no response
Response to psychiatric drugs	may worsen	often improvement
Personality profile	Variable, can occur in people from *normal* to all levels of psychopathology	Usually hysterical personality; the dissociated activity often has a rich symbolic meaning
Emotional reaction to symptom	Concern, worry	Usually indifferent
Secondary Gain	Variable	May be a prominent feature

5. During the period of postictal confusion, the patient may react with physical violence if excessively provoked.

6. It is very doubtful that the only manifestation of a temporal lobe seizure is a rage attack or an episode of directed violence.

7. EEG usually shows spikes, sharp waves or other paroxysmal discharges from the temporal areas.

8. If routine EEG is normal, then a sleep record-is best activating technique.

9. Table VIII-VIII (Temporal Lobe Seizure vs. Dissociative State) distinguishes these two conditions.

References

DeJong, Russell N.: *The Neurologic Examination,* 3rd ed. New York Hoeber Medical Division, Harper and Row, 1967.

Haymaker, Webb: *Bing's Local Diagnosis in Neurologic Disease,* 15th ed. St. Louis, C. V. Mosby Company, 1969.

Merritt, H. Houston: *A Textbook of Neurology,* 4th ed. Philadelphia, Lea and Febiger, 1967.

Brain, The Late Lord and Walton, John N.: *Brain's Diseases of the Nervous System,* 7th ed. London, Oxford University Press, 1969.

Chapter IX

SOMATIC TREATMENTS
IN PSYCHIATRY

A MONG THE MOST IMPORTANT therapeutic tools in Psychiatry are the two major forms of somatic treatment currently in use: psychotropic drugs and the convulsive therapies.
This chapter focuses upon the clinical application of these
forms of treatment.

The section devoted to psychopharmacology provides an
overall guide to clinical use of the five basic types of psychotropic agents: antipsychotic drugs, antiparkinsonism agents,
antidepressants, antianxiety drugs, and the sedative-hypnotics.
The use of lithium compounds in psychiatric practice is
detailed in a separate article. While certain specific commercially-available drugs within each general class of compounds have been selected as prototypes, this does not
represent an endorsement of one particular drug over any
other. The indications and dosages conform to practices
followed in the authors' medical communities but, because
such information is being continually revised, the reader
is advised to consult the latest manufacturers' data and
F.D.A. advisories.

The section devoted to the convulsive therapy outlines
the general indications and contraindications for this form
of treatment, followed by specific guidelines in the use of
both electro-convulsive therapy (ECT) and IndoKlon®.

The importance of accurate record-keeping in both drug
treatment and convulsive therapy is stressed and the reader
is provided with sample record-keeping systems for each
form of treatment.

PSYCHOPHARMACOLOGY

ARLIN BROWN, M.D.

Psychotropic drugs are among the most valuable therapeutic tools available to the psychiatrist. The skillful use of such drugs is based upon a sound understanding of their properties, clinical indications, side effects and other important information.

Equally important, if psychotropic drugs are employed, is an understanding of the purely psychological aspects of prescribing medication. The patient's clinical response to the drug (s) will depend to a large extent on these psychological factors. The clinician must be particularly aware of such dynamic factors as: (1) the psychological meaning of the drug to the patient, (2) the psychological meaning of the drug to the physician, (3) how drug-taking effects transference, (4) how drug-giving effects countertransference.

The following section on psychopharmacology provides a basic guideline to the current use of drugs in psychiatry. Obviously it is not possible to provide detailed, encyclopedic information on every drug currently available. Instead, the most commonly used drugs within each general category are described. For information on drugs not listed, or for further information on the drugs that are mentioned, the reader is referred to the references listed at the end of this section and to the manufacturers' data.

The drugs to be discussed have been divided into five major categories:

1. Antipsychotic drugs
2. Antiparkinsonism drugs
3. Antidepressant drugs
4. Antianxiety drugs
5. Sedative-hypnotic drugs

Antipsychotic Drugs

Probably the most important general category of drugs in psychiatry are the antipsychotic agents (or, *major tranquilizers*) . While there are a great many such drugs currently available, they fall basically into four groups. The clinician is advised that, rather than attempting to master all of the antipsychotic medications, he should select one drug in each major category and learn it well. He can then apply that knowledge in choosing a basic treatment course and may later select other specific drugs within any category as he finds necessary.

Listed below are the four major groups of antipsychotic medications and representative specific drugs within each group:

I. Phenothiazines
    A. Aliphatic Subgroup
        1. Thorazine® (chlopromazine)
        2. Sparine® (promazine)
        3. Vesprin® (triflupromazine)
    B. Piperidine Subgroup
        1. Mellaril® (thioridazine)
        2. Serentil® (mesoridazine)
        3. Quide® (piperacetazine)
    C. Piperazine Subgroup
        1. Stelazine® (trifluoperazine)
        2. Repoise® (butaperazine)
        3. Prolixin®; Permitil® (fluphenazine)
II. Thioxanthenes
    1. Navane® (thiothixine)
    2. Taractan® (chlorprothixene)
III. Butyrophenones
    1. Haldol® (haloperidol)
IV. Rauwolfia derivatives
    1. Serpasil® (reserpine)

The following outline focuses upon these four basic groups of major tranquilizers, with specific clinical information provided for the specific representative drugs.

I. Phenothiazines
    A. General Comments
        1. These drugs are effective in a variety of psychoses and, in particular, in the treatment of schizophrenia.
        2. The exact mechanism of action of these drugs is

not known; however, one of the more widely accepted theories is that the drug blocks access of dopamine from its receptor site at the post-synaptic membranes in the brain.

3. These drugs are contraindicated in CNS depression and in patients with previous hypersensitivity.

4. There is no evidence that one specific drug is better than another for one of the traditional subtypes of schizophrenia.

5. Minimal laboratory work should include a CBC and differential, SGPT and alkaline phosphatase as a baseline and subsequent studies should include WBC, differential, SGPT and alkaline phosphatase. With inpatients the subsequent studies may be obtained once a week for the first month, twice a month for the second month and then monthly until the first six months are over. (See Clinical Record-Keeping In Drug Therapy, this Chapter.)

   a. There are differing opinions as to how frequently laboratory tests should be obtained; however, the important thing to keep in mind is that laboratory tests do not preclude the necessity to closely follow patients clinically. In fact, even a weekly WBC could miss agranulocytosis because of its sometimes abrupt onset, whereas a sore throat, cervical lymphadenopathy and high fever would cause one to consider the possibility of agranulocytosis.

6. Although these drugs can often control psychotic symptoms such as hallucination or delusions and even produce remission in some cases, *they do not cure* the psychosis. Some researchers feel that with the schizophrenic patient a maintenance dose of medication should be continued indefinitely.

7. Precautions

      a. Phenothiazines increase the likelihood of seizures; consequently seizure medications should be increased for patients with a convulsive disorder.

      b. Phenothiazines potentiate CNS depressants

B. Side Effects

  1. Autonomic side effects such as

    a. dry mouth

    b. constipation

    c. urinary retention

  2. Hematologic side effects

    a. blood dyscrasias (i.e. leukopenia, etc.)

    b. agranulocytosis (uncommon)

      1. medication should be discontinued if this occurs.

  3. Cholestatic jaundice

    a. usually subsides upon withdrawing medication.

  4. Extrapyramidal side effects

    a. types

      1. acute dystonias

      2. akathisia

      3. parkinsonism

    b. See section on antiparkinsonism drugs for details of these side effects and how to treat them.

  5. Orthostatic hypotension

    a. rarely occurs to extent that a vasopressor is needed.

    b. If vasopressor is required levarterenol (Levophed®) should be used rather than epinephrine as the latter can paradoxically lower blood pressure further.

  6. Dermatologic side effects such as

    a. skin rash

    b. photosensitivity

C. Comments on administration

  1. Dosage

    a. medication can often be given b.i.d. or in one daily dose once the dosage for the specific patient has been well adjusted. In acute phase of illness use the drug t.i.d. or q.i.d.

    b. If one dose is given h.s. it may not be necessary to also prescribe sleeping medication.

  2. There is no good evidence that two or more antipsychotic drugs used in combination have any advantage over one antipsychotic drug by itself.

  3. If a patient is receiving a tricyclic antidepressant, the anticholinergic activity of the tricyclic itself should decrease the need for an antiparkinsonism drug.

  4. Abrupt discontinuation of medication will not lead to a physiological withdrawal syndrome.

D. Subclasses of phenothiazines
(Three subtypes of phenothiazines are derived on the basis of structural differences within the basic phenothiazine molecule.)

  1. The basic formula of the phenothines is:

  2. The three subtypes are grouped according to the type of side chain substituted as the R_1.

  3. Aliphatic subgroup (See Table IX-I.)

    a. Chlorpromazine (Thorazine) is the best known representative of this subgroup.

    b. Structural formula:

    c. Supposedly get greater sedation with this subgroup and therefore it is of use in more acute, agitated states.

    d. This subgroup is less potent (i.e. more mgs. of drug are needed for similar therapeutic effects) than the piperazines.

    e. Drowsiness, autonomic side effects, and hypotension are more common in this subgroup.

    f. Extrapyramidal side effects occur to a moderate degree.

2. Piperidine subgroup (See Table IX-II)

    a. Thioridazine (Mellaril®) is a good representative of this group.

    b. Structural formula:

    c. Potency of this drug is more like the aliphatic group.

    d. A good drug for outpatient and elderly patients in light of its low incidence of extrapyramidal and autonomic side effects.

    e. More likely to have hypotension with this medication than the piperazine group.

3. Piperazine subgroup (See Table IX-III.)

    a. Fluphenazine (Prolixin®) or trifluoperazine (Stelazine) are good representatives of this group.

    b. Structural formulae:

       1. Prolixin®

TABLE IX-I

ANTIPSYCHOTIC DRUGS: PHENOTHIAZINES (ALIPHATIC SUBGROUP)

Generic Name	Trade Name	How Supplied	Dosage	Special Comments
Chlorpro-mazine	Thora-zine®	Tabs:10,25, 50,100, 200mg Spansules: 30,75,150, 200,300mg Concentrate: 30mg/cc Injectable: 25mg/cc	Intensive Treat-ment:200–1600 mg daily Maintenance Treatment:100–300mg daily	Periodic ocular exams should be done to rule out corneal and len-ticular opacities if given in high doses or over a long period of time.
Proma-mazine	Sparine®	Tabs:10,25, 50,100, 200mg Concentrate: 30,100mg/ cc Injectable: 25,50mg/ cc	Intensive:600–1000mg daily Maintenance:100–300mg daily	IV route not recommended by author.
Triflupro-mazine	Vesprin®	Tabs:10,25, 50mg Concentrate: 10mg/cc Injectable: 10,20mg/cc	Intensive: 150–450mg daily Maintenance:50–150mg daily	

TABLE IX-II

ANTI-PSYCHOTIC DRUGS: PHENOTHIAZINES (PIPERIDINE SUBGROUP)

Generic Name	Trade Name	How Supplied	Dosage	Special Comments
Mesorida-zine	Serentil®	Tabs:10,25, 50,100mg Injectable: 25mg/cc	Intensive:150–400mg daily Maintenance:20–75mg daily	
Piper-aceta-zine	Quide®	Tabs:10, 25mg	Intensive:40–160mg daily Maintenance:20–160mg daily	Contraindicated in pregnant women
Thiorida-zine	Mellaril®	Tabs:10,25, 50,100,150, 200mg Concentrate: 30mg/cc	Intensive:200–800mg daily Maintenance:40–180mg daily	Doses above 800mg daily are to be avoided because of possibility of pigmentary retinopathy

2. Stelazine®

c. Potency relatively higher in this group.

d. Incidence of extrapyramidal side effects increased as compared to other subgroups of phenothiazines.

e. Hypotensive and sedative effects are felt to be somewhat less than other subgroups.

f. Frequently these drugs are more preferred for the chronic schizophrenic patient.

II. Thioxanthenes (See Table IX-IV)

A. Quite similar to phenothiazines in both structure and actions.

1. basic structural formula:

2. This structure differs from that of the phenothiazines in that the R_1 is double bonded to a carbon instead of a single bond to a nitrogen.

3. Knowledge of phenothiazine subgroup structures can be transferred to that of thioxanthenes according to sidechain differences.

B. Thiothixene (Navane) is a representative of this group.

C. Structural formula:

TABLE IX-III

ANTIPSYCHOTIC DRUGS: PHENOTHIAZINES (PIPERAZINE SUBGROUP)

Generic Name	Trade Name	How Supplied	Dosage	Special Comments
Aceto-phena-zine	Tindal®	Tab:20mg	Intensive:60–120mg daily Maintenance:40–60mg daily	
Buta-pera-zine	Repoise®	Tabs:5,10, 25mg	Intensive:30–100mg daily Maintenance:15–30mg daily	Do not exceed 100mg daily
Flu-phena-zine	Permi-til®	Tabs:0.25,1, 2,.5,10mg Chromotab: 1mg Concentrate: 5mg/cc	Intensive:6–20mg daily Maintenance:2–12mg daily	Monitor BUN for renal impairment with long term treatment. Persistent pseudo-parkinsonism syndrome may occur with chronic administration. Caution with doses greater than 20mg daily. Do not exceed 10mg daily by IM route.
	Pro-lixin®	Tabs:1,2.5, 5mg Elixir:0.5mg /cc Injectable: 2.5mg/cc		
Flu-phena-zine Enan-thate	Pro-lixin Enan-thate®	Injectable: 25mg/cc	Usual dose 25mg IM every 2 weeks Usual range 12.5–100mg every 2 weeks	This drug can be of benefit in chronic patient who is unreliable in taking oral medication; Required only every 2 weeks
Per-phena-zine	Trila-fon®	Tabs:4,8, 16mg Repetabs: 8mg Concentrate: 16mg/5cc Injectable: 5mg/cc	Intensive:12–48mg daily Maintenance:6–24mg daily	Do not exceed 64mg daily
Pro-chlor-pera-zine	Com-pazine®	Tabs:5,10, 25mg Spansule:10, 15, 30, 75mg Concentrate: 10mg/cc Injectable: 5mg/cc	Intensive:50–150mg daily Maintenance:15–60mg daily	

TABLE IX-III Continued

Generic Name	Trade Name	How Supplied	Dosage	Special Comments
Thio-propa-zate	Dartal®	Tabs:5,10mg	Intensive:60–90mg daily Maintenance:10–45mg daily	
Tri-fluo-pera-zine	Stela-zine®	Tabs:1,2,5,10mg Concentrate:10mg/cc Injectable:2mg/cc	Intensive:20–40mg daily Maintenance:4–30mg daily	

    D. Side effects compared to the phenothiazines
       1. Generally fewer side effects and less toxic.
       2. Increased incidence of extrapyramidal side effects.
       3. Decreased incidence of
          a. hepatotoxicity
          b. hematologic side effects
          c. photosensitivity type of reactions
III. Butyrophenones (See Table IX-V.)
    A. Pharmacologically similar but chemically different than the phenothiazines.
    B. Haloperidol (Haldol®) is the only butyrophenone available in the U. S. at this time.
    C. Appears to be at least as effective as the phenothiazines and provides an alternative when a patient develops an allergic reaction to any of the phenothiazines.
    D. Side effects compared to phenothiazines
       1. No evidence of liver damage with haloperidol.
       2. No evidence of significant blood dyscrasias with haloperidol.
       3. Lower incidence of autonomic side effects.
       4. Higher incidence of extrapyramidal side effects.
       5. Other types of side effects are similar for both classes of drugs.

TABLE IX-IV

ANTI-PSYCHOTIC DRUGS: THIOXANTHENES

Generic Name	Trade Name	How Supplied	Dosage	Special Comments
Chlor-prothi-xene	Tarac-tan®	Tabs:10,25, 50,100mg Concentrate: 20mg/cc Injectable: 25mg/2cc	Intensive:150– 600mg daily Maintenance:50– 150mg daily	Similar to aliphatic phenothiazines Postural hypotension possible
Thio-thixene	Navane®	Caps:1,2,5, 10mg Concentrate: 5mg/cc Injectable: 2mg/cc	Intensive:20–60mg daily Maintenance:10– 30mg daily	Similar to pipera-zine phenothia-zines Rarely get benefit with dose greater than 60mgm daily.

E. Like rauwolfia group it appears to have some po·tential to cause depression.

IV. Rauwolfia compounds (See Table IX-VI.)

A. This group is not as effective as phenothiazines and other antipsychotic agents and is chemically different than the phenothiazines.

B. Reserpine (Serpasil®) is a representative of this group.

C. Causes 10 to 15 percent of patients to become depressed.

D. High percentage (70 percent) of patients experience extrapyramidal side effects at therapeutic levels.

E. Rarely used except in patients who have allergic reactions to all other agents.

TABLE IX-V

ANTI-PSYCHOTIC DRUGS: BUTYROPHENONES

Generic Name	Trade Name	How Supplied	Dosage	Special Comments
Halope-ridol	Haldol®	Tabs:0.5,1,2, 5mg Concentrate: 2mg/cc Injectable: 5mg/cc	Intensive:3–15mg daily Maintenance:2– 6mg daily	Do not use epine-phrine for hypo-tension. Usually do not need to exceed 15mg daily.

TABLE IX-VI

ANTI-PSYCHOTIC DRUGS: RAUWOLFIA DERIVATIVES

Generic Name	Trade Name	How Supplied	Dosage	Special Comments
Reser-pine	Serpasil® (and others)	Tabs:0.1, 0.25,1mg Elixir: 0.2mg/4cc Injectable: 2.5mg/cc	25–50mg T.I.D. Intensive:1–5mg daily Maintenance:1–2mg daily	Contraindicated in peptic ulcer, ulcerative colitis, aortic insufficiency and patients receiving ECT. Depression may occur and may last several months after withdrawal of drug. Discontinue drug if depression occurs.

Antiparkinsonism Drugs

The antiparkinsonism drugs are commonly employed to control extrapyramidal side effects of the antipsychotic agents. Because they are not themselves primary therapeutic agents, the use of antiparkinsonism drugs tends to be imprecise and haphazard. The following outline presents important clinical information relating to the proper use of these drugs.

    I. Extrapyramidal symptoms can be roughly grouped into three categories. The most commonly encountered symptoms within each category are listed:

        A. Parkinsonian syndrome
1. Drooling
2. Flexed extremities
3. Mask-like facies
4. Muscle pain
5. Rigidity
6. Shuffling gait
7. Tremor

        B. Acute dystonias
1. Twisting spasms of head and neck
2. Oculogyric crises
3. Protrusion of the tongue

        C. Akathisia
1. Driven restlessness, particularly in the legs

2. Body rocking

3. Repetitive movements

D. When any of the above are present, one should consider employing antiparkinsonism agents.

E. In more dramatic reactions such as oculogyric crises, these drugs should be given IM so that onset of action will occur within minutes.

F. The possibility of both psychological and organic diseases causing such symptoms should be considered.

II. Mechanism of Action

A. The exact mechanism of action of these drugs is not known but it appears that it is their anticholinergic properties that are most important therapeutically.

III. Contraindications

A. In general, these drugs are contraindicated in:

1. Glaucoma.

2. Obstructive gastrointestinal disease.

3. Obstructive genitourinary tract disease.

IV. Further Guidelines on Usage

A. At present it is advised that these drugs *not* be used prophylacticly because:

1. They do not appear to prevent extrapyramidal side effects (although they do lessen them if they occur).

2. They may cause unnecessary anticholinergic side effects.

3. They may augment the anticholinergic side effects of the antipsychotic agents.

B. If the antiparkinsonism medication fails to control extrapyramidal symptoms, one should:

1. Reduce the antipsychotic medication, or

2. Discontinue the specific type of antipsychotic medication in favor of another one.

C. Many patients may be taken off antiparkinsonism agents without ill effect after three months; a minority of patients will require these medications continuously as long as they are receiving antipsychotics.

V. Side Effects
   A. Most side effects can be predicted on the basis of the anticholinergic activity of these drugs.
   B. The most common side effects include:
      1. Blurred vision.
      2. Dizziness.
      3. Gastric irritation.
      4. Lethargy.
VI. Table IX-VII outlines clinical information for the major antiparkinsonism drugs.

Antidepressant Drugs

Another important group of drugs in psychiatry are the antidepressants. There are two major types currently in use: the tricyclic group and the monoamine oxidase inhibitors. The use of psychostimulants such as the amphetamines is controversial and the potential of abuse is high (See Central Nervous System Stimulants, Chapter X); amphetamines are

TABLE IX-VII

ANTIPARKINSONISM DRUGS

Generic Name	Trade Name	How Supplied	Dosage
Benztropine Mesylate	Cogentin®	Tabs: 0.5,1,2mg Injectable:1mg/cc	1–8 mg daily; 2 mg IM or IV for acute dystonic reaction
Biperidin	Akineton®	Tab: 2mg Injectable: 5mg/cc	2–6 mg daily; 2mg IM or IV q. ½ hr. until symptoms abate, not to exceed four doses in 24 hrs.
Diphenhydramine	Benadryl®	Caps: 25,50mg Elixir:12.5mg/5cc Injectable:10,50mg/ cc	25–50mg t.i.d. 50 mg IM or IV for acute dystonic reaction
Orphenadrine	Disipal®	Tab; 50mg	150–250mg daily
Procyclidine	Kemadrin®	Tabs:2,5mg	6–20mg daily
Trihexyphenidyl	Artane® (and others)	Tabs;2,5mg Sequels: 5mg Elixir:2mg/5cc	5–15mg daily

not generally considered to be a drug of choice in the treatment of depression by psychiatrists. Drugs such as antianxiety agents (minor tranquilizers) and antipsychotics (major tranquilizers) are occasionally employed by themselves or in combination with antidepressants in cases of agitated or psychotic depression.

The following outline summarizes the proper use of all of these drugs and combinations.

I. Tricyclic Agents (See Table IX-VIII.)
   A. Classified according to structure:
      1. Dibenzazepines
         a. structural formula:

$$CH_2-CH_2$$

$$N$$

$$CH_2-CH_2-CH_2-N\begin{array}{c}R\\CH_3\end{array}$$

         b. note similarity to phenothiazine nucleus
         c. different from phenothiazine in that S atom is replaced by an ethylene group as a bridge between the two benzene rings
         d. imipramine (Trofranil,® Presamine®) : R = CH_3
         e. desipramine (Norpramin®, Pertofrane®): R = H
      2. Dibenzocycloheptenes
         a. structural formula:

$$CH-CH_2-CH_2-N\begin{array}{c}R\\CH_3\end{array}$$

         b. note similarity to thioxathene nucleus
         c. bridge between two benzene rings is ethylene group instead of S atom

    d. amitriptyline (Elavil®) : $R = CH_3$
    e. notriptyline (Aventyl®) : $R = H$
    f. protryptyline (Vivactil®) : like nortriptyline except there is a double bond (shown as the dashed double bond above) .
  3. Dibenzoxepins
    a. structural formula:

    b. note similarity to amitryptiline but ethylene bridge between two benzene rings is replaced by $-CH_2-O-$.
    c. doxepin (Sinequan®) is prototype
B. Indications
  1. Depression
  2. It is generally believed that antidepressants are more effective in cases of endogenous (nonsituational) depression than in reactive (situational) depression. Clinically, it is not always easy to distinguish clearly between the two. Selection of antidepressant medication, then, is usually best made on the basis of the presenting symptom constellation.
  3. Look especially for following symptoms:
    a. depression experienced as physical illness
    b. blunted affect
    c. psychomotor retardation
    d. insomnia
    e. anorexia
    f. social withdrawal
  4. Use of established rating scales can be helpful in diagnosis and management (See Self-Rating Depression Scale, Chapter III.)
C. Contraindications
  1. Comatose states

2. Glaucoma
3. Urinary retention tendency (such as prostatic hypertrophy)
4. History of agranulocytosis
5. Hypersensitivity to these medications
6. Recent myocardial infarct

D. Precautions
1. Patient may become greater suicidal risk as he begins to emerge from severe, retarded depression.
2. Severe constipation.
3. Latent schizophrenia (may become floridly psychotic).
4. Mania may occur as patient emerges from depression.
5. Pregnancy (risks should be outweighed by benefits).
6. Monoamine oxidase inhibitors.
   a. most researchers feel that these drugs should not be used in combination with tricyclics.
   b. do not use tricyclics until MAO inhibitors have been discontinued for at least two weeks.
   c. do not use MAO inhibitors until tricyclics have been discontinued for at least three days.

E. Mechanism of actions
1. Exact mechanism is not known but most widely accepted hypothesis is that tricyclics increase norepinephrine (NE) at critical brain receptors.
2. Tricyclics act at adrenergic nerve endings both centrally and peripherally.
   a. they inhibit the reuptake at the nerve ending of NE released into the synaptic space.
   b. this action allows NE to act longer at post synaptic receptor sites.

F. Side effects
1. Common side effects
   a. dry mouth
   b. constipation

       c. blurred vision

       d. excess perspiration

   2. Other side effects

       a. heartburn or nausea

       b. drowsiness

       c. mild agitation

       d. hypotension (if severe do *not* treat with epinephrine but with levarterenol (Levophed®.)

       e. cholestatic jaundice (rare)

       f. agranulocyrosis (rare)

G. Comments on administration

   1. Tricyclics lower seizure threshold so additional anticonvulsant medications should be given to epileptics.

   2. Physical dependence does *not* occur but headache, nausea and malaise may occur if drug is abruptly discontinued.

   3. Dosage should be decreased for elderly and debilitated.

   4. These drugs carry a greater suicidal risk than the phenothiazines and should be prescribed in small amounts for patients with significant suicide potential.

   5. Drugs may take from three days to three to four weeks to take effect.

   6. Begin treatment with a low initial dose and build up to higher dosage levels gradually over several days.

   7. If a specific drug has no effect after several weeks, it should be discontinued in favor of another tricyclic or other therapy.

   8. Keep patient on medication for about three to six months (hopefully for at least the amount of time one would estimate to be on normal course of the depression).

   9. When the medication is discontinued, it should be tapered gradually over several weeks.

a. During this time the physician must be alert for signs of recurrent depression.

10. Amitriptyline (Elavil®) and imipramine (Tofranil®, Prosamine®) are drugs that should be considered prototypes and known well; most clinical experience has been with these drugs.

11. Amitriptyline (Elavil) and nortriptyline (Aventyl®) have more sedative effect than other tricyclics; doxepin (Sinequan®) has antianxiety action.

12. Intramuscular forms of these medications are not commonly used; Parenteral use is reserved for the uncooperative patient. Treatment should be converted to the oral route as soon as feasible.

II. Monoamine Oxidase Inhibitors (See Table IX-IX)
   A. Indications
      1. These drugs are indicated for the same disorders as the tricyclics but the tricyclics are the drugs of first choice since they are more effective and have fewer dangerous side effects than MAO inhibitors.

TABLE IX-VIII

ANTIDEPRESSANT DRUGS: TRICYCLIC AGENTS

Generic Name	Trade Name	How Supplied	Dosage
Amitriptyline	Elavil®	Tabs:10,25,50mg Injectable:10mg/cc	Inpatients:75–225mg daily Outpatients:50–150mg daily
Nortriptyline	Aventyl®	Pulvules:10,25mg Liquid:10mg/5cc	Inpatients:40–100mg daily Outpatients:20–100mg daily
Protriptyline	Vivactil®	Tabs:5,10mg	Inpatients:15–60mg daily Outpatients:10–40mg daily
Imipramine	Tofranil®	Tabs:10,25,50mg Injectable:25mg/cc	Inpatients:75–225mg daily Outpatients:50–150mg daily
	Presamine®	Same as above	
Desipramine	Norpramin®	Tabs:25,50mg	Inpatients:75–200mg daily Outpatients:75–150mg daily
	Pertofrane®	Caps:25,50mg	
Doxepin	Sinequan®	Caps:10,25,50mg	Inpatients:75–225mg daily Outpatients:50–150mg daily

2. Three situations in which MAO inhibitors may be used:
   a. patient has not responded to an adequate trial of tricyclics
   b. allergic reaction to tricyclics
   c. previous episode of depression that responded well to MAO inhibitor

B. Contraindications
   1. Cerebrovascular defect
   2. Cardiovascular disease
   3. Advanced liver damage
   4. Hypersensitivity to these drugs
   5. Manifest mania
   6. Pheochromocytoma

C. Precautions
   1. Avoid using with the following medications
      a. anticholinergic medications
      b. tricyclics (see under precautions of tricyclics)
      c. other MAO inhibitors
         1. wait ten days before switching from one MAO inhibitor to another
      d. amphetamines or sympathomimetics
      e. MAO inhibitors potentiate CNS depressants such as:
         1. barbiturates
         2. narcotics
         3. general anesthetics
      f. insulin
      g. antihypertensive agents
   2. In pregnancy possible benefits should outweigh risks
   3. Latent schizophrenia (may become floridly psychotic)
   4. Patient may become greater suicidal risk as he begins to emerge from severe retarded depression
   5. Mania may occur as depression lifts
   6. Can lower seizure threshold

7. Certain foods taken with MAO inhibitors may precipitate a hypertensive crisis (see side effects) :
   a. alcohol
   b. cheese
   c. chicken liver
   d. pods of broad beans
   e. pickled herring
   f. caffeine (patient should not drink more than six cups of coffee per day)
D. Mechanism of action
   1. MAO inhibitors act at sympathetic nerve endings to inhibit monoamine oxidase, an enzyme
   2. This inhibition results in less norepinephrine being metabolized, which in turn makes more available for synaptic transmission
E. Side effects
   1. Autonomic side effect include:
      a. dry mouth
      b. constipation
   2. Drowsiness.
   3. Dizziness.
   4. Orthostatic hypotension.
   5. Insomnia.
   6. Agitation.
   7. Hepatocellular jaundice.
   8. Hypertensive crisis.
      a. MAO inhibitors prevent metabolism of other amines (such as tryptophan or tyramine).
      b. Consequently when such amines are taken into the body from certain food sources (see precautions), they build up to excessive levels and cause hypertensive crisis.
F. Comments on administration
   1. Physician should instruct patient in:
      a. dietary restrictions.
      b. dangers of other medications that may be harmful

     1. Common over-the-counter preparations should be avoided (e.g. nose drops, cold pills, etc.).

     c. informing physician of any side effects, especially headache.

  2. In general a priming dose is initiated and this is then cut back to a maintenance dose.

  3. Duration of treatment is similar to tricyclics.

  4. These drugs can be used for suicidal purposes; thus, they should be prescribed in small quantities for patients with significant suicidal potential.

  5. Medication should be slowly tapered when discontinued.

  6. Drug dependence does not occur although abrupt withdrawal may cause a blood pressure rise, precordial discomfort, and tachycardia.

III. Other Drugs Used in Treatment of Depression

  A. Phenothiazines

    1. Drugs such as chlorpromazine (Thorazine)

TABLE IX-IX

ANTIDEPRESSANT DRUGS: MAO INHIBITORS

Generic Name	Trade Name	How Supplied	Dosage
Isocarboxazid	Marplan®	Tabs:10mg	initially use 30mg daily; with clinical improvement decrease to 10–20mg daily.
Nialamide	Niamid®	Tabs:25,100mg	initially use 100–150mg daily; with improvement decrease to maintenance dose of 50–75mg daily. Do not exceed 500mg daily.
Phenelzine	Nardil®	Tabs:15mg	Initially 45mg daily if improvement decrease to maintenance of 15mg daily. Do not exceed 75mg daily.
Tranylcypromine	Parnate®	Tabs: 10mg	initially 20mg daily; if no improvement in 2 weeks may increase to 30mg daily; if improvement maintain on 10mg daily.

and thioridiazine (Mellaril) are of value in agitated depressions.

2. The combination of a phenothiazine and a tricyclic may be used where the distinction between a psychotic depression and schizoaffective reaction with depression is clouded and in the depressive phase of schizophrenia that sometimes follows the acute psychotic break.

    a. Perphenazine in combination with amitriptyline is available in fixed dosages (Triavil®, Etrafon®)

        1. There is less freedom of adjustment with such fixed combinations but they can be used if a maintenance level can be established in dosages available.

        2. Available fixed dosages include combinations of perphenazine two and four mg with amytriptyline 10 and 25 mg. (Further information is available about each of these drugs where they are discussed separately.)

B. Antianxiety agents

  1. Antianxiety agents such as diazepam (Valium) may be of value in mild depressions that are associated with anxiety, tension or mild agitation.

C. Psychostimulants

  1. The use of such medications as amphetamine in the treatment of depression is controversial and not well established.

    a. the potential for abuse of these drugs is a substantial argument against their use. (See Central Nervous System Stimulants, Chapter X.)

D. Electroconvulsive therapy

  1. In severe depressions with a high suicide potential ECT is often the treatment of choice since antidepressant medications customarily re-

quire a period of a few days to as long as three to four weeks to become effective.

2. Antidepressants, if appropriate, can be used concurrently with ECT.

3. See section on the convulsive therapies in this chapter.

Antianxiety Drugs

The antianxiety drugs (also called *minor tranquilizers*) produce mild sedation at doses which are unlikely to have a hypnotic effect, unlikely to adversely affect psychomotor performance, or to adversely affect clarity of consciousness. These agents, therefore, have largely replaced the sedative-hypnotics for use as tranquilizers.

Currently there are many such drugs available commercially. The following outline focuses upon the two major groups of antianxiety drugs currently in use (the propanediol derivatives and the benzodiazepines) and offers basic clinical information on some of the other more widely used tranquilizers.

Table IX-X summarizes important prescribing information for representative drugs within each major group.

I. Propanediol Derivatives
   A. Representative Members
      1. Miltown® (meprobamate)
      2. Solacen® (tybamate)
   B. Indications
      1. Anxiety in psychoneuroses and psychosomatic illnesses.
      2. Agitation.
      3. Nervous tension and restlessness.
      4. Not indicated in psychosis.
   C. Contraindications
      1. Previous hypersensitivity to drugs of this class.
      2. Acute intermittent porphyria.
   D. Precautions

  1. Possible benefits should outweigh risks in pregnancy.
  2. Ability to operate machinery or automobile may be impaired.
  3. Can potentiate and be potentiated by other CNS depressants.
  4. Psychological and physical dependence has occurred with meprobate (Miltown) and although this has not occurred with tybamate (Solacen), the possibility of this occurring with these drugs should be kept in mind.
  5. Administer cautiously in patients with impaired renal function and liver disease.
E. Clinical effects of importance
  1. Sedative effect.
  2. Muscle relaxant activity.
F. Mechanism of action
  1. Unknown.
G. Side effects
  1. Drowsiness.
  2. Confusion (more commonly in the elderly).
  3. Ataxia
  4. Dizziness
  5. Headache
  6. Blood dyscrasias (rarely)
  7. Jaundice (rarely)
H. Comments on administration
  1. Minimal effective dose should be established in order to prevent oversedation in the elderly or debilitated.
  2. There is large individual variance in response to these medications and dosage should be individualized within the ranges stated.
  3. Minimal amount of drug should be given to minimize the suicide risk.
  4. Medication should be tapered slowly over 2 weeks if patient has been receiving excessive medication.

II. Benzodiazepines
  A. Representative members:
    1. Librium® (chlordiazopoxide).
    2. Valium (diazepam).
    3. Serax® (oxazepam).
  B. Indications
    1. Same as propanediol derivatives.
    2. Treatment of delirium tremens.
    3. Not indicated in psychosis.
  C. Contraindications
    1. Previous hypersensitivity to these drugs.
  D. Precautions
    1. Possible benefits should outweigh risks in pregnancy.
    2. Can potentiate and be potentiated by other CNS depressants.
    3. Like propanediols, if taken in excessive doses for long periods of time, psychological and physical dependence can occur.
    4. Ability to operate machinery or automobile may be impaired.
    5. For long term use, periodic CBC, SGPT and alkaline phosphatase should be obtained.
  E. Mechanism of action
    1. Unknown.
  F. Side effects and clinical effects
    1. See propanediol derivatives.
  G. Comments on administration
    1. See comments on administration of propanediol derivatives.
  H. Miscellaneous comments
    1. The benzodiazepines are the most widely prescribed antianxiety agents at the present time.
    2. As with other antianxiety agents, they are believed to have a much wider margin of safety than barbiturates in the event of an overdose.
III. Other Agents
  A. Diphenylmethane Derivatives

1. Representative of group:
   a. Vistaril® (hydroxyzine).
   b. This is a rather heterogeneous group and the following information is related specifically to this representative, which is most widely used drug of this group.
2. Indications
   a. same as propanediol derivatives.
3. Contraindications
   a. early pregnancy.
   b. previous hypersensitivity to this drug.
4. Precautions
   a. can potentiate CNS depressants such as
      1. narcotics.
      2. barbiturates.
   b. injectable should only be given IM, not intravenously.
5. Clinical effects
   a. mild sedation.
   b. antihistaminic.
   c. anticholinergic.
6. Mechanism of action
   a. unknown.
7. Side effects
   a. drowsiness.
   b. dry mouth.
   c. tremors and convulsions (rarely).
8. Comments on administration
   a. There is large individual variance in response to this medication and dosage should be individualized within the ranges stated.
   b. Physical dependence is not reported with this medication.

Sedative-Hypnotic Drugs

The sedative-hypnotics are drugs that in small doses have the effect of reducing anxiety, tension and agitation; in larger doses they induce sleep. Once used for their tran-

TABLE IX-X

ANTIANXIETY DRUGS

Generic Name	Trade Name	How Supplied	Dosage (in divided doses)	Special Comments
Mepro-bamate	Mil-town® (and others)	Tabs:200, 400mg Spansules: 200,400mg	usually 1200–1600mg daily; Do not exceed 2400mg daily.	
Tyba-mate	Solacen® (and others)	Caps:250, 350mg	usually 750–2000mg daily; Do not exceed 3000mg daily	
Chlor-diaze-poxide	Lib-rium®	Caps:5,10, 25mg Tabs:5,10, 25mg Injectable: 100mg to be dis-solved	usually 10–100mg daily; Try not to exceed 300mg daily	For delirium tre-mens: 50–100mg IM q.2 to 4 hours prh
Diaze-pam	Valium®	Tabs:2,5, 10mg Injectable: 5mg/cc	usually 4–40mg daily	Contraindicated in acute narrow an-gle glaucoma. For delirium tre-mens: 10mg IM q3–4 hours prn.
Oxaze-pam	Serax®	Caps:10,15, 30mg Tabs:15mg	usually 30–120mg daily	For delirium tre-mens: 15–30mg t.i.d. to q.i.d.
Hydrox-yzine	Vistaril®	Caps:25,50, 100mg Suspension: 5mg/cc Injectable: 25,50mg/cc	usually 75–400mg daily	

quilizing properties, they have been largely replaced by the newer antianxiety agents in this area and currently are used in psychiatry almost exclusively as hypnotic agents (sleepers).

The sedative-hypnotics can be classified into two major groups: the barbiturates and the nonbarbiturates.

The following outline summarizes the proper use of these drugs.

I. Barbiturates (See Table IX-XI)
    A. Indications
        1. Insomnia.

2. Same as propanediol derivatives.
3. Amytal interview (See Barbiturate Interview, Chapter III).

B. Contraindications
1. Hypersensitivity to barbiturates.
2. Acute intermittent porphyria.

C. Precautions
1. Physical and psychological dependence can develop.
    a. This is one of the major factors against using barbiturates as daytime sedatives or tranquilizers.
    b. See Central Nervous System Depressants, Chapter X.
2. Potentiate CNS depressants.
3. Can induce enzyme production in the liver which can increase the rate of metabolism of such drugs as:
    a. diphenylhydantoin (Dilantin)
    b. warfarin (Coumadin®)
4. Hepatic and renal impairment.
5. Avoid long-term use.

D. Mechanism of action
1. Depression of cerebral cortex.

E. Side effects
1. Drowsiness.
2. Lethargy.
3. Residual sedation (hangover).
4. Paradoxical excitement (rarely).
5. Skin eruptions.

F. Comments on administration
1. In treating outpatients, small amounts of the drug should be prescribed at any one time because of the dangers of abuse, dependence and overdose.
2. Have been replaced as sedatives by antianxiety drugs and are now primarily used as hypnotics.
    a. Amytal is still considered a very effective

sedative in more emergent situations and can be given IM to a combative or severely agitated patient.

3. Taper dose slowly in patients who have been on the medication for long periods in order to avoid withdrawal syndrome (See Central Nervous Systems Depressants, Chapter X, for step-by-step method of withdrawing patients from barbiturates).

4. There is great variability in effective individual dosage and suggested dosages are merely rough guidelines for sedation.

II. Nonbarbiturates (See Table IX-XII.)

A. General comments

1. These medications represent a rather heterogeneous group chemically but are similar in that they all produce a reversible nonspecific depression of the CNS.

2. Because of their heterogeneity only a few general statements will be included in the following tables.

a. Indicated for same states as propanediol derivatives and insomnia.

b. These drugs have been largely replaced as sedatives by the antianxiety agents and are now primarily used as hypnotics.

c. Contraindicated in those who have shown previous hypersensitivity to a specific drug.

d. Potentiate other CNS depressants.

e. Decreased doses should be used in the elderly and debilitated.

f. Minimal amounts of drugs should be prescribed because of danger of abuse or overdose.

g. Physical and psychological dependence has occurred with most of these drugs; the others should be considered to have such potential until proven otherwise.

h. Avoid long-term use.

TABLE IX-XI

SEDATIVE-HYPNOTIC DRUGS: BARBITURATES

Generic Name	Trade Name	How Supplied	Dosage	Special Comments
Amo-bar-bital	Amytal (and others)	Tabs:15,30, 50,100mg Pulvules:65, 200mg Elixir: 440mg/ 100cc, 880mg/ 100cc Injectable: concentra-tion de-pends on amount of sterile wa-ter added.	Seadtive:30–50mg b.i.d.–q.i.d Hypnotic:100–200mg h.s.	for emergency sedation: 250mg IM Is shortest-acting barbiturate. Do not exceed 500mg IM in one dose. More commonly used as sedative than for sleep.
Pheno-bar-bital	Lum-inal® (and others)	Tabs:16, 32mg Injectable: 130mg/cc	Sedative:15–30mg b.i.d.–q.i.d Hypnotic:100–200mg h.s.	Do not exceed 600mg in 24 hours. more commonly used for seda-tion than sleep.
Pento-bar-bital	Nem-butal® (and others)	Caps:30,50, 100mg Tabs (long release form) : 100mg Elixir:20mg/ 5cc Supposito-ries:30,60, 120,200mg Injectable: 50mg/cc	Sedative:30–60mg b.i.d.–q.i.d Hypnotic:100–200mg h.s.	more commonly used as a hypnotic
Seco-bar-bital	Seconal®, Tui-nal®, (and others)	Caps:30,50, 100mgm Supposito-ries:30,60, 120, 200mgm Elixir: 22mgm/ 5cc Injectable: variable concentra-tions	Sedative:30–50mgm b.i.d.–q.i.d Hypnotic:100–200mgm h.s.	More commonly used as hypnotic. Injectable form can also be given rectally.

TABLE IX-XII
SEDATIVE-HYPNOTIC DRUGS: NONBARBITURATES

Generic Name	Trade Name	How Supplied	Dosage	Contraindications	Side Effects	Precautions	Special Comments
Chloral betaine	Beta-Chlor®	Tabs:870mg	Hypnotic:1–2 tabs 15–30 minutes before h.s.	marked liver or renal impairment	gastric irritation, excitement	severe cardiac disease; may need to increase dose of other medications	rapid, reliable, and inexpensive; can avoid unpleasant taste with capsule
Chloral hydrate	Noctec® (and others)	Caps:250,500mg Syrup:100mg/cc	Sedative:250mg t.i.d. p.c. Hypnotic:500–1000mg h.s.	marked liver or renal impairment	gastric irritation, excitement	Do not exceed 2000mg daily caution in using simultaneously with warfarin (Coumadin®)	less predictable than chloral hydrate
Ethchlorvynol	Placidyl®	Caps:100,200, 500,750mg	Hypnotic:500–750mg h.s.	porphyria	nausea, vomiting, hypotension, blurred vision, aftertaste, dizziness, facial numbness, urticaria	Toxic amblyopia may occur with long term use; Not recommended for first 6 months of pregnancy.	
Ethinamate	Valmid®	Tabs:500mg	Hypnotic:500–1000mg h.s.		mild G.I. symptoms, skin rashes	Not recommended in pregnancy	good for mild degrees of insomnia

Generic	Trade	Forms	Dose	Side effects	Precautions	Comments
Flurazepam	Dalmane®	Caps:15,30mg	Hypnotic:30mg h.s.	lightheadedness, drowsiness, ataxia, dizziness, headache, G.I. symptoms, joint pain, nervousness, chest pain, genitourinary complaints	In pregnancy use only if benefits outweigh risks; Get periodic blood counts, liver and renal function tests if use is prolonged.	relatively new but effective hypnotic
Glutethimide	Doriden®	Caps:500mg Tabs:125,250, 500mg	Sedative:125–250mg t.i.d. p.s. Hypnotic:250–500mg h.s.	skin rash, other side effects rare	In pregnancy use only if benefits outweigh risks	difficult to remove from the body in the event of overdose; not dialyzable. Margin of safety less than barbiturates.
Methaqualone	Quaalude® (and others)	Tabs:150,300mg	Sedative:75mg t.i.d.-q.i.d. Hypnotic:150–300mg h.s.	Pregnancy minor gastric upset, nausea, headache, dry mouth, drowsiness, acroparesthesias of extremities, fatigue	Do not give more than 3 months; be careful when liver damage present	
Methyprylon	Noludar®	Tabs:50,200mg Caps:300mg	Hypnotic:200–400mg h.s.	mild to moderate gastric upset, rash, dizziness, paradoxical excitement, headache, hangover	Be careful when liver or renal damage present. In pregnancy use only if benefits outweigh risks.	

References

1. *AMA Drug Evaluations.* AMA Council on Drugs, Chicago, 1971.
2. Ban, Thomas: *Psychopharmacology.* Baltimore, Williams & Wilkins, 1969.
3. Dimascio, Alberto and Shader, Richard I. (Eds.) : *Clinical Handbook of Psychopharmacology.* New York, Science, 1970.
4. Dimascio, Alberto: Toward a more rational use of antiparkinson drugs in psychiatry. *Drug Therapy, 2:* 23, 1972.
5. Domino, Edward F.: Antianxiety drugs. In DePalma, Joseph R.: *Drill's Pharmacology in Medicine,* 4th ed., New York, McGraw Hill, 1971.
6. Hollister, Leo E.: Mental disorders, antipsychotic and antimanic drugs. *N Engl J Med, 286:* 984, 1972.
7. Hollister, Leo E.: Mental disorders, antianxiety and antidepressant drugs. *N Engl J Med, 286:* 1195, 1972.
8. Katz, Ronald L.: Sedative and tranquilizers. *N Engl J Med, 286:* 757, 1972.
9. Kiev, Ari: The chemotherapy of depressive illness. *Drug Ther, 1:* 9, 1971.
10. Kiev, Ari: Minor tranquilizers: perceptive management of the anxious patient. *Drug Ther, 2:* 105, 1972.
11. Kline, Nathan S.: What every doctor should know about drug therapy for psychotics. *Hosp Physician, 8:* 32, 1972.
12. *Physician's Desk Reference: To Pharmaceutical Specialties and Biologicals,* 26th ed., New Jersey, Medical Economics, 1972.

USE OF LITHIUM IN CLINICAL PRACTICE

Joseph R. Novello, M.D.

The use of lithium compounds in the treatment of manic forms of manic-depressive illness is now firmly established in the United States. There remain, however, many misconceptions about the clinical use of the drug. The following outline is provided to give the psychiatrist a convenient reference to the clinical application of lithium compounds. Further information is available in manufacturer's data.

I. Indications

    A. Manic phase of manic-depressive illness

II. Contraindications

    A. Cardiovascular and/or renal disease

    B. Evidence of brain damage

    C. Caution in pregnancy and women of child-bearing potential

    D. Children under 12

III. Side-effects Related to Dosage Level

A. While side effects are seldom seen at serum lithium levels below 1.5 meq/l they can (and do) occur at therapeutic levels (0.5 to 1.2).

B. Below 2.0 meq/l (mild, may be transient or persist throughout treatment).

    1. Diarrhea, nausea, vomiting, anorexia.

    2. Drowsiness, muscular weakness.

    3. Lack of coordination, tinnitus, blurred vision, slurred speech.

    4. Coarse tremor, increased deep tendon reflexes.

    5. Polydipsia, polyuria, hematuria

    6. See manufacturers' data for other (less common) side effects.

C. Complex, multiple-organ involvement at higher serum levels (above 2.0 meq/l).

IV. Side-effects Not Related to Dosage Level

    A. Thyroid toxicity

        1. Goiter, lowering of PBI, increased I^{131} uptake

    B. EKG changes

        1. Reversible flattening, isoelectricity, or inversion of T-waves

    C. EEG changes

        1. Diffuse slowing

    D. Other

        1. Headache

        2. Pruritis with or without skin rash

        3. Metallic taste

        4. Swollen ankles, wrists

        5. Leg ulcers

        6. Transient hyperglycemia

V. Initial Workup

    A. Complete physical exam

    B. Urinalysis, complete blood count

    C. Stool guiac

    D. SGPT, Alkaline Phosphatase, Bilirubin

    E. EKG

    F. BUN, serum creatinine

    G. PBI, T_3

VI. Treatment
   A. Serum lithium levels must be closely monitored
   B. Therapeutic levels: 0.5 to 1.2 meq/1
      1. Do not exceed 2.0 meq/1 in acute phase.
      2. Do no exceed 1.5 meg/1 in maintenance therapy.
   C. Dosage
      1. Adjust per serum assay and clinical picture
      2. Acute phase
         a. 600 mgm tid (usual starting dose)
         b. Patients in acute phase may require higher doses but must be monitored closely
      3. Maintenance therapy
         a. 300 mgm tid (usual maintenance dose)
   D. Major tranquilizers can be used simultaneously with lithium
      1. The usual drawbacks, however, of combined drug therapy are observed
         a. Uncertain efficacy of each agent in treatment response.
         b. Difficulty in distinguishing side effects.

VII. Laboratory Followup
   A. Lithium levels
      1. Serum, clotted blood.
      2. Blood to be drawn 9 to 12 hours after last dose and before first dose of the day.
      3. Week No. 1; determine lithium levels on fourth and seventh day.
   B. Other tests
      1. Use guidelines suggested in Table IX-XIII (Laboratory Followup in Lithium Therapy) but repeat tests at any time they are clinically indicated.
      2. In long term maintenance the entire laboratory profile listed in Table IX-XIII should be repeated at least every three months.

VIII. Special Precautions

TABLE IX-XIII

Laboratory Follow-Up In Lithium Therapy

	Week # 1	2	3	4	5	6	7	8	9	10	11	12	Maintainence to be done Once/Month
Serum Lithium	•	•	•	•	•	•		•		•		•	•
CBC	•	•	•	•	•	•		•		•		•	•
Urinalysis	•	•	•	•	•	•		•		•		•	•
Stool guiac	•	•	•	•	•	•		•		•		•	•
PBI, T_3	•			•				•					
SGOT, Alkphos	•			•				•					
Bilirubin	•			•				•					
BUN, Creat	•			•				•					
EKG	•	•		•				•					

A. Facilities for determining prompt and accurate serum lithium levels must be available.

B. Assure adequate diet, especially NaCl intake.

C. Toxic symptoms may appear on less than 1800 mgm per day or serum levels less than 1.5 meq/1. These usually are not cause for serious concern or discontinuing treatment.

D. Appearance of mild symptoms does *not* always herald the onset of severe intoxication.

E. Dangerously high lithium serum levels can occur without the symptoms of intoxication.

F. 300 mgm lithium carbonate is rough equivalent of 8 mgm lithium.

IX. Treatment of Severe Toxicity

A. Discontinue drug immediately.

B. No specific antidote available.

C. Can usually restart treatment 24 hours later at lower doses.

X. Commercially-available Lithium Products. (See Table IX-XIV.)

TABLE IX-XIV

COMMERCIALLY-AVAILABLE LITHIUM PRODUCTS

Drug	Manufacturer	Generic	How Supplied
Eskalith®	Smith,Kline,&French	Lithium Carbonate	300 mgm caps
Lithane®	Roerig	Lithium Carbonate	300 mgm caps
Lithonate®	Rowell	Lithium Carbonate	300 mgm caps
Lithium Carbonate	Phillips-Roxane	Lithium Carbonate	300 mgm caps

CLINICAL RECORD-KEEPING IN DRUG THERAPY

JOSEPH R. NOVELLO, M.D.

Precise record-keeping for patients who are being treated with psychotropic drugs is a vital part of the treatment effort. Not only are accurate records necessary in following response to treatment but they can also aid the psychiatrist in recognizing the earliest manifestations of side effects and idiosyncratic reactions.

There is a tendency to minimize the importance of undesirable side effects with psychotropic drugs. Although it is true that, by and large psychotropic drugs generally have a high margin of safety, there exist a wide spectrum of side effects ranging from relatively innocuous nausea, skin rash, etc., to life-threatening agranulocytosis, cardiovascular collapse and other emergencies.

When a decision is made to begin a patient on a course of psychotropic medication, the psychiatrist is well-advised to ask about any history of drug reaction and, before starting treatment, to obtain baseline blood studies including: CBC, liver function, renal function and urinalysis.

This information should then be carefully entered directly into the patient's psychiatric record. Table IX-XV (Drug Therapy Record) provides an example of the type of clinical record keeping system that might be established for patients who are receiving psychotropic medication.

The clinician can adjust the record-keeping system to

TABLE IX-XV

Drug Therapy Record

NAME: _____

IDENTIFYING NO.: _____

	Date			
Drug (s)				
Dosages (s)				
No. Prescribed				
Patient's Status				
Side Effects				
Laboratory Data*				
Hematocrit				
Hemoglobin				
WBC				
Differential				
Alk. Phos.				
SGPT/SGOT				
BUN				
Urinalysis				
Other				
Next Visit				
Doctor's Signature				

*Obtained as baseline prior to treatment, then at 3 weeks, 6 weeks, 3 months, 6 months, and one year after beginning drug therapy.

his own needs; he can make changes in the type of tests that are requested and their repetition frequency based on the specific drug (s) employed and the patients' clinical course. As a minimum, however, it is useful to obtain basic laboratory data at three weeks, six weeks, three months, six months and one year. For patients who are being maintained on long-term medication (such as major tranquilizers in chronic schizophrenia), it is wise to order such tests every four to six months on a routine basis.

In addition to the purely medical aspects, such a record keeping system should include basic psychiatric information as well. If both parameters of the patient's case are followed in one central record it is less likely that one will be neglected in favor of the other.

The psychiatric status of the patient can adequately be recorded in the space marked Patient's Status, in Table

IX-XV. A short, succinct statement is generally adequate. If the patient is being scored periodically on one of the psychiatric rating scales (see Chapter III), the scores can be entered in this space.

This type of clinical record can be easily adapted for use on a problem-oriented record-keeping system. See Chapter VI, The Problem-Oriented Record-Keeping System in Hospital Psychiatry.

BASIC INFORMATION ON THE USE OF CONVULSIVE THERAPY

Joseph R. Novello, M.D.

The subject of convulsive therapy in psychiatry continues to raise controversy. Opponents of convulsive therapy maintain that CT is an inelegant, indiscriminate treatment method and charge that it is used far too excessively. Proponents tend to excesses in the opposite extreme. The truth, of course, lies somewhere between the two poles. Although the precise mechanism of action is unknown, convulsive therapy if used appropriately, can be life-saving and is still among the most important therapeutic tools available in psychiatry.

There are basically two methods of convulsive therapy in use today: electroconvulsive therapy and IndoKlon therapy. These have largely replaced Metrozol® and insulin which are rarely used.

The following outline summarizes basic information about convulsive therapy in general. It is followed by outlines detailing the use of electroconvulsive therapy and IndoKlon convulsive therapy.

   I. Indications
     A. Depression
       1. Best results are obtained in involutional depression (melancholia), depressive phase of manic-depressive illness, recurrent (nonreactive) depression and psychotic depressive reactions.
       2. Neurotic (reactive) depression response less reliable.

a. Use antidepressants for reactive depression unless other indications (below) exist.

B. Suicide risk

1. Immediate use of CT in patient who is strong suicide risk can be life-saving. (See Evaluation of the Suicidal Patient, Chapter IV.)

C. Time Factor

1. Patient's need to quickly return to work, lack of hospitalization insurance, etc.

D. Schizophrenia

1. Chronic schizophrenia does not respond well to CT.

2. Acute schizophrenia is now adequately treated with major tranquilizers.

3. Therefore use of CT in treatment of schizophrenia is now limited to occasional use in acute schizophrenia where drug therapy is unsuccessful or medically contraindicated.

E. Postpartum psychosis

1. CT may give dramatic results

F. Other

1. CT has been used in almost every conceivable type of psychiatric disorder, but those conditions listed above are generally considered the only present indications for this type of treatment.

II. Contraindications

A. Brain tumor

B. Recent myocardial infarction

C. Cerebral aneurysm, subdural hematoma

D. All other conditions are relative contraindications and the possibility of undesirable side effects must be weighed against the potential benefits of treatment. In general, CT is quite safe. For example, it has been used successfully in the following conditions:

1. Peptic ulcer

2. Aortic aneurysm

       3. Retinal detachment

       4. Glaucoma (Avoid use of succinyl choline, however, which can cause increase of intra-occular pressure.)

       5. Cardiac arrhythmia

         a. Cardiac consult is desirable prior to treatment

         b. Increase oxygenation during treatment

   E. Age of patient is of little concern, though results are generally better with older patients. CT has been reported successful with patients ranging in age from 8 to 92.

III. Complications of Treatment

   A. Vertebral fractures

       1. Incidence is much decreased with use of muscle relaxants

       2. Usually between T4 and T8

       3. Clinically of little or no importance and patient may be entirely asymptomatic

       4. Usually not an indication to interrupt treatment

   B. Fractures of long bones

       1. Incidence is much decreased with use of muscle relaxants

       2. Usually of head of humerus or head of femur.

       3. Are clinically important and usually an indication to interrupt treatment.

   C. Fatalities

       1. Very rare, fewer than one per 10,000 treatments.

       2. Often related to anesthesia or underlying disease i.e. barbiturate anesthesia is a risk in any patient with myocardial disease.

   D. There is no conclusive evidence that CT creates any form of permanent brain damage.

IV. Treatment Course

   A. There is no absolute limit to the number of treatments that may be given. The clinician should continuously evaluate the patient's response to treatment and terminate or modify it as indicated.

   B. Generally, for depressed patients some significant response should be seen within six to ten treatments.

C. Acute schizophrenics may require 10 to 20 treatments before response is noted.

D. Classic method is to give treatments every other day.

V. Modifications of Technique

  A. Unilateral ECT

    1. Electroshock is delivered to the nondominant hemisphere only.

      a. results in less memory loss than bilateral ECT.

    2. Usually requires more treatments for an adequate response but should be strongly considered under the following circumstances:

      a. no pressure of time (no suicide risk, etc.).

      b. patients with pre-existing memory deficits.

      c. outpatient ECT where the patient will be ambulatory and going about the activities of daily living.

  B. Concurrent use of antidepressants

    1. There is no contraindication to this except that the patient's response to treatment may be difficult to ascribe to either one of the two treatment modalities.

    2. One caution: MAO inhibitors potentiate barbiturates. Consult with anesthesiologist.

  C. Maintenance CT

    1. Patients who, in the past, have shown a predisposition to recurrence soon after CT may be maintained on periodic (weekly, etc.) CT as outpatients.

    2. Treatment may be discontinued when there has been no recurrence in three to four months.

  D. Multiple CT (MCT)

    1. Recently it has been reported that subjecting the patient to multiple convulsions, each immediately succeeding the last, has led to an increased rate of treatment response. This has not been well documented and, to this time, the advantages, if any, are unclear.

VI. Legal Factors

A. The psychiatrist performing CT should be well-qualified to do so and should be familiar with all of the legal requirements associated with it in his state of residence.

B. Patient's written consent is almost always required. In many cases it is desirable to request written consent from next of kin.

C. Where the patient is unable to give legal consent state laws vary and the psychiatrist should be familiar with his legal obligations.

D. Many states require a qualified anesthesiologist or anesthetist to administer the anesthesia. Where they are not required the psychiatrist must be competent in intubation and resuscitation and have a nurse or trained assistant available to aid him.

References

Kalinowsky, L. B.: The convulsive therapies. In Freedman, A. and Kaplan, H. (Eds.): *Comprehensive Textbook of Psychiatry*. Baltimore, Williams and Wilkins, 1967.

Kalinowsky, L. B. and Hoch, P. H.: *Somatic Treatment in Psychiatry*. New York, Grune and Stratton, 1961.

Sargant, W. and Slater, E.: *An Introduction to Physical Methods of Treatment in Psychiatry*. London, E. and S. Livingstone, 1963.

ELECTROCONVULSIVE THERAPY

The following outline for performing electroconvulsive therapy is the general protocol used at the Neuropsychiatric Institute of the University of Michigan Medical Center. The outline is purposefully brief and is not intended to be an exhaustive discussion of ECT.

I. Workup prior to ECT:

A. Thoracic and lumbar spine x-ray.

B. EKG for patients over 40 years of age or any patients suspected of having a cardiovascular disorder.

C. Hemoglobin and hematocrit.

D. Complete blood count, urinalysis.

    E. SGP Transaminase and alkaline phosphatase.

    F. A thorough physical examination and medical history including a complete review of systems and a neurological examination with especially funduscopic examination.

    G. Permission for ECT signed by patient and next of kin.

    H. Operation permit (for anesthesia) signed by the patient.

  II. NPO after midnight (minimum of eight hours NPO).

 III. Atropine 0.4 mg subcutaneously 30 minutes before induction of anesthesia. (If patient has increased oral-pharyngeal secretions, use 0.6 mg atropine.)

 IV. Before the patient is taken to the treatment room, make sure that all dentures and metal objects are removed from the patient's person as well as removal of fingernail polish and facial makeup. The patient should be dressed in a hospital gown and if the patient is female, her brassiere should be removed so as not to interfere with deep respiratory movements and monitoring of heart action.

  V. Before bringing the patient into the treatment room, allow the power to be on in the ECT machine for at least five minutes and test the machine before putting the patient to sleep. Set the ECT machine at 120 volts and 0.6 seconds for an unknown patient; for later treatments this can be adjusted on the basis of the patient's response.

 VI. Put the electrode discs in the elastic headband 9 to 12 notches apart. (This varies with the configuration and size of the patient's head.) Then put EKG electrojelly on the electrode discs. Make sure that the electrode discs are completely covered with the electrojelly so as to avoid loss of current through the skin surface.

VII. While the patient is awake wash the temples with soap and wipe off with alcohol being sure to swab dry with cotton. The patient at this time should be lying flat on the treatment table. It is very important to maintain contact with the patient both verbally and physically at this time through conversation, explanation of the procedure, reassurance that the patient will be asleep during the procedure, etc. Physical contact can be maintained through washing the temples as already described and personally taking the blood pressure and pulse of the patient. This is very important in order for the patient to recognize the electrotherapist as a real person.

VIII. The anesthetist will then give the patient Brevital® intravenously 80 to 150 mg for the average sized patient until they are asleep. (They will not respond to brushing of the eyelashes.)

IX. After the patient is asleep wrap the elastic headband with the electrode discs firmly around the head and connect to the machine. (Do not allow the elastic headband to impinge closely on the eyebrows or eyelids. With seizure movements of the facial musculature around the eyes if this musculature is already placed on the stretch a ptosis of the lid could result.)

X. Next place the combination mouth gag and rubber airway into place.

XI. Be sure that No. 9 and No. 10 are completed before next asking the anesthetist to give the patient Anectine® I.V. 20 to 60 mg. (This of course is succinylcholine chloride, a muscle relaxant.) This will induce fasciculation and when this is completed as adjudged by an endpoint of the ceasing of fasciculation of the skeletal muscles, then the psychiatrist is ready to give the treatment.

XII. When the fasciculation of the skeletal muscles ceases, give the shock. In order to make sure that one gives the entire voltage indicated hold the treatment button down for a full five seconds. This will avoid a reflex releasing the button too quickly before full voltage is delivered to the patient. The patient must have a grand mal seizure (indicated by twitching of the orbicularis oculi muscles, tonic-clonic motion of toes or fingers or goose pimples). If a grand mal seizure does not occur, increase the duration and voltage in step-wise fashion and reshock until successful a total of two more times.

XIII. The anesthetist will then bag-breathe the patient until he begins to breathe on his own. Incidentally it is useful after the administration of the Anectine and prior to giving of the shock stimulus to hyperventilate the patient briefly before giving the treatment.

XIV. When the blood pressure, pulse and respiration are stabilized and the patient is conscious, he may then be returned to the ward. A useful position is to have the patient lie on one side with a pillow to the small of the back. Having the head to the side will also avoid problems of regurgitation and aspiration of stomach contents.

XV. One of the most frightening aspects of electroconvulsive therapy to the patient is the period of acute confusion just after the treatment has taken place and the patient has regained consciousness after administration of anesthesia. It is often helpful, as the patient is first awakening, to reorient him by calling him by name, identifying yourself as Dr. So-and-So, telling him that he has just had a treatment, he is at such-and-such a hospital, he is doing fine and he will be going back to the ward, etc.

XVI. After the series of ECT has been completed, one should take an x-ray of the thoracic and lumbar spine to rule out possible compression fractures.

XVII. Brief mention will be made of another technique occasionally used at N.P.I. for electroconvulsive therapy. This is the unilateral technique in which the shock stimulus is applied to the nondominant hemisphere (as determined by right or left handedness). This technique is useful in those patients where the acute organic brain syndrome and memory loss would not be clinically useful. This technique is felt to minimize these aspects. Technique is basically the same as for the one mentioned above with the exception that the electrodes are applied by hand and are gauze covered, soaked in a saline solution. One electrode is applied to the temporal area, the other is applied to the frontal parietal area on the same side (over the nondominant hemisphere). The assistant holding the patient's head should have on an insulated (shock resistant) glove at the time of treatment.

Outpatient Electroconvulsive Therapy

ECT may be administered adequately and safely to outpatients. The following general guidelines have been established at the Neuropsychiatric Institute of the University of Michigan Medical Center:

   I. Routine Workup
      A. Complete physical and neurological exam
      B. Complete blood count, urinalysis
      C. Thoracic and lumbar spine x-rays
      D. SGP Transaminase, alkaline phosphatase
      E. EKG for all patients over 40 (and others if indicated)
  II. Permission for ECT signed by patient and next of kin before each treatment.
 III. Operation permit signed by patient before each treatment.
  IV. Patient to be fasting for at least eight and preferably ten hours.
   V. Patient to be accompanied to hospital by relative or other responsible adult.
  VI. Patient to come to hospital an hour before induction. Bed assigned to him. Change clothes. Atropine 0.4 mg subq. 30 minutes before induction.
 VII. ECT
VIII. Patient may return home after he is fully awake, in

the company of some person. If traveling by automobile, the other person must drive. The patient is not to act as driver.

IndoKlon Convulsive Therapy

IndoKlon (flurothyl) was discovered during work with the anesthetic properties of aliphatic fluorinated ethers. Given to laboratory animals, it was seen to cause grand mal seizures from which the animals recovered quickly and without significant side effects. It was then adapted for use as a convulsive therapy agent.

Administration is now limited to inhalation techniques. Intravenous use causes venous sclerosis.

I. General Information
    A. Indications, precautions, side effects, efficacy, etc., are all roughly equivalent to bilateral ECT.
    B. It is generally believed, however, that there is somewhat less acute memory loss with IndoKlon.
II. Specific Indications
    A. Same as CT in general
    B. Use in place of ECT if patient has been unsuccessfully treated with ECT in past.
    C. Many patients accept the idea of a treatment in which they inhale something much better than they accept the idea of having electrodes placed on their skulls.
III. Type of seizure
    A. Characteristically myoclonic movements initially, followed by brief tonic phase, then prolonged clonic phase.
    B. If only the myoclonic phase is observed, suspect a poor fitting mask.
IV. Technique
    A. Preparation and premedications as per ECT
    B. Special equipment
        1. 5-liter breathing bag
        2. oxygen supply

C. Connect breathing bag to vaporizer and to a face mask
D. Partially fill bag with oxygen
E. Pour 0.25 to 1.00 cc of liquid IndoKlon into vaporizer
F. Anesthesia administered as per ECT technique
G. Face mask is placed tightly on patient's face and the bag is squeezed once every three seconds (avoid breathing the fumes yourself)
H. The patient rebreathes into the bag
I. Technique usually requires four to nine inhalations
J. Usually see seizure within 40 seconds
K. Post-treatment technique as per ECT
L. Treatment, similar to the one suggested for ECT, should be constructed.

References

Fink, M. (Ed.) : *Seminars in Psychiatry,* Vol. IV, No. 1. February, 1972.
Freedman, A . M. and Kaplan, H. I.: *Comprehensive Textbook of Psychiatry.* Baltimore, Williams and Wilkins Co., 1967.
Kafi, A. and Dennis, M. S.: Advantages of IndoKlon Convulsive Therapy. *Hospital and Community Psychiatry,* October, 1966.

CLINICAL RECORD-KEEPING IN CONVULSIVE THERAPY

As in other aspects of psychiatric treatment, efficient record-keeping is important in documenting treatment-response in convulsive therapy.

Table IX-XVI (ECT Treatment Record) is an example of the type of official record that is in use at the Neuropsychiatric Institute, University of Michigan Medical Center.

Although most items in the record are self-explanatory, some explanation is required. *Current* refers to the number of milliamp of electrical current applied as the convulsive stimulus. *Time* refers to the amount of time (in seconds) over which the electric current is applied. *Meds* refer to the type, amount and route of administration of the *pre-op* medications. *Seizure* refers to whether or not a seizure resulted; a note can also be made regarding the nature of the seizure,

TABLE IX-XVI

ECT Treatment Record

Patient's Name: _____

Registration (or identifying) Number: _____

Date	Current (Milliamps)	Time (Sec.)	Meds	Seizure	Remarks	Physician

Pre-Treatment Check-off List

☐ Signed Consent

☐ Spine X-rays

☐ Physical Exam

☐ Routine Lab

☐ EKG

i.e. *Grand mal, clonic, tonic,* etc. The remarks column can be used for miscellaneous information but should also make some note of the patient's response to treatment. For example, if the patient's clinical depression is being periodically assessed by the use of a rating scale (see Chapter III, Aids to Diagnosis in Psychiatry, for information regarding clinically useful rating scales), the scores should be entered under remarks.

With obvious minor changes, this record can be adapted for use where IndoKlon is the convulsive agent employed.

Chapter X

THE PSYCHIATRIST'S ROLE IN THE DIAGNOSIS AND TREATMENT OF DRUG ABUSE

ONE OF THE GREATEST CHALLENGES facing medicine and psychiatry today is the problem of widespread drug abuse. The problem exists in many and diverse forms ranging from street freak acid heads, to ghetto bound heroin addicts, to middle and upper class individuals who abuse tranquilizers, barbiturates, amphetamines and alcohol. Drug abuse knows no boundaries. It has invaded every age group and every level of society.

In most communities it is the psychiatrist who is turned to as the expert in this arena. His involvement may be at several levels. It may range from responsibility for front-line emergency medical-psychiatric treatment of acute intoxication, to a more-or-less classic psychotherapy model, to consultation to teachers, parents' groups, etc. Therefore, he must be knowledgeable and prepared on several levels.

This chapter is designed to aid the psychiatrist in this task. It focuses upon the most commonly abused drugs, and while emphasis is placed upon matters of practical, clinical importance, other background information is added to aid the psychiatrist in his role as consultant to medical colleagues and as resource person for community groups.

The chapter includes six articles: I. The General Clinical Approach to Diagnosis and Treatment of the *Unknown* Ingestion, II. Differential Diagnosis in Drug Abuse, III. Hallucinogens, IV. Central Nervous System Stimulants, V. Central Nervous System Depressants (including alcohol) and VI. Narcotics.

I. THE GENERAL CLINICAL APPROACH TO DIAGNOSIS AND TREATMENT OF THE *UNKNOWN* INGESTION

H. J. SCHULTE, M.D.

In the emergency room setting the psychiatrist's first job is to distinguish a toxic drug reaction from an acute functional psychotic reaction. (See Chapter I, Table I-IV, Differential Diagnosis: Organic Psychosis vs. Functional Psychosis). Assuming a drug reaction, the psychiatrist's next step is to determine the basic category of the drug involved (hallucinogen, stimulant, depressant, narcotic). In cases of severe acute intoxications with accompanying medical problems, treatment will usually be in the hands of the internist. However, the psychiatrist should be able to treat the majority of the problems, and he will be called upon to be a knowledgeable consultant.

A. History taking

Taking a careful history is important although emergency situations may require intervention with less than ideal information.

1. If patient is conscious:
    a. Ask his friends not to leave until his condition is known. It is helpful to allow friends to stay with the patient who is in a strange anxiety-producing environment.
    b. Interview patient.
        1. Reassure the patient that this information is confidential (only if indeed it is!), that the authorities or his parents will not be called unless his medical condition necessitates it, and then only after discussing it with him. Trust is essential if the doctor is to establish a therapeutic relationship.

   2. Inquire what type of drug was taken and when.
      Take a complete medical history. Has he ever
      been in a psychiatric hospital or experienced se-
      vere emotional problems?
   3. Information regarding any recent behavior
      changes should be specifically sought from the
      patient and accompanying friends, relatives, etc.
      Have there been any changes in the person's
      usual life-style, work performance, physical ap-
      pearance or personality? What is his current
      social setting, and what is the drug usage pattern
      in that setting?
   c. It is noteworthy that aside from allergic and idio-
      syncratic drug reactions, the same drug may not
      effect everyone in the same way. An individual's
      response may vary widely, depending on his imme-
      diate situation (How tired is he? How anxious?
      Where he is? Who he is with? Past history of drug
      reactions?). For example, it is not uncommon to
      observe a panic reaction, and subsequent bad trip,
      caused by a long-time user simply becoming sep-
      arated from his friends at something like a rock
      concert or other gathering.
2. If the patient is unconscious:
   a. Retain friends who brought the patient for all rel-
      evant information such as: names and telephone
      numbers of parents, friends, medical history, drug
      history, etc.
   b. If physical examination and history indicate drug
      use and other medical cause is absent, then give
      appropriate treatment (see treatment under each
      class heading that follows).
   c. In a case of drug abuse resulting in loss of con-
      sciousness, avoid labeling it as a suicidal attempt
      until the patient's motive is known. Many such
      cases, especially when heroin is involved, are ac-
      cidental.

3. Indiscriminate notification of parents or authorities will only further alienate the youthful patient. Check the requirements of state laws for reporting narcotic abuse. In some states, i.e. Massachusetts, acute poisoning need be reported by occurrence only; and even with the chronic use of narcotic drugs, which requires reporting, there is some leeway. The general requirement for reporting to the authorities is that the street drugs abused must be narcotic drugs. (Zarafonetis, 1972)

B. Diagnosis
   1. For differential diagnosis, see Section II of this chapter, Differential Diagnosis in Drug Abuse.
   2. Because of frequent impurities, incomplete drug synthesis, inaccurate dosages and mixtures of drugs (see II, C), there is often much uncertainty in the diagnosis and treatment of acute drug intoxications. The physician must combine the history with his observations of the physical and behavioral changes and his knowledge of the local drug scene in order to make the diagnosis. It must be stressed again that the best one can generally do (and all that is really necessary from a practical, clinical standpoint) is to identify the general class of drug involved: hallucinogen, CNS stimulant, CNS depressant or narcotic.

C. General treatment considerations
   1. If the patient is comatose, refer to Internal Medicine
   2. General medical treatments (for specifics, see treatment of each drug)
      a. Supportive care is the main treatment of choice for most acute intoxications except:
      b. Amphetamine overdose, use Thorazine, I.M., 1 mg/kg.
      c. Narcotic overdose, use Narcan®, I.V., 0.4 to 0.8 mg; or Nalline®, I.V., 10 mg
      d. Atropine overdose, use Physostigmine, I.M., 4 mg, q 1–½h for severe symptoms

  e. Strychnine poisoning, use Amytal®, 0.5 gm, I.V. in
     20 ml of water to prevent convulsions and succinyl-
     choline (Anectine)
  f. *In general, avoid phenothiazines and other major
     tranquilizers for unknown ingestions,* (may cause
     fatal cardiovascular collapse).
3. The treatment of choice for bad trips and panic reactions is to talk the patient down (see III, A, 4).
4. Usually it is best to refrain from drug treatment of
   bad trips, but if necessary, due to agitation or verbally
   uncontrollable behavior, use Valium®, I.M., 5 to 15 mg.
   This may be repeated every ½ hour p.r.n. until symptoms subside. In some patients a 10 mg oral dose will
   be less frightening and should be used instead.
5. Be knowledgeable about resources in the local community. Friends, community drug workers and hospital personnel are invaluable for helping to talk
   down a bad trip and to stay with the patient.
D. Physician's attitude

The physician should maintain a calm, tolerant approach,
realizing that these patients often tend to see him as an
authority figure, representing the establishment. It is not
uncommon that the individual will respond positively to
reassurance, but it also is true that a peer with a previous
bad trip experience is invaluable. Maintain an open mind.
Remember that in these problems more harm may be done
by overtreatment than by undertreatment.

II. DIFFERENTIAL DIAGNOSIS IN DRUG ABUSE

Table X-I (Differential Diagnosis in Drug Abuse) provides the clinician with a quick reference to aid in the diagnosis of drug abuse. By carefully noting certain behavioral
and physical signs the physician should, in most cases, be
able to determine in what general class (hallucinogen, stimulant, depressant, narcotic) to place his diagnosis. Treatment, then, proceeds accordingly.

In some cases, however, not even a general class diagnosis
will be possible. The individual may have ingested a com-

bination of drugs; certain contaminants may have been added; unusual, idiosyncratic reactions may occur, etc. In these cases the physician should exercise extreme caution. As a general rule it is wise to avoid using phenothiazines in the treatment of the unknown abuse. Similarly it is wise to avoid abuse-specific drugs such as phisostigmine and the narcotic antagonists which may be hazardous themselves in the hands of the inexperienced.

III. HALLUCINOGENS

H. J. SCHULTE, M.D.

These drugs produce a toxic delirium characterized by hallucinations and visual illusions. These effects include mood alteration, as well as changes in sensory perception. They are usually taken orally on a sugar cube, paper, cookie, etc. Occasionally they are injected intravenously. The psychodelics will be discussed first in their pure forms and then in their street forms, which are the result of incorrect synthesis, end product breakdown and adulterants. This section will also include information concerning cannabis (marijuana) abuse. These drugs will be covered under three basic categories: hallucinogens, street substitutions and marijuana. Hallucinogens include: LSD, mescaline, psilocybin, DOM, MBA, DMT, DET. Street substitutions (i.e. drugs which are not hallucinogens but which are often sold on the street as hallucinogens or that appear in combination with true hallucinogens) include amphetamines, phencyclidines, strychnine, belladonna.

A. LSD (D-lysergic acid diethylamide)
   1. Slang names: acid, sunshine, dots
   2. Pharmacology: Synthesized from lysergic acid found in the fungus, ergot and in morning glory seeds. An indoleakylamine derivative, structurally similar to serotonin. Central nervous system effects: alterations in mood, perception and body image. Sensory illusions: colors heard, sounds seen. Autonomic nervous system: sympathomimetic (constricts smooth muscle). Sites of action: facilitates sensory input into the brain stem

TABLE X-I

DIFFERENTIAL DIAGNOSIS IN DRUG ABUSE *

Signs and symptoms are variable depending on purity, combinations used and individual reaction. The terms designated reflect the *usual* reaction to one type of drug. Exceptions are frequent but not included in the list.

CODE: X—Acute Phase   W—Withdrawal Phase

Signs and Symptoms	Hallu-cinogens	Central Nervous System Stimulants	Central Nervous System Depressants	Narcotic Analgesics
Aggressive Behavior	X	X	X	
Anorexia		X		
Areflexia			X	
Ataxia	X	X	X	X
Circulatory Collapse		X		
Coma (Overdose)			X	X
Confusion		X	X	
Cramps		W	W	W
Depression		W	X	
Disorientation	X	X	X	
Drowsiness	X (Occ. Marij.)		X	X
Drunken Behavior	X (Occ. Marij.)		X	
Euphoria	X	X	X (Solvents)	X
Fever		X	W	
Gooseflesh			W	W
Hallucinations	X	X	X	
Hyperreflexia, Convulsions		X	W	
Hypotension			X, W	X
Inattentiveness			X	X
Increased Appetite	X			
Irritability		X	X	
Lacrimation	X		X (Solvents)	W
Needle Tracks		X	X	X
Nystagmus			X	
Paranoia, Panic Reaction	X	X	W	
Parkinsonian			X (Tranquilizers)	

TABLE X-I Continued

Signs and Symptoms	Hallu-cinogens	Central Nervous System Stimulants	Central Nervous System Depressants	Narcotic Analgesics
Psychotic Symptoms	X	X	W	
Pupils—Pinpoint				X
Dilated			X (Scopolamine) (Doriden®)	W
Normal			X	
Reaction to Pain Reduced	X	X	X	X
Respiratory Depression		X (Cocaine)	X	X
Restlessness	X	X	W	W
Runny Nose			X (Solvents)	W
Skin Rash		X	X (Bromides)	
Slurred Speech			X	X
Tachycardia	X	X		W

* Copyright 1970, revised 1971, New York State Department of Health. Reprinted with permission.

reticular formation; reduces transmission over some axodendritic synapses and enhances transmission over some axosomatic synapses. Mechanism: 5-HT agonist and antagonist; increased 5-HT levels; cholinesterase inhibitor (unknown relation to mental effects). Biotransformation occurs in the liver. (Zarafonetis, 1972) Usual dose: 50 to 400 micrograms. Onset in two hours and duration of action eight to twelve hours. Potential for tolerance leading to increased dose: occurs but disappears in several days. Potential for physical dependence: none.

Long term effects: Reactivation or precipitation of schizophrenic reaction in susceptible individual. Possible organic brain syndrome with chronic abuse. Possible chromosomal breakage similar to stress. Possible birth defects if taken early in pregnancy. Flashbacks. Psychotic depression.

3. Diagnosis
   a. Behavioral factors
      1. Frank hallucinations: visual, tactile, auditory; confusion, disorientation, depersonalization.
      2. Psychotic state can lead to self mutilation, suicide, homocide (rare).
      3. Panic reaction present for some; for others, a lessened anxiety and feelings of a deep and transcendental experience.
   b. Physical factors
      1. Sympathomimetic: increased blood pressure, tachycardia, mydriasis, piloerection.
      2. Other: nausea, fine tremor, metallic taste
      3. Hyperventilation syndrome not uncommon
      4. Synthesis failures and substitutions are common, making possible ergot poisoning with vomiting and diarrhea.
   c. Laboratory: no lab tests generally available.
   d. Street substitutions for LSD are common: amphetamine, phencyclidine, strychnine, atropine and JB compounds. (see III, C, D)
4. Treatment
   a. Acute intoxication
      1. Psychological aspect: Talking down a bad trip. Anyone can have a bad trip, it is not necessarily an indication of an underlying psychosis. Many factors such as dosage, personal history, immediate situation contribute. Talking down is the treatment of choice if patient is not overly aggressive, convulsive or showing respiratory depression. Goal is to counteract the panic, disorientation, paranoia and depression of the bad trip.
         a. *Panic:* most common reaction. Be reassuring and friendly. Repeatedly inform patient that drug's effects are causing the distortions and that it will wear off. It is helpful to put person in touch with himself by discussing the

experience, concentrating on relaxed breathing. The major advantage of this is that it provides a focus of attention and helps the person feel more in control. Tell the person to stop fighting the experience, to relax and to let it happen. One possible metaphor that may be used to help the person relax is the suggestion that he watch the flow of images as if he was viewing a movie.

b. *Disorientation:* common. Put the individual back in touch with his own reality testing. Focus on the here and now such as familiar objects in the room, who he is, where he is, what is happening. This assists in the process of self-identification and reality identification.

c. *Problem solving.* Listen for clues to anxieties that are present. Drug may have uncovered important psychic material. Explain that the drug magnifies and distorts problems. Discuss the problems in nonexploratory, noninterpretive fashion. Allay guilt feelings, and quietly, but firmly, oppose self-derogatory comments. Patient must feel the attendant is sympathetic, understands and will stay with him no matter how long a time is required. (Lampe, 1972)

d. Differences of opinion as to who should treat. Generally nonprofessional peers with similar prior experiences are most successful. Physicians represent authority and establishment figures. Also it would be difficult for them to stay with the person for the duration of the experience.

2. Medications
   a. Should be used only as last resort for bad trip. Only when patient is otherwise unmanageable. Decreased incidence of flashbacks if person deals with trip without meds. Using a drug to sedate a bad trip reinforces drug taking

behavior, i.e. the answer to problems is simply to find the right drug.

    b. Thorazine (and other phenothiazines) are contraindicated because of interaction with possible adulterants; use of Thorazine can lead to increased respiratory depression or cardiovascular collapse if STP, strychnine, belladonna or phencyclidine are present.

    c. Use Valium, 5 to 15 mg, I.M. or orally, 5 to 10 mg, q ½h, p.r.n. (It is safer and preferred, especially in treating unknown ingestions.)

  b. Unmasking of an underlying psychosis by drug abuse. Presumptive if psychotic state persists for longer than 24 hours without other drugs being used. Psychiatric hospitalization indicated.

  c. Flashbacks: re-experiencing of bad trip without drug or while using marijuana, etc. Treatment consists of talking down.

  5. Medical complications of LSD abuse

    a. Major adverse effects of LSD are psychiatric in nature. Besides the panic reaction, flashback phenomenon and potential precipitation of psychosis, chronic hallucinogen abuse may lead to a thought disorder. This thought disorder, which appears reversible, consists of difficulties with memory, concentration and expressing thoughts. This is accompanied by a change in self confidence. (Lampe, 1972)

    b. There is much conflicting data concerning the possibility of chromosomal damage secondary to LSD use. Anyone using this drug should be clearly aware of the potential genetic risk. (Zarafonetis, 1972)

B. Other hallucinogens

    These drugs differ from LSD only in potency and duration of action; the quality of their CNS effects are similar. Diagnosis and treatment are virtually identical. It is not often possible to distinguish clinically the ingestion of one hallucinogen from another. Fortunately, for treatment purposes such a differentiation is not necessary. These other hallucinogens can be divided into two classes: phenethylamines, (amphetamine-like psychotomimetics) and other delusional drugs.

    1. Phenethylamines

        a. Mescaline (3,4,5-trimethoxyphenethylamine)

            1. Slang names: mesc, peyote

            2. Pharmacology: Made synthetically or from cactus plant, *Lophophora williamsii* (peyote buttons). Central nervous system: psychic alterations of visual hallucinations of brightly colored geometric shapes, increased arousal, altered color and space perception. Autonomic nervous system: sympathomimetic. Sites of action: stimulates brain stem activating system. Mechanism of action: unknown. Assumed related to catecholamines such as dopamine or 5-HT. Cross tolerance with LSD.

Biotransformation: oxidation by MAO and demethylation. Usual dose: 250 to 600 mg. Onset of action: one to three hours. Duration of action: eight to twelve hours. (Zarafonetis, 1972) Diagnosis: Behavior essentially as per LSD. Nausea and vomiting are more common, especially with peyote.

            4. Treatment same as LSD.

        b. Psilocybin (4-phosphoryloxy N, N-dimethyltryptamine)

            1. Slang name: Silly

            2. Pharmacology: Derived from magic mushroom of Mexico, *Psilocybus Mexicanus.* Can be extracted or synthesized.

            3. Diagnosis and treatment, same as LSD.

        c. DOM (Dimethoxy Methylamphetamine)

            1. Slang name: STP

            2. Pharmacology: synthetic. Related to mescaline and amphetamine. Dose: 3 to 10 mg. Duration

8 to 12 hours at normal doses, may last for two days in higher doses.

    3. Diagnosis and treatment, same as LSD.

    4. *Avoid Phenothiazines.* As they may accentuate the adverse mental effects and induce lethal cardiovascular collapse.

  d. MDA (Methylene Dioxyamphetamine)

    1. Pharmacology: similar to LSD. Usual dose: 75 to 100 mg. Higher doses are very toxic. Fewer perceptual distortions, more noted for stimulation of empathic feelings (love drug) and talking.

    2. Diagnosis and treatment, same as LSD.

    3. Avoid phenothiazines.

  e. DMT (Dimethyltryptamine)

    1. Pharmacology: A synthetic derivative of tryptamine. Dose: 75 to 100 mg. Duration of action one-half to four hours. Smoked with tobacco or injected.

    2. Diagnosis and treatment, same as LSD.

  f. DET (Diethyltriptamine): Duration two to three hours. Smoked or injected.

 2. Other delusional drugs include: atropine, phencyclidine and Ditran (see III, D).

C. Hallucinogens: street forms and impurities

Drugs sold on the street are often not what they are advertised to be by the sellers. They may be blatently counterfeit or contain varying amounts of impurities. The reasons for this vary from the greed of some illicit marketeers, the difficulties in syntheses, as well as the ignorance of those involved: chemist, seller, user. Street forms can be divided into several groups: those substances whose syntheses were incomplete, incorrect or whose products have degraded; and those which have had extra ingredients added or substituted for the named drug. After a brief comment on the former, there will follow a discussion of the adulterants.

  1. LSD: Street forms of LSD may represent both synthesis failure (the predominating factor) and substi-

tutions. LSD is more difficult to synthesize than is commonly thought. The product which is consumed consists mostly of ingredients that did not quite make it into LSD or those that have degraded over time from LSD (refrigeration and other care is necessary to maintain the purity). There is some danger of ergot poisoning due to the contaminants, but this is rare because of the small amounts of ergot substances present in most street products. LSD substitutions are most commonly amphetamines, phencyclidine, atropine and (fortunately much rarer) strychnine. (See part D of this section.)

2. Mescaline and Psilocybin: These drugs are much more difficult to make than LSD, and thus the chances of failure and of substitutions are greater. A Combined Drug Help—University of Michigan (Department of Pharmacology) study of mescaline sold on the streets of Ann Arbor revealed that none of the purported mescaline sold on the street between July, 1970 and January 1971 contained any mescaline at all! What was consumed as "mescaline" actually contained a combination of phencyclidine (a sizeable percentage), amphetamine (less) and LSD (most). The situation is similar with psilocybin. (Lampe, 1972)

D. Hallucinogens: street substitutions

The drugs most commonly substituted for hallucinogens include: Amphetamines, phencyclidine, strychnine, belladonna and Ditran.

1. Amphetamines are commonly added to street hallucinogens (Lampe, 1972) because they are cheap, available and their stimulant actions enhance the effects of the hallucinogens. CNS stimulants are discussed in Section IV.

2. Phencyclidine (Arylcycloalkylamines)

a. Trade name: PCP, Sernyl®

b. Pharmacology: Class known as cataleptoid-anesthetics. Not used in man because of its psychotomimetic effects. In animals produces mixed excitement-sedative effects and cataleptoid anesthesia. Central nervous system: moderate doses are analgesic and anesthetic; cataleptoid motor phenomena; large doses produce convulsions. Autonomic nervous system: sympathomimetic, potentiates catecholamines; hypertension. Sites of action: thalamoneocortical system; limbic system. Mechanism of action: unknown. Biotransformation: mostly hydroxylated derivatives which are more convulsant than PCP. Dosage: 10 mg, orally gives slight drunken feeling; 0.2 mg/kg, I.V. is anesthetic. Duration: 3 to 18 hours. (Zarafonetis, 1972)

  c. Diagnosis:

    1. Behavioral factors: small doses produce a drunken state. Larger doses produce delusional behavior, hallucinations and agitation. The person feels very stoned, termed a psychadelic down.

    2. Physical:

      a. Sympathomimetic symptoms of tachycardia, hypertension, sweating. Injected conjunctiva. Notable numbness in face and extremities.

      b. Large doses produce convulsions which do not interfere with respiration.

      c. When combined with other depressants such as chlorpromazine or alcohol, may lead to coma and respiratory arrest. Mis-syntheses of PCP may also lead to respiratory depression.

      d. Treatment

        1. Monitor vital signs.

        2. Numbness is very striking and may lead to fear of dying. Treat as bad trip (see LSD).

        3. Supportive, symptomatic approach.

  3. Strychnine: Its inclusion in street drugs is fortunately very rare. Also found as an occasional adulterant in marijuana, especially on the West Coast. It has been used as a rat poison since the sixteenth century and has been used with success in suicide attempts. Not a drug of demonstrated therapeutic value.

a. Pharmacology: A very strong stimulant of all portions of CNS. A convulsant. Increases the level of neuronal excitability by selectively blocking postsynaptic inhibition, leading to increased reflexes in response to sensory input.

b. Diagnosis
  1. Physical factors:
     a. No direct effect on blood pressure or pulse.
     b. First effect is stiffness in the face and neck muscles. Any sensory stimuli may poduce violent motor response. Early stages: coordinated, symmetrical extensor thrust. Later stages: tetanic convulsion, opisthotonos. Death results from respiratory paralysis.
  2. Drug is rapidly eliminated from the body by urinary excretion, complete in ten hours. (Goodman & Gilman, 1970)

c. Treatment: acute intoxication
  1. If receive a phone call regarding person in this condition, recommend that the person be kept still in a quiet, dark room until medical help can arrive.
  2. Prevent convulsions with Amytal 0.5 gm, stat, in 10 to 20 ml of water, slowly I.V. Repeat in 30 minutes if necessary.
  3. Control convulsions with succinylcholine (Anectine)
  4. Support respiration. Endotracheal intubation, if necessary, and oxygen.
  5. If possible, gastric lavage with potassium permanganate 1:1000 concentration.
  6. Minimize tactile and auditory stimulation.
  7. General measures: give charcoal or tannic acid in water, or strong tea. May quiet the patient by inhalation of ether or chloroform. (Krupp, *et al.,* 1972)

4. Belladonna Alkaloids: Since ancient times, it has been well known that belladonna plants can produce marked psychic changes which resemble an organic brain syn-

drome. One synthetic atropine derivative, member of a group known as the glycolate esters, is a potent hallucinogen. This is known as Ditran (JB-329). Stramonium is found in Asthmador cigarettes which are readily available to the public.

Belladonna		Atropine
Scopalamine		Homatropine
Hyoscyamine		Ditran (JB-329)
Datura Stramonium (Jimson weed)

a. Pharmacology: Central nervous system: auditory hallucinations, clouding of conscious, marked memory loss in comparison to LSD. Autonomic nervous system: antagonizes most muscarinic cholinergic actions of acetylcholine. Sites of action: brain stem activating system, neocortex, limbic system. Mechanism of action: central and peripheral muscarinic cholinergic blockade. Dosage: 0.4 mg/kg body weight; high dose of atropine: 500 mg; Duration of action: dose related, in high doses, up to 48 hours, some symptoms may persist for a week. (Zarafonetis, 1972)

b. Diagnosis
  1. Behavioral factors
     a. Acute intoxication characteristics; mad as a wet hen, hot as a hare, dry as a bone, and red as a beet. Similar to a toxic delirium or organic psychosis with gross memory disturbances and difficulty orienting oneself.
     b. This organic brain syndrome is associated with auditory hallucinations (visual hallucinations predominate with LSD).
     c. This madness is not easily differentiated from delirium tremens of chronic alcoholism.
  2. Physical factors:
     a. The skin is flushed, mydriasis and cycloplegia, tachycardia, dryness of mouth and of mucous membranes of respiratory tract.
     b. In high doses, may get significant hyperthermia, respiratory depression, coma.

  c. Treatment (same as for atropine overdose)

    1. Severe hyperthermia constitutes a serious medical emergency. Symptomatic treatment with ice packs or sponge bath.

    2. Minimize external stimulations (sound, light).

    3. May need physical restraints to control delirium reaction.

    4. Valium®, I.M., 5 to 15 mg to calm the delirium. *Do not use* major tranquilizers (phenothiazines) or barbiturates as these drugs may potentiate atropine induced respiratory depression.

    5. Supportive care for respiratory depression (mechanical assistance for respiration, if needed).

    6. With severe symptoms, may reduce the central effects with a cholinesterase inhibitor, such as physostigmine, I.M., 4 mg, q 1–1½ hours. Tetrahydroaminoacridine is more effective against Ditran.

    7. Sominex® overdose is treated as above. Its active ingredient is scopalamine.

E. Marijuana (Cannabis)

Derived from the flowering tops of *cannabis sativa,* a hemp plant, and used for its psychic effect since 2700 B.C. Marijuana consists of the chopped plant, is smoked or eaten and varies considerably in potency (1 to 4 per cent THC). Hashish is derived from the flowering top of female plants and is more potent (10 per cent THC).

  1. Slang names: grass, pot, hash, etc.

  2. Pharmacology: Active ingredient is Δ 9 tetrahydrocannabinol (THC) which can be synthesized by a difficult process and is very unstable in its pure synthesized form (although it is claimed that pure THC is sold on the streets, this is unlikely). Central and peripheral nervous system: dose dependent. Sites of action: mild depression of brain stem activating system; reduction of polysynaptic spinal cord reflexes. Mechanism of action: unknown. Dosage: in cigarettes: 50 micrograms/kg of THC is a mild social high, 250 micrograms/kg of THC is psychotomimetic;

orally: 5 to 30 mg. Duration of action two to five hours. Half life of seven days. Tolerance occurs with large amounts of THC, but not associated with cross tolerance to LSD or mescaline, although flashbacks can be produced by THC. It is not a narcotic; no addiction or abstinence syndrome. No substantiated cause-effect correlation with narcotic abuse. No proven direct association with violent crime; on the contrary the user is usually more passive than aggressive during the drug state. Prolonged use may lead to loss of interest in assigned vocational tasks but not substantiated that leads to chronic dementia. (Zarafonetis, 1972)

3. Diagnosis
   a. Behavioral factors:
      1. Euphoria, or accentuation of other affective phenomena, increased tactile and auditory awareness, distortion of space (diminished depth perception) and time (slowed); mild sedation.
      2. Environment, personality factors and amount of THC determine reaction by user. Usually does not produce an intense psychological effect.
      3. Larger doses may produce hallucinations.
   b. Physical factors: dryness of mouth, tachycardia, hypertension, drowsiness, injected conjunctiva.
4. Treatment:
   a. Acute intoxication; rare, but must be taken seriously.
      1. Panic is most common. Reactions of the user to effects of the drug. Treat as bad trip (see LSD).
      2. A toxic psychosis may be seen; an overdose syndrome usually following ingestion of large amount of hashish. May persist for 12 to 14 hours followed by a severe hangover up to 48 hours. Treat as a bad trip.
      3. Use of medication rarely indicated in marijuana reactions, but if person is very overexcited, give Valium, orally, 10 mg, q 2h as indicated.

IV. CENTRAL NERVOUS SYSTEM STIMULANTS

H. J. SCHULTE, M.D.

The general effect of these drugs is to bring about increased wakefulness and alertness, feelings of increased ability and initiative, and suppression of appetite. This excited state is followed by a depression which often leads to repeated use. Not uncommonly one will encounter a concomitant barbiturate addiction. The barbiturates are used to lessen the undesirable agitation and restlessness and to allow the heavy user a down period for sleep. Excessive dosage, especially by intravenous administration, may produce a psychosis (amphetamine psychosis).

Usually the drugs are ingested, but they may also be sniffed (cocaine) or used intravenously (speed freak).

A. Amphetamines and amphetamine-like stimulants

1. *Chemical Name*	*Generic Name*	*Slang Names*
Amphetamine	Benzedrine®	Bennies, beans, whites, cross tops, truck drivers
Dextroamphetamine	Dexedrine®	Dexies, oranges
Dexedrine & Amobarbital	Dexamyl®	Christmas trees (Spansule form)
D-amphetamine & Amphetamine	Biphetamine®	Black Beauties
Methamphetamine	Methedrine®, Desoxyn®	Meth, crank, crystal, speed
Phenmetrazine	Preludin®	
Diethylpropion Hydrochloride	Tenuate®	
Benzphetamine Hydrochloride	Didrex®	

2. Pharmacology: Amphetamine is a sympathomimetic amine, with actions like norepinephrine. Central nervous system: it affects cortical stimulation and possibly stimulation of the reticular activating system. It stim-

ulates the respiratory center. Autonomic nervous system: peripheral alpha and beta actions common to sympathomimetic drugs. Mechanism of action: peripherally it acts indirectly by releasing norepinephrine from peripheral adrenergic stores. Produces its central adrenergic effects by displacing norepinephrine and dopamine from intraneuronal storage sites and inhibiting their uptake by nerve terminals. Amphetamine also competitively inhibits the oxidative deamination of norepinephrine and dopamine, thus prolonging their effects in the CNS. In high doses it may be related to decrease breakdown of endogenous 5-hydroxytryptamine. Usual single dose: 2.5 to 5 mg. Duration of action: four to six hours. High potential for psychological dependence and for tolerance leading to increased dosage. Occurrence of physical dependence with clear-cut abstinence syndrome is questionable. (Zarafonetis, 1972) Lethal dose: 25 mg/kg; Lethal blood level: 0.2 mg per cent.

3. Diagnosis
    a. Behavioral findings:
        1. General: increased alertness, insomnia. Increased drive to undertake tasks, accompanied by a euphoric high. Progresses to increased psychomotor activity, restlessness, tremors, sterotypic behavior, irritability and paranoia.
        2. Amphetamine psychosis is a state of extreme paranoia with auditory and/or visual hallucinations, but it lacks certain features of an organic delirium since there is no disorientation or true confusion. This can follow a single dose of 50 mg but is more common among chronic abusers. Even without therapy, the symptoms of amphetamine psychosis usually disappear in three to six days after discontinuation of the drug, but may last up to a week.
    b. Physical findings of amphetamine poisoning:
        1. Restless, insomnia, hyperreflexia, tremor, sweating, mydriasis

    2. Hypertension, tachycardia, extrasystoles

    3. Delirium, mania, hyperpyrexia, arrythmias, marked hypertension, tachycardia

    4. All of the above plus convulsion, coma, circulatory collapse, death (Espelin and Done, 1968.)

  c. There is some debate whether a well-defined abstinence syndrome exists. Upon withdrawal there occurs a period of profound sleep (the crash which may last for two to three days) but little physical danger. Kramer, *et al.* (1967) suggests that this represents a true abstinence syndrome. After this there is a profound sense of lethargy, irritation, frustration and a severe depression which may lead to suicide.

  d. Laboratory: identifiable in blood and urine samples.

4. Treatment: watch for concomitant barbiturate addiction

  a. Amphetamine poisoning (see physical findings 3, 4).

    1. Thorazine, 1 mg/kg, I.M., given to patients with 2 or greater findings; decrease to 0.5 mg/kg if barbiturates are involved, repeat in 30 minutes if necessary.

    2. If hypertension or other sympathomimetic symptoms are severe, use an alpha-adrenegic blocking agent such as phenoxybenzamine (Dibenzyline®). Exercise caution and careful maintaining of blood pressure and other vital signs.

    3. Empty stomach by emesis or in comatose patient by gastric lavage (after endotracheal intubation only) because of delayed emptying time.

    4. Supportive care as necessary: seizure precautions, maintain open airway; I.V. fluids may be necessary to support circulation.

    5. Avoid stimulation as much as possible; quiet, dark room.

    6. Peritoneal dialysis if patient fails to respond to the above procedures (Espelin & Done, 1968).

b. Amphetamine psychosis
1. *Do not use phenothiazines if an atropine-like drug is also involved.*
2. Thorazine, I.M., 1 mg/kg, decrease to 0.5 mg/kg if barbiturates are involved.
3. Psychiatric hospitalization is indicated with continued use of phenothiazines if necessary.
4. Definitive treatment and supportive aftercare are necessary because relapse to abuse of amphetamine is frequent.
c. Withdrawal: three phases
1. User should be hospitalized
2. With pure amphetamine abuse, the drug may be completely withdrawn in one step (cold turkey). Be alert to possibility of combined amphetamine-barbiturate addiction. In that case, withdrawal of the barbiturate must be gradual, however the amphetamine can still be abruptly stopped.
3. Allow the patient to sleep undisturbed during the crash phase (two to three days).
4. During the early abstinence phase, try to resist medicating the patient and work with him psychologically; be supportive with a willingness, not an insistence, to be of help.
5. Chronic amphetamine users, even when down from their high, may exhibit hyperactivity, agitation and a need to keep busy. Devise activity programs to direct this energy.
6. Firmly block further drug availability in the hospital.
7. Rehabilitation phase: If there is severe underlying depression, transfer to a psychiatric facility. If appropriate, consider environmental changes. Psychotherapy of some sort is essential (Novello, 1972).
d. Chronic abuse constitutes the major problem with these drugs (see VIII).
5. Medical complications of CNS stimulant abuse

    a. Acute medical complications of amphetamine poisoning are noted above (3 b.).

    b. Necrotizing angiitis has been described after I.V. usage.

    c. Organic brain syndrome may occur after chronic, heavy use of central stimulants. (Zarafonetis, 1972)

B. Cocaine (Benzoylmethylecgonine)

    1. Slang names: coke, snow, flake, candy

    2. Pharmacology: Obtained from the leaves of *Erythroxylon coca* and other species of *Erythroxylon*. Has been used for centuries in Bolivia and Peru, especially by the mountain people, to increase endurance (central stimulation). It has the fundamental structure of the synthetic local anesthetics, and its most important clinical application is its ability to block nerve conduction upon local application. Central nervous system: stimulates the CNS from above downward. Stimulation of lower motor centers is probably the result of depression of inhibitory neurons. Acts on the medulla to increase respiration. Higher doses depress the respiratory center leading to death by respiratory depression. Autonomic nervous system: potentiation of both the excitatory and inhibitory responses of sympathetically stimulated organs. Hyperpyrexia due to increased muscular activity, and to autonomic and central effects. Small doses result in bradycardia; large doses produce tachycardia; a large I.V. dose can cause cardiac failure by a direct toxic action on the myocardium. Mechanism of action: similar to amphetamine. It is the only local anesthetic to interfere with epinephrine uptake by the nerve ending, and in this fashion produces sensitization to epinephrine and norepinephrine resulting in vasoconstriction and mydriasis (not used in ophthamology because of corneal scarring). Predominantly detoxified rapidly in the liver; some excreted unchanged in the urine. Dose: 20 to 300 mg, although it is reported that some users have taken as much as 10 gms in series of injections over 24-hour

periods. Duration: four hours. (Goodman & Gilman, 1970) Route of administration: poorly absorbed orally so usually injected or sniffed. Potential for psychological dependence: high. No tolerance develops to the excitatory effects of this drug; no physical dependence. Availability: rarest and most expensive stimulant available on the street. May be injected with heroin (speed ball). A pure cocaine user is exceedingly rare.

3. Diagnosis:
  a. Behavioral findings:
    1. Restless, garrulous, feelings of increased muscular strength and mental capacities.
    2. Most potent antifatigue agent known.
    3. Decrease in hunger, indifference to pain.
  b. Physical findings:
    1. Generalized sympathetic stimulation; hyperactivity.
    2. Emesis common.
    3. Sniffing usually results in perforations of the nasal septum due to intense vasoconstriction.
  c. Cocaine poisoning: usually results from a large dose giving a toxic syndrome similar to amphetamines. Visual auditory, tactile hallucinations. Paranoid ideations and persecutory delusions to which the person may respond violently. Hyperpyrexia is a striking characteristic, as well as vasoconstriction. Convulsions and death from respiratory depression.

4. Treatment:
  a. General: usually only need supportive care, may require artificial respiration and oxygen.
  b. Talk down a bad trip if necessary (see LSD).
  c. Gastric lavage with tap water or induce vomiting. Remove drug from skin or mucous membrane.
  d. Sedation:
    1. Nembutal® 0.2 to 0.5 gm, I.V. or I.M., repeat as indicated.
    2. May consider sedatives used for amphetamine

intoxication: Thorazine 1 mg/kg, I.M. (only if certain adulterants are not involved).

3. If convulsion, Valium, I.V., 2 to 10 mg given slowly. Monitor respirations. Or Phenobarbital, initial dose: 5 mg/kg, I.V. given slowly; additional dose 3 mg/kg, I.V., given slowly. (Conn, 1972)

e. Chronic abuse constitutes the major problem with these drugs.

V. CENTRAL NERVOUS SYSTEM DEPRESSANTS

H. J. SCHULTE, M.D.

This section includes information on those CNS depressants that have the greatest abuse potential. These include: A. Barbiturates and other sedative-hypnotics (includes some minor tranquilizers), B. Alcohol, and C. the Volatile hydrocarbons.

A. Barbiturates and other sedative-hypnotics

1. Pharmacology: The sedative-hypnotic drugs produce general progressive depression of the central nervous system, characterized by sedation and sleep. They are general depressants and in large doses cause depression of activity of the nerves, smooth muscle (leading to decreased effective blood volume), skeletal muscle and cardiac muscle. In a stimulating environment most of these drugs produce excitement and disinhibition resembling that seen in acute alcoholic intoxication. Such excitement may be due to the depression of inhibitory nervous connections rather than to direct stimulation. Central nervous system: effects restricted almost entirely to the CNS except in high doses. Drug-induced sleep generally produces fewer rapid-eye movements (REM) episodes and may inhibit dreaming. Relatively nonselective in action, in contrast to the hallucinogens, CNS stimulants and narcotics. However, the CNS depressants do not depress all neuronal connections to the same extent. The ascending reticular formation, which provides a neuronal stimulation

background for wakefulness, is depressed by small doses of sedative-hypnotic drugs that have no effect on the classical afferent pathway. Respiratory area is more resistant to depression by sedative-hypnotic drugs, but when its reflexes are lost, death ensues unless supportive care is initiated. Mechanism of action: major action is postsynaptic, reducing transmitter effects. They diminish excitatory and inhibitory postsynaptic potentials. Also impaired release of transmitters at nerve endings. After absorption, distributed throughout total body water. All are extensively metabolized largely in the liver (except barbital and phenobarbital). Tolerance develops as well as high potential for psychological and physical dependence. Dose varies. Duration of action: two to five hours. Cross tolerance and cross dependence exist among the drugs in this class. The effects of these drugs, including alcohol, are mutually additive. (Zarafonetis, 1972)

2. Table X-II provides an overview of the abuse potential of barbiturates and several of the nonbarbiturate sedative-hypnotics.
3. Diagnosis
   a. Behavioral factors:
      1. A person having taken a hypnotic dose of barbiturates and not going to sleep will present with euphoria or confusion resembling alcoholic intoxication.
      2. Drowsiness, drunken behavior, such as a staggering gait and slurred speech without alcoholic breath.
      3. Memory impairment, confused thinking, irritability
   b. Sedative-hypnotic drug poisoning
      1. May constitute a major medical emergency. May be accompanied by large quantities of alcohol or another sedative-hypnotic with additive effects. Physical exam alone will not determine the different agents involved. Circumstantial evidence of empty medicine bottle, color of capsules, blood

chemistry, gastric contents and information from relatives or friends concerning dosage and time of ingestion are helpful.

2. Lab: urine gives qualitative determination; blood sample for quantitative level.
3. Signs and symptoms:
   a. Mild poisoning: drowsiness, mental confusion, headache, euphoria or irritability.
   b. Moderate or severe poisoning:
      1. Hyporeflexia with positive Babinski sign. Delirium, stupor or coma. Pupillary changes are not specific until later, and then are dilated and nonreactive to light. Changing level or neurological status noted with barbiturates, Doriden®, Placidyl®, Miltown.
      2. Respiratory changes occur early: rapid and shallow or slow respirations: Cheyne-Stokes rhythm may be present; decreased respiratory minute volume (resulting in hypoxemia and respiratory acidosis). (Doriden has unpredictable sudden onset of respiratory failure.)
      3. Hypotension developing into circulatory collapse (due to direct drug depression of medullary vasomotor center, myocardium, sympathetic ganglia and vascular smooth muscle; hypoxemia).
      4. Shock syndrome: above plus cold, clammy skin, cyanosis; weak, rapid pulse.
      5. Pulmonary complications (atelectasis, pulmonary edema, and bronchopneumonia) and renal failure are not uncommon in severe sedative-hypnotic poisoning.
   c. Abstinence syndrome. Symptoms following discontinuation of the various sedative-hypnotic drugs are similar to each other and to barbiturate abstinence. Hospitalization is indicated.
   1. Minor abstinence findings (can include one or

TABLE X-II

SEDATIVE-HYPNOTIC DRUGS: THEIR ABUSE POTENTIAL, FATAL DOSE, AND OTHER INFORMATION
(Adapted from DeGross, 1970; Smith, 1967; Wesson, 1972; and Krupp, 1972)

Trade Name	Generic Name	Slang Name	Oral Sedating Dose (mg)	Oral Hypnotic Dose (mg)	Dependence Producing Dose (gm/day)	Time Needed to Produce Dependency (Days)	Withdrawal Comments	Fatal Dose Gm.	Total Blood Level Mg%	Symptoms Upon Abrupt Withdrawal and Other Information
Seconal®	Sodium secobarbital	Red devils, reds	30	100	0.80–2.2	35–37	Convulsions within 2 to 3 days	3	3.5	Generally for short-acting barbiturates, the lethal serum level is 3.5 mg/100 ml; 8 mg/100 ml for long-acting barbiturates
Nembutal®	Sodium pentobarbital	Yellow jackets, yellows, nembies	30	100	0.80–2.2	35–37	Same	3	3.5	
Tuinal®	50% Amobarbital 50% Secobarbital	Rainbows, tuies	30	100						
Luminal®	Phenobarbital	Phennies	30	100			Onset of convulsions later	5	8	
Doriden®	Glutethimide	Goofers	250	500–1000	2.5		*	10–12		Like barbiturates (Essig, 1964)
Miltown® Equinil®	Meprobamate		400	800–1200	3.2	40	*	0.15 gm/kg		As per barbiturates (Essig, 1964)

Noctec®	Chloral Hydrate		500	1000–1500		*		Marked gastric irritations and vomiting
Noludar®	Methyprylon		50–100	200–300	2.4	*	6	Hallucinations, schizophreniform reactions, convulsions, death (Berger, 1961)
Quaalude®	Methaqualone	Sopers, Qs, Ludes	75	150–300		*		Delirium, convulsions (Kato, 1969); increase in recent abuse. Taken to obtain drunk effect.
Placidyl®	Ethchlorvynol		100–200	500	1.0	*		Hallucinations, delirium, convulsions
Valmid®	Ethinamate			500		*		Minor abstinence signs, delusions, hallucinations, convulsions (Ellinwood and Ewing, 1962)
Carbrital®	Sodium Pentobarbital + Carbromal			100–250	13			

TABLE X-II Continued

Trade Name	Generic Name	Slang Name	Oral Sedative Dose (mg)	Oral Hypnotic Dose (mg)	Dependence Producing Dose (gm/day)	Time Needed to Produce Dependency (Days)	Withdrawal Comments	Fatal Dose Gm.	Total Blood Level Mg%	Symptoms Upon Abrupt Withdrawal and Other Information
Valium	Diazepam		5–10	15–25	(80–120 mg.)	42	Convulsions within 5 to 8 days			Seizures (Hollister, 1963); (maximum overdose with recovery in an adult is 1500 mg. single dose)
Librium®	Chloridiazo- poxide HCL		25	75–100	0.35–0.60	60–180	Same			Seizures (Hollister, 1961); (Maximum overdose with recovery in an adult is 2500 mg. single dose; also a case with suspected dose of 3750 mg.) Onset of abstinence may be delayed 3 to 4 days and seizures may not occur until the eighth day. This abstinence syndrome requires very high doses.
Dalmane	Flurazepam		15	30						No overdoses reported yet

* Clinical data not available. Clinical experience has shown that many of these drugs do indeed produce a withdrawal syndrome.

more of the following) : anxiety, apprehension, agitation, nausea, vomiting, excessive sweating, tachycardia, syncopal episodes, tremulousness, muscle twitches, hyperactive reflexes, insomnia, polyuria.

2. Major abstinence findings

    a. Generalized convulsions, hyperpyrexia, delirium or psychotic behavior, and sometimes death.

    b. The seizures are like idiopathic grand mal seizures; can occur anytime from 12 hours to 12 days after withdrawal. Not all patients develop seizures; dose related; may develop status epilepticus. If a delirium occurs, it may include delusions, confusion and auditory or visual hallucinations. This may be indistinguishable from delirium tremens and death may occur. Some patients develop seizures not followed by a delirium, and for others the opposite occurs. The abrupt onset of seizures or an acute psychosis in an adult should raise the suspicion of sedative-hypnotic addiction.

    c. Sedative-hypnotic abstinence syndrome is potentially more serious than opiate withdrawal. If convulsions or delirium occur with opiate withdrawal, the person has probably been abusing depressants as well.

4. Treatment of sedative-hypnotic poisoning

    a. The critical factor is constant medical and nursing attendance to maintain physiologic responses until the danger of circulatory depression and respiratory failure have passed.

    1. Mild poisoning

        a. Induce vomiting with syrup of ipecac, 30 ml orally and large amounts of warm water.

        b. Symptomatic and supportive nursing care with observation of vital signs until out of danger; hospitalize.

    c. Psychiatric consultation and treatment for suicidal patient.

2. Moderate or severe poisoning:

    a. Hospitalize and institute antishock measures; closely monitor vital signs.

    b. The majority of patients will survive days of unconsciousness if the airway is kept open (endotracheal intubation or may require a tracheostomy) and artificial respiration with pulmonary toilet is maintained (IPPB, tank respirator, etc.). Serial blood gases are helpful.

    c. Gastric lavage with two to four liters of warm water or isotonic saline using Ewald tube. Caution: danger of aspiration pneumonia is great in stuperous or comatose patients, and lavage should be performed only if cough reflex is intact or patient is intubated.

    d. Alkalinize urine with $NaHCO_3$; promote diuresis with mannitol or Lasix® and I.V. fluids. This is most useful with phenobarbital (30 per cent excreted in the urine). Do not force diuresis with Valium, Librium or Thorazine overdose.

    e. Indwelling bladder catheter; urine and blood studies.

    f. I.V. fluids; monitor central venous pressure. In the event of shock, give volume expanders to maintain blood pressure.

    g. Do not use CNS stimulants (analeptics or convulsants) such as amphetamine, Picrotoxin, bemegride (Meginide®), ephedrine or strychnine. They have been used, but are not true antidotes, do not shorten the duration of poisoning and have possible severe complications (cardiac arrythmias, convulsions, hyperthermia, psychotic episodes).

    h. Peritoneal or hemodialysis may be indicated if above measures fail.

5. Treatment of sedative-hypnotic abstinence syndrome
   a. This should be undertaken in the hospital. There are several methods available for managing sedative withdrawal. (Bakewell and Ewing, 1969; and Wesson, *et al.*, 1972) The general aim is to maintain a good balance between intoxication and withdrawal symptoms.
   b. Use the following equation to determine an adequate schedule for the withdrawal (phenobarbital method) :

$$\frac{\text{Amount of drug reported taken daily}}{\text{Oral hypnotic dose of that drug (see Table X-II)}}$$

$$\times$$

30 mg phenobarbital = Total daily phenobarbital dosage needed to initiate withdrawal (Wesson, 1972).

1. The method is to substitute 30 mg of phenobarbital for every hypnotic dose of barbiturate the patient reports taking.
2. Advantages: phenobarbital is relatively long-lasting, produces only moderate fluctuations in barbiturate blood level, the fatal dose far exceeds the toxic dose, and the signs of phenobarbital toxicity are easily detected (sustained nystagmus, ataxia, slurred speech).
3. If intoxication occurs, may omit next dose, or, if necessary, cut the next daily dose in half and closely monitor the patient's withdrawal.
4. If withdrawal symptoms develop; may increase daily dosage until signs of intoxication occur. If advanced withdrawal symptoms such as tremors, muscular weakness, hyperreflexia or postural hypotension occur, increase daily dosage and give phenobarbital 200 mg, I.M., stat. May repeat in two hours, if needed.
5. After the patient's condition has been stabilized, decrease the daily dose of phenobarbital by 30

mg. The withdrawal should proceed smoothly. (Wesson, 1972)

c. Combined amphetamine and CNS depressant abuse;
   1. Hospitalize the patient; observe closely.
   2. The amphetamine itself may be abruptly stopped.
   3. Stabilization with barbiturates (using the method of Wesson, *et al.*, 1972, or that of Bakewell, *et al.*, 1969), followed by gradual barbiturate withdrawal.

d. Combined barbiturate and narcotics abuse:
   1. Hospitalize patient; observe closely.
   2. Stabilization with both a barbiturate and a narcotic (methadone).
   3. Withdraw the methadone by approximately 10 percent per day (Wesson, 1972).
   4. After the withdrawal of the methadone is complete, begin the reduction schedule for the barbiturates (Bakewell, 1972).

B. Alcohol

This is by far the most commonly abused drug today. Alcohol is considered a CNS depressant with many qualities in common with the sedative-hypnotic drugs discussed above.

1. Diagnosis of major alcoholic manifestations
   a. Acute intoxication: drunkenness
      1. Varying degrees of exhilaration, disinhibition, loquacity, slurred speech, incoordination of movement and gait, irritability, drowsiness. In advanced cases, stupor and coma. Blood level to be legally drunk is 150 mg/100 ml (with minor variations from state to state).
      2. On rare occasions, acute intoxication may present as combative, destructive, irrational: acute alcoholic paranoid state (Wintrobe *et al.*, 1970).
      3. Coma due to alcohol may be a difficult differential diagnosis. The diagnosis of alcoholic coma is made only partially on the basis of a flushed face, stupor and the odor of alcohol; all the other causes of coma must carefully be excluded (espe-

cially head trauma and subdural hematoma). This coma is not always benign. Respiratory depression (preceded by loss of corneal and pupillary reflexes) and peripheral vascular collapse may occur (for treatment see V, A, 4, a).

b. The abstinence syndrome. There must be a sustained period of chronic intoxication preceding a period of relative or absolute abstinence from alcohol during which the symptoms become manifest. Although the major symptoms usually appear in various combinations, they may appear individually and will be described one by one: tremulousness, hallucinatory, epileptic and delirious states. The individual most likely to be vulnerable is the periodic or spree drinker, although the steady drinker may also experience these symptoms if he abruptly stops drinking.

There is a significant prognostic difference between alcoholic hallucinosis and delirium tremens. As noted, the tremulous-hallucinosis-epilepsy-delirium states depend on chronic alcoholic intoxication and relative or absolute withdrawal to be manifested. The mildest degree of this syndrome, the tremulousness and nausea, may appear after only several days of alcohol ingestion and after a relatively short period of abstinence. Alcoholic hallucinosis occurs usually in the first 12 to 48 hours after withdrawal. Alcoholic epilepsy, which occurs in the discrete time interval of the first 12 to 48 hours, appears in long time drinkers as does delirium tremens. One third of alcoholic epilepsy patients proceed to develop delirium tremens. Delirium tremens requires several months of inebriaation and does not occur until several days after abstinence. Any given patient may display one or all of the symptoms of withdrawal. If all the symptoms of abstinence are present in a patient, they become manifest in a predictable sequence; first tremulousness and hallucinosis (and/or seizures), followed by delirium tremens (Wintrobe, *et al.*, 1970).

1. Tremulousness: the shakes or the jitters
   a. The symptoms appear in the aftermath of several days of drinking. Often first seen when the person awakes from sleep (abstinence) with the shakes, general irritability and gastrointestinal symptoms, especially nausea and vomiting. This is relieved by more alcohol. Generally the symptoms become increasingly pronounced and reach their peak intensity 24 to 36 hours after the drinking stops.
   b. Stage of 24 to 36 hours: Patient alert and easily startled. Facial flush, injected conjunctiva, tachycardia, anorexia, nausea, vomiting; insomnia and irritability; mild confusion regarding the last few days of the spree but no serious disorientation; notable generalized tremor worse with activity and emotional stress.
   c. The tendency to startle and tremulousness may persist for a week or more. Uneasy feelings and insomnia may persist for two weeks.
2. Alcoholic hallucinosis:
   a. Most common form of disordered sense perception in the alcoholic.
   b. Described as bad dreams which are difficult to separate from real experience. Sounds, shadows, familiar objects assume distorted forms. More commonly associated with animated (human, animal, insect) than inanimate. Scant evidence to support the popular belief that certain visual hallucinations are specific to alcoholism.
   c. Occurs in about one quarter of tremulous pa-

tients. Hallucinations may be visual, auditory, mixed and occasionally tactile or olfactory.

3. Auditory hallucinosis: An alcoholic psychosis which occurs in the face of an otherwise clear sensorium—patients are not confused, disoriented, obtunded and display no memory loss.

   a. Acute form: vocal hallucinations where one hears voices, often reproachful, to which the person responds appropriately, e.g. call for police protection or attempt suicide to avoid the threat of the voices. Full recovery is possible.

   b. A small number go on to become chronic. Ideas of reference and other poorly systemized paranoid delusions become prominent. At this late stage, the picture resembles symptoms of schizophrenia. However, there is no family history; age of onset is considerably later than that of classic schizophrenia, and symptoms develop in close temporal relationship to a drinking bout.

4. Alcoholic epilepsy (rum fits)

   a. During abstinence following chronic alcoholic abuse, there is a high likelihood of developing seizures.

   b. A discreet period, usually 12 to 48 hours after cessation of drinking.

   c. Distinctive features: abnormal EEG which returns to normality in a few days; usually a burst of four to six grand mal seizures; may develop status epilepticus; one third go on to develop delirium tremens.

   d. If seizures are focal in nature, then a focal lesion (usually traumatic) will likely be found in addition to the alcohol factor.

   e. The postictal confusion may blend with the onset of delirium tremens or there may be a clearing of the postictal state over several hours to several days before the delirium sets in.

f. Distinguish from other causes of adult onset epilepsy.

5. Delirium tremens: most dramatic and grave of all alcoholic complications.

a. Symptoms: profound confusion, delusions, visual hallucinations, tremor, agitation, insomnia. Increased autonomic nervous system activity: dilated pupils, tachycardia, fever, profuse perspiration.

b. Onset: following a long spree, the person may experience several days of tremulousness and hallucinosis or one or more seizures, and may be recovering when he suddenly develops delirium tremens. A long-time steady drinker may be admitted to the hospital for an unrelated illness or accident, and three to four days later delirium tremens appears.

c. Course: The majority of cases are benign, short-lived and end abruptly. If there is only a single episode, duration is usually 72 hours. After several days of hyperactivity, the patient sleeps and awakens with no memory of the delirious period. Less commonly, the delirium gradually subsides. Rarely, one or more relapses with lucid intervals; the whole process may last for two to three days or as long as five weeks (rarely). 15 percent fatality. Death from hyperthermia or peripheral vascular collapse.

c. Korsakoff's Psychosis

1. Usually occurs in patients following an episode of delirium tremens; also may be caused by cerebral atherosclerosis or other toxic conditions. The hallucinations, insomnia and inattentiveness have cleared; the patient is alert and talkative.

2. Symptoms: retrograde and anterograde amnesia; disorder or retentive memory which is impaired out of proportion to other cognitive functions. Inability to learn. Becomes apathetic and inert. Confabulation (found in other confusional states as well) is absent in the late stages.

3. Course: One quarter of these patients attain partial or complete recovery. More commonly there is some improvement over a year or longer. The person is left with large memory gaps and inability to sort out events temporally. Common diagnosis at this time is organic brain syndrome due to alcohol.

4. The same clinical features as found in Korsakoff's psychosis may occur in other diseases: ruptured saccular aneurysm and subarachynoid hemorrhage, subdural hematoma, tuberculous meningitis and tumors in the walls of the third ventricle.

d. Wernicke's Disease

1. Due to Thiamine deficiency and results in degeneration of the basal ganglia. When found in the chronic alcoholic with malnutrition, it may often be accompanied by other nutritional diseases of the nervous system.

2. Course and symptoms:

   a. Sudden onset with mental disturbance, paralysis of eye movements (ophthalmoplegia) and ataxic gait. In Wernicke's (1881) original description, all three of his patients progressed to coma and death.

   b. Occular symptoms: Crucial, for diagnosis. Nystagmus (either horizontal or vertical or both) and/or *any degree* of lateral rectus muscle weakness or paralysis. This sixth nerve palsy is bilateral, although not always symmetric, and accompanied by internal strabismus and diplopia. The eye signs and ataxia preceed the mental disturbance by a few days to two weeks.

c. Symptoms of deranged mental function are found in over 80 percent of the patients and take one of several forms. A small proportion have the symptoms of delirium tremens (hallucinations, confusion, autonomic overactivity) which are mild and clear without treatment. The majority of patients are listless, apathetic and severely confused. In this latter state, the patient is inattentive, cannot concentrate, suspends conversation in the middle of a sentence, is disoriented and his remarks have no consistency from one moment to another. Some patients display the symptoms of Korsakoff's syndrome from the time they are first seen.

d. In advanced states, indications of high output cardiovascular failure occur.

e. It appears that in the chronic alcoholic who is nutritionally deficient, Wernicke's disease and Korsakoff's psychosis represent different aspects of the same disease (Wintrobe, *et al.,* 1970).

2. Treatment

a. Acute alcohol intoxication

1. Examine for possible trauma (especially head trauma), pulmonary and abdominal emergencies. Rule out diabetic crisis.

2. Gastric lavage or emesis

3. $NaHCO_3$, 1 tsp to 1 pt water, q 1 to 2 h, to prevent acidosis. $NaHCO_3$, I.V. for acidosis.

4. Stimulants; caffeine, sodium benzoate or strong coffee.

5. *Avoid depressant drugs* (many sedative hypnotic drugs interfere with alcohol metabolism) and potent respiratory stimulants (Conn, 1972).

6. If the patient is comatose and areflexic, treat as for barbiturate poisoning.

7. For intractable retching or acute alcoholic excitation, give phenothiazine tranquilizer (e.g. Thorazine 25 to 50 mg, I.M.; be aware of orthostatic hypotension) (Krupp, *et al.*, 1972).

8. Start during acute phase and continue for several days; Vitamin B complex, orally; antacids.

b. Alcohol withdrawal seizures

1. Treat acutely with parenteral phenobarbital (Luminal®). Decrease phenobarbital over ten-day period if no history of repeated withdrawal seizures (Conn, 1972).

c. Delirium

1. Etiology: drug ingestion (sedatives, alcohol); may also accompany metabolic, infectious and other diseases.

2. Treatment of the delirium is no substitute for correct diagnosis and specific treatment of the underlying cause.

3. Patient should be in a quiet room.

4. Observe closely; monitor vital signs and fluid intake and output. Explain all procedures to patient before they are performed.

5. Restraints may be necessary if the patient is combative, if he is receiving I.V. fluids or if he is in danger of falling out of bed.

6. Do not write continuing sedative medication orders. Order each time only after being informed of the patient's immediate clinical status.

7. Sedation medication:

a. Librium®: I.M., 25 to 100 mg, for those who will not take oral meds; repeat dose q 4 to 6 h, p.r.n. *Do not give I.V.* Occasionally, repeated doses produce cumulative effects which result in the patient becoming oversedated.

   b. Paraldehyde, orally, 5 cc in milk or orange juice; can be increased by 1 to 3 cc as necessary, repeat dose q 4 to 6 h, p.r.n. May combine with 0.5 to 1.0 gm doses of chloral hydrate. Effective and safe, but occasionally objected to because of its odor; sterile absesses may occur with I.M. paraldehyde. Rectal and I.M. routes are not as effective.

   c. Valium® orally or I.M., 5 to 10 mg, q 2 to 6 h, p.r.n. Less cumulative effects than Librium.

8. Do not use phenothiazines because of possible additive effects and hypotension.

9. In the alcoholic patient:

   a. Give multivitamins and Thiamine 100 mgm I.V. or I.M. Q.D. x three to ten days (Conn, 1972).

   b. Treatment of Wernicke-Korsakoff syndrome

     1. *Wernicke's disease is a medical emergency. Immediate treatment with thiamine,* 50 mg, I.V., and 50 mg, I.M.; repeat the latter dose each day until the patient resumes a normal diet. (Even a delay of a few hours may be crucial in preventing an early picture of Wernicke's disease from developing the mental signs or preventing the progression to Korsakoff's psychosis.)

     2. Give other B vitamins orally or I.V. if necessary.

     3. Continuous medical observation

     4. Add B vitamins to all glucose I.V. solutions (because the glucose solution may exhaust the already-depleted

B vitamin reserve in these patients precipitating Wernicke's disease by causing a rapid thiamine deficiency or causing circulatory collapse and death).

5. If signs of cardiovascular failure (pulmonary edema, faint heart sounds or gallop, tachycardia, low blood pressure) are present, rapid digitalization is indicated.

6. After recovery from the acute phase of the illness, assess the predominance of the amnestic psychosis. Disposition of the patient to family, nursing home or mental institution must be determined (Wintrobe *et al.*, 1970).

c. Chronic alcohol abuse: There are a multitude of approaches and specific techniques which have been used with varying degrees of success in the treatment of alcoholism. Here only a few guidelines will be mentioned.

1. Psychosocial approach

a. When a patient comes to a physician for emotional problems and it becomes clear that alcoholic abuse plays a central role, the physician should clearly state to the patient his impression of the person's alcohol abuse. It is crucial that the individual see his drinking as a problem (disease, etc.) that needs to be worked on or else nothing will be done. The physician should be alert to other indications of alcoholism (car accidents, the social drinker, etc.) and inquire specifically.

b. Undoubtedly the most successful

approach to date is Alcoholics Anonymous. They employ the method of group social pressure, as well as group reinforcement in order to help the person stay dry. Central to this approach is the necessity of the individual to admit that he has a drinking problem (disease, etc.) .

c. Supportive psychotherapy of various methodologies.

2. Drug approach: Antabuse® (disulfiram) is a helpful adjunct for those selected alcoholic patients who want to remain in a state of enforced sobriety so that supportive and psychotherapeutic treatment may be best utilized. It is not a cure for alcoholism, and is not effective without proper motivation and supportive therapy. This drug in combination with alcohol produces an unpleasant and potentially severe reaction. Prescribe carefully, only after reading thoroughly about this drug. One may consult the *Physician's Desk Reference,* 1972, or manufacturer's data for further information.

3. The Michigan Alcoholic Screening Test (MAST) is a useful instrument in the diagnosis of chronic alcoholism. (See Chapter III, Aids To Diagnosis In Psychiatry) .

C. The volatile hydrocarbons

These CNS depressants are not as widely abused as the sedative hypnotic class of drugs, but present a severe threat of acute organ damage and are very dangerous. With chronic abuse, they are more likely to induce changes not unlike an organic brain syndrome. They are sniffed to induce a high. The most commonly abused volatile hydrocarbons include:

Glue	Aerosols
Benzene	Lighter fluid, gasoline
Carbon tetrachloride	Paint
Nail polish remover	Lacquer & varnish thinner

1. Diagnosis
   a. Behavioral findings:
      1. Hazy euphoria, slurred speech; impaired perception coordination and judgment.
      2. The initial excitement may be followed by depression and stupor.
      3. Hallucinations in 50 percent of cases. Psychotic episodes occasionally occur.
   b. Physical findings:
      1. Odor on patient's breath and clothing.
      2. Rapid pulse; anoxia by replacing pulmonary air.
      3. Death has occurred secondary to freezing of larynx, laryngospasm, and asphyxiation.
      4. Damage of liver, brain, kidneys, bone marrow and myocardium (potential ventricular tachycardia or fibrillation).
2. Treatment
   a. General: Similar to acute barbiturate intoxications. If severe hypotension occurs, treat with volume expanders.
   b. Specific:
      1. If swallowed, gastric lavage may be performed, but do not use emetics.
      2. If inhaled, treat with fresh air, or 95 percent oxygen and 5 percent carbon dioxide.
      3. *Do not inject epinephrine because of the possibility of myocardial sensitization and arrythmias* (N.Y. Department of Health, 1971).
3. Medical complication of volatile hydrocarbon inhalation
   a. If the substance is inhaled in a plastic bag pulled over the head, suffocation may result.

b. Glue sniffing may result in fatal, acute cerebral edema; severe bone marrow depression attributed to the benzene base in the glues; and death due to cardiac arrythmias (Zarafonetis, 1972).

VI. NARCOTICS

H. J. Schulte, M.D.
AND
S. J. Wilson, M.D.

These substances are medically used primarily for the control of pain. Opium, derived from poppy juice, was used before history was recorded. Its active ingredient is morphine, an alkaloid which gives opium its analgesic action and remains the standard against which new analgesics are measured. Morphine, other natural alkaloids of opium, semisynthetic opiate derivatives and synthetic morphine surrogates (opioids) are all considered narcotics, in that they produce sleep as well as analgesia. They are all addicting to one degree or another, producing physical and psychological dependence.

The abuse of these drugs has become a serious psychosocial problem. Illicit trade has become a big business and criminal activity to pay for the addict's fix is a major urban crisis. "It should be emphasized, however, that the action of the drug itself is to reduce hunger, pain and aggressive and sexual drives; it is the need for the drug rather than its effects that motivates criminal activity." (Goodman and Gilman, 1970).

To appreciate the growing abuse of these drugs one must try to understand the immense relief (though short-lived) from anxiety, tensions and problems that the user experiences. The high obtained from these drugs becomes a fixed memory of a most pleasurable reprieve from the apparently unsolvable psychosocial problems of the user. This is a strongly reinforcing experience, and to achieve abstinence one needs psychological as well as physical supportive treatment. A crucial aspect must be the learning and integration of new problem-solving behaviors.

Table X-III presents an overview of commonly abused narcotic drugs.

A. Heroin and heroin-related drugs
  1. Street usage and some implications.
     a. The user receives heroin with adulterants added. Each time heroin (and most other drugs as well) change hands the seller decreases the quantity of heroin per dose (spoon, bag, etc.) by adding (cut with) one of the following substances:

  Heroin + Lactose + quinine +/— a sedative-
          (common) (common)   hypnotic
             or   or   (to give
          Dextrose   Mannitol   the user
          (tastes   (rare)   what he
          bitter)   believes
                                  to be the
                                  nods)

     b. Implications:
        1. Because of adulteration, the amount of heroin per dose varies widely. For example in New York there is approximately 5 to 10 percent heroin per dose, while in Detroit the same market may only have 1 to 2 percent heroin. In Vietnam a similar market dose may have 98 percent heroin in it (unpublished data).
        2. This makes it difficult to determine how much an addict may have taken to cause an overdose or to determine the amount that brought about addiction (many other factors involved here; see 4 c of this section).
        3. It is important to note this factor when reading the literature concerning heroin addiction or methadone withdrawal or replacement. Often not clearly stated is the actual amount or purity of the heroin involved. By omitting this information many of the conclusions must be qualified.
  2. Pharmacology of morphine (a prototype narcotic)
     a. Central nervous system:

TABLE X-III

NARCOTICS

Nonpropriety Name	Trade Name	Slang Name	Usual Dose Mg*	Method of Administration	Duration of Action-Hours	Withdrawal Symptoms	Distinguishing Features
Opium		O, OP	1 to 2 pipes	Smoking, sniffed	5	Mild	Possession illegal in U.S.
Morphine (diacetylmorphine)		MS, Miss Emma, white stuff	10	Oral, IM, SQ, IV, sniffed	4	See Dx of Abstinence Syndrome	
Heroin	Diacetylmorphine	H, horse, smack, junk jones, hairy, jive	spoon (varies amount) 2 to 8	IV, SQ,† sniffed	4	Like Morphine	Manufacture or possession illegal in U.S.
Hydromorphone (dihydromorphone)	Dilaudid® etc.		2	Oral, IM, IV	4 to 5	Like Morphine	
Codeine		Fours	30 to 65	Oral, IM, IV	4 to 6	See Dx of Abstinence Syndrome	
Oxycodone (dihydrohydroxycodeinone)	Percodan®		10 to 15	Oral (tab)	4 to 5	Close to morphine	
Levorphanol	Levo-Dromoran®		2 to 3	Oral, IM, IV	4 to 5	Like Morphine	Synthetic Analgesic
Methadone	Dolophine®	Mets	10 to 40	Oral, IV, IM	3 to 4	See Dx of Abstinence syndrome	Cummulative effects on repeated dosage. Withdrawal does not begin until 72 hours after last oral dose.

		Dose* (mg)	Route	Duration (hrs)	Abstinence Syndrome	Notes
Meperidine	Demerol® etc.	50 to 100	Oral, IM, IV, SQ	4	See Dx of Abstinence Syndrome	Retains much of its potency when given orally
Anileridine	Leritine®	30 to 40	Oral, IM, IV	2 to 3	Like Meperidine	Retains much of its potency when given orally,
Codeine	Cough Syrups: Romilar AC® Robitussin AC® Turpin Hydrate Elixir® Turpin Hydrate with Codeine® Cheracol® Hycodan®, others	2 to 4 oz. for euphoria: 1 oz. for cough	Oral (Liquid)	2 to 4	Variable Between morphine and codeine	Many obtainable without prescription.
Propoxyphene HCL	Darvon® or Darvon compound® Not a narcotic but abused by narcotic addicts	32, 65	Oral, IV			Diagnosis: Symptoms resemble heroin overdose with gastric irritation being prominent. Treatment is similar to that for heroin overdose. Nalline or Lorfan are effective antagonists. Lethal blood level: 6 mg. %

† Heroin is rarely used I.M., but is used subcutaneously (skin popping).

* Dose shown is the amount given subcutaneously that produces approximately the same analgesic effects as 10 mg of morphine given SQ. Duration of action shown is for SQ administration; following IV use, peak effects are somewhat more pronounced but overall effects are of shorter duration.

(Reference: Goodman & Gilman, 1970; Smith, 1967; New York Department of Health, 1971).

1. Analgesia, (often without sleep), drowsiness, changes in mood (euphoria; although it is not uncommon to experience dysphoria upon initial abuse), mental clouding, miosis, nausea and vomiting (addicts refer to this as a good sick because it is associated with the desired euphoria).
2. The pain threshold is raised. The user experiences pain sensations, but the ability to tolerate it is markedly increased.
3. Polysynaptic reflexes are depressed at doses that have little effect on two neuron arcs such as the knee-jerk. This may be due to a depressant action on the mechanism involved in temporal summation.
4. Physiological effect on the hypothalamus is to decrease afferent stimulation and release of anti-diuretic hormone.
5. In high doses (which would cause death by respiratory depression) all narcotics and antagonists are CNS stimulants and can cause convulsions. Rarely, meperidine (Demerol®) can cause seizures at lower, intoxicating doses. The stimulation felt after a lower dose is probably due to disinhibition like that felt with alcohol and similar depressants. However, the central depressant action of morphine is unlike that of barbiturates.
6. Morphine has a depressant effect on the brain stem causing respiratory depression.

b. Cardiovascular effects:
1. Decreased capacity to respond to the stress of gravitational shifts; orthostatic hypotension; peripheral vasodilatation.
2. The concurrent use of a narcotic and a phenothiazine potentiates respiratory depression and hypotension.

c. Gastrointestinal effects:
Opium has been used for relief of diarrhea for

centuries. Decrease in propulsive contractions and decrease in secretions. Constipation. Increase in biliary tract pressure.

d. Skin: vasodilation

e. Dextoxified mainly by conjugation with glucuronic acid in the liver.

f. Tolerance: Develops to the respiratory depressant, analgesic, sedative and euphoriant effects, but not to miosis or the gastrointestinal effects. With intermittant use it is possible to limit tolerance. Some addicts are able to maintain social productivity and a stable life style for many years. A more or less continuous usage is required for tolerance. High degree of cross tolerance is present.

g. Potential for physical and psychological dependence is high (Goodman and Gilman, 1970).

3. Narcotic antagonists:

a. Naloxone (Narcan®)
   Nalorphine (Nalline®)
   Levallorphine (Lorfan®)

b. Nalorphine is a semisynthetic congener of morphine. Their pharmacological effects differ according to their use:

   1. If given to a person who has no narcotics in his body, the antagonists produce analgesia, respiratory depression, (except Naxolone®) miosis and usually dysphoria (euphoria is rare).

   2. If given to an individual who is depressed by an overdose of a narcotic, they act as narcotic antagonists and are specific therapy for narcotic poisoning, stimulating respiration, counteracting lethargy.

   3. If given to someone who has developed tolerance to a narcotic, they cause an abrupt short-lived abstinence syndrome.

4. Diagnosis of narcotic analgesic abuse

a. Acute intoxication:

   1. Behavioral findings:

Euphoria, drowsiness, nodding, altered personality and activity, constipation.

2. Physical findings:

Pinpoint pupils (less in chronic abusers and with some opioids), needle tracks of extremities, abdomen, groin (may resemble pock marks when subcutaneous route used), nausea and vomiting, itchy nose, slow pulse and respiration.

b. Acute poisoning:

Triad: pinpoint pupils, depressed respirations and coma usually indicate acute narcotic poisoning. (This may be seen with phenothiazines, also with anticholinergic drugs.) The patient may be asleep, in a stupor or coma. Apnea may lead to respiratory death. Cyanosis may be present. As respiratory exchange decreases, blood pressure may fall. Pupils are equal and miotic. If hypoxia is present, pupils may be dilated. In the experience of Sapira and McDonald (1970), one third of heroin overdose patients presenting with coma may have normal or even increased respirations and will not have marked miosis.

c. Acute abstinence syndromes:

1. This is an agonizing but rarely life-threatening illness, usually lasting from three to five days, but some symptoms persist for as long as seven to ten days. Its severity depends on many factors including the specific drug used, the total daily dose and interval between doses, the duration of use and the personality and health of the individual involved.

2. Morphine and heroin abstinence syndrome

a. Shortly before the time of the next scheduled dose the person begins to experience early signs of withdrawal and his behavior becomes oriented solely toward getting more drugs. This reaches its peak at 36 to 72 hours after the last dose and then gradually subsides.

b. 8 to 12 hours after last dose symptoms: lacrimation, rhinorrhea, yawning and perspiration.

c. At 12 hours: addict may have a restless sleep known as the yen lasting for a few hours.

d. At 48 to 72 hours symptoms reach their peak. Severe expression of earlier symptoms, as the syndrome progresses, symptoms include: dilated pupils, anorexia, gooseflesh (cold turkey), restlessness, increasing irritability, insomnia, marked anorexia, weakness and depression, nausea, vomiting, diarrhea, tachycardia and hypertension, marked chills alternating with flushing (hot and cold flashes), abdominal cramps, muscle spasms and pain in the bones and muscles of the back and extremities.

e. Because of the failure to take in food and fluids along with the above losses, the individual experiences marked weight loss, dehydration, ketosis and acid-base disturbance. Occasionally cardiovascular collapse occurs.

f. Most of the observable symptoms disappear in seven to ten days, but insomnia and some restlessness persist. If a suitable narcotic is taken at any point the symptoms abate dramatically.

3. Meperdine abstinence syndrome: (Demerol®)
Shorter course: peaks in eight to twelve hours and over in four to five days. Fewer autonomic signs (nausea, vomiting, diarrhea), but more severe muscle twitching and nervousness.

4. Methadone abstinence syndrome:
Less intense. Develops more slowly and more prolonged than for heroin. Symptoms begin on the third day, peak on the sixth day and minimal by the tenth to fourteenth day.

5. Codeine, semisynthetics and synthetics abstinence syndromes:
Usually similar but less intense than that for

heroin. General rule: A shorter duration of drug action leads to shorter but more intense withdrawal.

6. Antagonists stimulate withdrawal in a matter of minutes and peak in one half hour. The intensity of Naloxone-precipitated withdrawal is often more severe than if the opiate itself were abruptly withdrawn. Methadone withdrawal produced by an antagonist is especially severe (Goodman and Gilman, 1970).

5. Treatment
   a. Acute narcotic intoxication:
   The user (on a typical high) may arrive at the emergency room because of an unrelated medical problem which may require treatment. Be aware of signs and symptoms of acute narcotic intoxication. Although treatment for this problem will probably not be requested, methadone withdrawal may be recommended.
   b. Acute narcotic poisoning (overdose):
   1. Hospitalization. Observe vital signs and respiration closely. Supportive treatment. May need to assist ventilation.
   2. Narcotic antagonists: improves respiratory state, may not affect consciousness.
      a. Naloxone (Narcan); (10 to 30× as potent as Nalline®). Dosage: 0.4 to 0.8 mg, I.V.; repeat 0.4 mg, I.V., q 5 min. ×2, if no response. Then discontinue this drug. Advantage over Nalline is that it does not produce respiratory depression and therefore can be given with minimal risk in situations where etiology of respiratory depression is unclear. If the coma is misdiagnosed, Narcan is safe whereas other antagonists may worsen the situation. In infants a dose of 5 micrograms/kg of body weight has been recommended. Dosage in pregnancy has not been established.

    b. Nallorpine (Nalline) : Dosage: 10 mg, I.V., may repeat dose in 20 to 30 minutes if necessary.

    c. Levallorphan (Lorfan®) : (10× as potent as Nalorphine). Dosage: 1 to 2 mg, I.V. If no effect after 15 to 20 minutes, poisoning is not narcotic overdose. Dosage should not exceed 3 mg.

    d. *Administer with caution to those suspected of physical addiction because may precipitate an acute abstinence syndrome.*

    e. *It is important to remember that the duration of the narcotic antagonists is shorter than the duration of the narcotic analgesics themselves and therefore, the patient must be kept under observation for a period of at least six hours as they may relapse into coma.*

c. Treatment approaches to chronic narcotic addiction

  1. Milieu of total involvement:

    Treatment consisting of drug withdrawal and psychological rehabilitation is done in milieu settings by exaddicts in conjunction with professional personnel. Involvement in a total therapeutic community and progression through a series of levels or stages during which a form of relearning to adapt to society takes place, are the concepts used in this approach. The most well known of these facilities are Synanon, Daytop Village and the Mendocino Family.

  2. Use of methadone:

    Methadone came into use at the end of World War II. Its pharmacological properties are qualitatively similar to morphine even though its chemical structure only remotely resembles morphine. Its outstanding properties are: effective analgesia, oral efficacy and its extended duration of action in physically dependent individuals. Central nervous system: cumulative sedative effects, analgesia, respiratory depression. It stimulates smooth muscle, resulting in constipation and biliary tract spasm. Cardiovascular effects are not prominent. Biotransformation occurs largely in the liver by N-demethylation. In those physically dependent on methadone, withdrawal symptoms do not begin for 72 to 96 hours after the last oral dose. Subjects are completely comfortable with a single dose as infrequently as every 72 hours (Goodman & Gilman, 1970).

a. Methadone dosage equivalent:
Methadone equals morphine if S.Q. or I.V.; only half as potent P.O. It is usually impossible to ascertain the purity of the heroin which is self-injected as the purity varies markedly from sample to sample.

b. Side effects and adverse reactions to methadone: Precautions must be taken with the following: asthmatic patients in acute attack, chronic obstructive pulmonary disease or cor-pulmonale, head injury or increased intracranial pressure in conjunction with other narcotic analgesics, anesthetics, phenothiazines and other tranquilizers, sedative hypnotics, tricyclic antidepressants and other central nervous system depressants and with monoamine oxidase inhibitors. Adverse reactions include: respiratory depression, light-headedness, dizzyness, sedation, nausea, vomiting and sweating. Side effects may include:

CNS—euphoria, dysphoria, weakness, headache, insomnia, agitation and visual disturbances.

GI—dry mouth, anorexia, constipation, biliary tract spasm.

G-U—urinary retention or hesitancy, reduced libido and/or potency, antidiuretic effects.

Allergic—prurutis, urticaria and other skin rashes.

With the above data, a dosage level adequate to blockade the effects of narcotics should be prescribed. Usually adequate maintenance in smaller cities away from distribution points is 40 to 60 mgm of methadone q.d. in a single dose delivered in a fruit juice vehicle. In larger cities, however, 60 to 80 mgm methadone q.d. is usually required.

c. Methadone withdrawal treatment:

Withdrawal treatment differs from maintenance in that methadone is first substituted for the drug to which the patient is addicted and then detoxification with methadone is undertaken. Patients should be told to expect some discomfort as detoxification progresses because though the methadone abstinence syndrome is mild, it may produce discomfort.

Methadone withdrawal symptoms differ from morphine or heroin withdrawal by being less intense, occurring later (third through tenth day following last dose) and producing prolonged lethargy and anorexia.

Detoxification dosages empirically should begin with approximately 20 to 50 mgm methadone q.d. and be reduced 20 percent of the total dose per day. Detoxification can be accomplished as rapidly as three days or more slowly over seven to ten days. The more rapid the detoxification, the more severe the withdrawal symptoms.

Preference for both methadone maintenance and withdrawal treatment is the use of liquid methadone or Diskets. (The tablets are easily dissolved and injected and are therefore more readily abused.) As adjuncts in controlling insomnia, muscle cramps, and irritability, tranquilizers may be used. Chlordiazepoxide (Librium) 25 mgm Q.I.D.: diazepam (Valium) 5 mgm Q.I.D.: or doxepin (Sinequan) 25 mgm Q.I.D. are effective.

d. During the withdrawal period, group and/or individual psychotherapy have been helpful in maintaining a drug free patient. In methadone programs, the main difficulties in psychotherapy include involvement of the patient and maintenance of therapeutic contact even though the patient may relapse to drug use.

e. Methadone maintenance treatment:

Treatment of hard core addicts using Methadone Maintenance was first accomplished by Done and Nyswander (1968). The approach consisted of the following: Addicts were placed on 80 to 120 mgm of oral methadone in a fruit juice vehicle once daily, and maintained at that level indefinitely. The treatment goal is to permit the former addict to function in the community as a productive citizen. Approach to methadone maintenance: An adequate physical examination prior to initiation of therapy to determine whether any complication of narcotic addiction such as hepatitis, cellulitis or subacute bacterial endocarditis are present. If they are, hospital treatment is advised.

Three urine samples should be taken serially from the patient under direct observation (someone observes the patient urinating) to determine the presence or absence of narcotic breakdown products present (some individuals *say* they are addicts and might not be). An attempt to determine the strength of heroin in the area should be made. This will have some bearing on the dosage of methadone to be employed, as described above.

f. Methadone poisoning

As methadone is used more frequently as a maintenance therapy for heroin addiction, there is increasing danger of ingestion by nontolerant subjects who are not on a methadone program. This constitutes a medical emergency and is especially dangerous to children who may ingest a parent's methadone dose. It is important that patients on methadone maintenance be informed about the safe custody of the drug.

1. Diagnosis:

   a. Essential to have a history of a close contact of the patient being in a methadone program. Often methadone dispensed in an orange juice-like mixture.

   b. Patient may present in comatose state. Coma onsets in overdose cases from one half to three hours.

   c. Increasing respiratory depression.

2. Treatment

   a. Maintain respiration. May need airway tube, or endotracheal intubation. Start I.V. infusion of glucose and saline.

   b. Observe vital signs q 15 minutes for at least 24 hours. Methadone effects may persist for 24 to 48 hours whereas an antagonist may last only two to three hours.

   c. Narcan, use 0.4 mg/kg, I.V. as the antidote of choice. If this is not available use Nalline, 10 mg I.V. or Lorfan 1 to 2 mgm I.V. The danger of the latter two drugs is that they will increase respiratory depression if the diagnosis is barbiturate intoxication. Narcan will not do this.

   d. If the status of the patient improves,

may repeat the antagonist in five minutes and again in ten minutes. If the patient's status does not improve, may repeat Narcon but do not repeat Nalline or Lorfan because the diagnosis may be barbiturate intoxication.

e. If the respirations are adequate, do not use the antagonists.

f. Once resuscitation is successfully underway, the antagonist may be given I.M. with double the I.V. dose.

g. If the patient is seen more than one hour after ingestion, gastric lavage is not indicated.

h. The amount of methadone in the blood is negligible, therefore dialysis is not indicated.

i. Do not use central nervous system stimulants. They do not change the depressive effect of methadone and may be synergistic to the harmful stimulant effects of the drug (Reference: New York Department of Health, 1971).

c. Newborn infant of mother addicted to narcotics. The intensity of the newborn's withdrawal is dependent on the mother's dose and the length of time from her last dose to delivery of the infant. There is a significant infant mortality if this condition is not treated.

1. Diagnosis:

a. Hyperactivity, tremors, and shrill, constant cry are notable.

b. Irritability, flushing, sweating, yawning, sneezing, lacrimation, vomiting, diarrhea, poor food intake, excess mucous secretion, signs of respiratory distress (rarely apnea), fever and convulsions.

c. Differential diagnosis:

Hypoglycemic tetany, intracranial hemorrhage, tetanus and sepsis.

2. Treatment
   a. Paregoric is the first drug of choice; 5 drops orally, q 3 to 4 h, may need 10 to 20 drops in q 3 to 4 h, in severe cases. This drug controls all symptoms.
   b. If oral paregoric is vomited, then use Luminal® (phenobarbital) 4 mg (1/5 grain), subcutaneously, q 4 to 6 h, may need up to 8 to 15 mg (1/8 to 1/4 grain), q 4 to 6 h.
   c. Thorazine may be used only if attempts with paregoric fail. Thorazine 0.7 mg to 1.3 mg/kg, I.M., P.R.N.; later, oral doses.
   d. Rarely and only as an emergency measure, may use Lorfan, 0.05 to 0.10 mg, I.V., into the umbilical cord.
   e. Supportive sedation:
      Over a period of 30 to 60 days, or longer if necessary, the supportive sedation is gradually withdrawn as tolerated (New York Department of Health, 1971).

6. Medical complications of heroin abuse
   a. Overdose Syndromes: There are at least three different clinical syndromes associated with an overdose of heroin.
      1. Profound respiratory depression may occur (breathing rate of less than ten per minute; at times apnea).
      2. Cardiac arrest or conduction aberrations may be seen. They are most likely due to the adulterant, quinine, and not from the heroin.
      3. Pulmonary edema. The disparity between the roentgenologic finding of a diffuse pulmonary infiltrate (should stimulate tachypnea via the Herring-Breuer receptors) and the anticipated breathing rate is commonly diagnostic of opiate overdose.

b. Endocarditis (report of case studies)
  1. May involve a bacterial (usually staph) endo-
     carditis of the tricuspid valve. This may be first
     evidenced by pulmonary embolization. May only
     display insignificant murmur. Embolism to other
     organs (kidney, spleen, brain) is possible.
  2. A normal aortic valve may be the site of a *Strep-*
     tococcus viridans infection. This organism is
     common in subacute endocarditis of nonaddicts
     but unusual for a normal valve.
  3. Endocarditis with gram-negative and fungal in-
     fections. Endocarditis in addicts is associated
     with a high mortality rate; with *Candida species*
     it is almost always fatal.
c. Hepatitis: up to 80 percent of chronic addicts have
   hepatitis even if not clinically apparent.
d. Subcutaneous injection (skin popping) may result
   in tetanus, scarring, cellulitis and abscesses. There
   is a high mortality rate among addicts if tetanus
   occurs (Zarafonetis, 1972).

References

Ausubez, David P.: *Drug Addiction: Physiological, Psychological and Socio-*
  logical Aspects. New York, Random House, 1958.
Bakewell, W. E. and Ewing, J. A.: Therapy of non-narcotic psychoactive
  drug dependence. *Curr Psychiatr Ther,* 1969.
Berger, H.: Addiction to Methyprylon, *JAMA, 177:* 63–65, 1961.
Conn, H. F. (Ed.) : *Current Therapy 1972.* Philadelphia, W. R. Saunders Co.
DeGross, J.: Emergency treatment of drug abuse and poison ingestion.
  Resident and Staff Physician, February, 1970.
Desk Reference on Drug Abuse. Department of Health, New York, 1971.
Dole, V. P. and Nyswander, M. Warner: Successful treatment of 750 criminal
  addicts, *JAMA, 206:* 2708–2711.
Done, A. K.: Getting Rid of the Poisons, *Emergency Medicine.* New York,
  Fischer-Murray, Inc., 1972.
Ellinwood, E. H., Ewing, J. A. and Hoaken, P. C. S.: Habituation to
  Ethinamate. *N Engl J Med, 266:* 185–186, 1962.
Espelin, D. E. and Done, A. K.: Amphetamine poisoning: effectiveness of
  chlorpromazine. *N Engl J Med, 278:* 1361, 1968.

Essig, C. F.: Addiction to nonbarbituate sedative and tranquilizing drugs. *Clin Pharmacol Ther, 5:* 334-343, 1964.

Goodman, L. S. and Gilman, A.: *The Pharmacological Basis of Therapeutics.* New York, The Macmillan Co., 1970.

Harms, Ernest: *Drug Addiction in Youth.* London, Permagon Press, 1965.

Hollister, L. E., *et al.*: Diazepam in newly admitted schizophrenics. *Dis Nerv Syst, 24:* 746–750; Dec., 1963.

Hollister, L. E.; Motzenbecker, F. P. and Degan, R. O.: Withdrawal reactions from chlordiazepoxide (Librium). *Psychopharmacologia,* (Berlin) *2:* 63–68, 1961.

Kato, M.: An epidemiological analysis of the fluctuation of drug dependence in Japan. *Int J Addict, 4:* 591–621, 1969.

Koumons, A. J.: *Manual for the Treatment of Acute Drug Intoxications.* Massachusetts Medical Society, Committee on Mental Health, July, 1970.

Kramer, J. C.; Fischman, V. S. and Littlefield, D. C.: Amphetamine abuse, patterns, and effects of high doses taken intravenously. *JAMA, 201:* 305, 1967.

Krupp, M. A.; Chatton, M. J. et al.: *Current Diagnosis and Treatment.* Los Altos, California, Lange Medical Pub, 1972.

Krystal, Henry and Raskin, H.: *Drug Dependence: Aspects of Ego Function.* Detroit, Wayne State University Press, 1970.

Lampe, Matthew: *Drugs: Information for Crisis Treatment.* Beloit, Wisconsin, The Student Association for the Study of Hallucinogens, (STASH Press), 1972.

Lynn, E. J.: Effects of commonly abused drugs and emergency treatment of their effects. *Mich Med,* February, 1972.

Novello, J. R.: Management of amphetamine withdrawal in the general hospital setting. *Univ Mich Med Cent J,* Ann Arbor, 1972.

Nyswander, M.: *The Drug Addict as a Patient.* Grune and Stratton, New York, 1956.

Pollard, J. C.: *Some Commonly Abused Drugs.* Department of Psychiatry, University of Michigan, 1970 (unpublished).

Physician's Desk Reference: New Jersey, Medical Economics, Inc., 1972.

Resource Book for Drug Abuse Education: Washington, D.C. U.S. Department of Health, Education and Welfare, Public Health Service, National Institute of Mental Health, 1969.

Sapira, J. D. and McDonald, R. H., Jr.: Drug Abuse, *Disease of the Month,* 1970.

Smith, D. E. (Ed.): *Journal of Psychadelic Drugs.* Volume I: Issues 1 and 2; Volume II: Issue 2, San Francisco, Haight-Ashbury Medical Center, 1967–1968.

Wesson, D. R.; Gay, G. R. and Smith, D. E.: Managing narcotic and sedative withdrawal. *Hosp Physician,* January, 1972.

Wilson, C. W. M.: *The Pharmacological and Epidemiological Aspects of Adolescent Drug Dependence*. London, Pergamon Press, 1968.

Wintrobe, M. W.; Thorn, G. W.; Adams, R. D.; Bennett, Jr., I. L.; Braunwald, E.; Isselbacher, K. J.; Petersdorf, R. G. (Ed.) : *Harrison's Principles of Internal Medicine*. New York, McGraw-Hill, 1970.

Wittenborn, J. R.; Wittenborn, S. A.; Brill, H. and Smith, J. P.: *Drugs and Youth*. Springfield, Charles C Thomas, Pub., 1969.

Zarafonetis, C. J. D. (Ed.) : *Drug Abuse: Proceedings of the International Conference*. Philadelphia, Lea & Febiger, 1972.

Dr. Schulte wishes to acknowledge R. A. Winfield, M.D., Dept. Internal Medicine, University of Michigan, whose advice and assistance was invaluable in the preparation of this chapter.

PART TWO:

A GUIDE TO
CONTINUING EDUCATION

Chapter XI

THE PSYCHIATRIST'S BOOKSHELF

THIS CHAPTER IS INTENDED as a guide to the psychiatric literature. The first article, Basic Reading Lists in Psychiatry, presents three separate reading lists: (1) the ten books that residents in psychiatry find to be most useful, (2) the 18 books that are most recommended *to* residents *by* their training programs, (3) an expanded version of the second list, 104 books, that includes all books that appeared on 20 percent or more of the reading lists submitted by 87 separate residency programs.

The second article, Journals in Psychiatry is a compendium of 91 journals currently in publication that are of special interest to the psychiatric profession. Each journal is briefly described and information regarding subscription (for potential subscribers) and manuscript submission (for authors) is provided.

BASIC READING LISTS IN PSYCHIATRY

JOSEPH R. NOVELLO, M.D.

The psychiatric literature is rich and voluminous. In fact, a major difficulty facing professionals in the field is the very enormity of the literature. No one can be expected to know the entire literature, yet most psychiatrists strive, as a minimum, to be knowledgeable in the basic psychiatric literature.

But what *is* the basic literature? This section is designed to help answer that question and to provide the reader with a manageable reading list that can be considered both basic and useful.

Three short reading lists are provided.

The first list (Residents' Reading List of Most Useful Books) grew out of a study that the author conducted in 1972. Residents in four large and representative training programs were asked to select those books from among their entire professional reading that they actually found to be most useful to them in their training.

The second list (Books Most Recommended by Residency Training Programs) is the research product of Woods, Pieper and Frazier (1967). They canvassed training programs in psychiatry and asked chairmen and directors of training for a list of the books that were being recommended to residents in training. Several rank orders were determined for the 2,800 different books that were recommended. All rank-orders agreed on the single most recommended book and on the following 17 books. These books appear as the second list.

The third list (Basic Psychiatric Literature as Determined from the Recommended Reading Lists of Residency Training Programs) is also derived from the work of Woods, Pieper and Frazier. It can be considered a basic reading list in that it is composed of all books that appeared in 20 percent or more of the reading lists submitted by 87 residency programs that participated in the study. A total of 104 books is cited.

I. Residents' Reading List of Most Useful Books
(in order of preference)

1. Freedman and Kaplan — *Comprehensive Textbook of Psychiatry*
2. Brenner, C. — *An Elementary Textbook of Psychoanalysis*
3. Colby, K. M. — *Primer for Psychotherapists*
4. DeWald, P. A. — *Psychotherapy, A Dynamic Approach*

5. Greenson, R. R.	*The Technique and Practice of Psychoanalysis*
6. Sullivan, H. S.	*The Psychiatric Interview*
7. Tarachow, S.	*An Introduction to Psychotherapy*
8. Fromm-Reichmann, F.	*Principles of Intensive Psychotherapy*
9. Erickson, E.	*Childhood and Society*
10. Noyes and Kolb	*Modern Clinical Psychiatry*

II. Books Most Recommended by Residency Training Programs
(Woods, Pieper, Frazier, 1967)

| 1. Noyes and Kolb | *Modern Clinical Psychiatry* |

Others (in alphabetical order)

Aichhorn, A.	*Wayward Youth*
Alexander and Ross (Eds.)	*Dynamic Psychiatry*
Arieti, Silvano (Ed.)	*American Handbook of Psychiatry*
Bleuler, Eugen	*Dementia Praecox or the Group of Schizophrenias*
Brenner, C.	*An Elementary Textbook of Psychoanalysis*
Colby, K. M.	*Primers for Psychotherapists*
Erickson, Erik	*Childhood and Society*
Fenichel, Otto	*Psychoanalytic Theory of Neurosis*
Freud, Anna	*Ego and the Mechanisms of Defense*
Fromm-Reichmann, F.	*Principles of Intensive Psychotherapy*
Kalinowsky, L. and Hoch, P.	*Somatic Treatments in Psychiatry*
Kanner, Leo	*Child Psychiatry*
Munroe, Ruth	*Schools of Psychoanalytic Thought*
Stanton, A. and Schwartz, M.	*The Mental Hospital*

Sullivan, H. S.	*The Psychiatric Interview*
Wolberg, Lewis	*Technique of Psychotherapy*
Zilboorg, G.	*History of Medical Psychology*

III. Basic Psychiatric Literature as Determined from the Recommended Reading Lists of Residency Training Programs
(with permission: Woods, Pieper, Frazier)

Alphabetically by subject

I. General

A. Dictionaries

Hinsie, Leland Earl (Ed.), and Campbell, Robert Jean (Ed.): *Psychiatric Dictionary: with encyclopedic treatment of modern terms,* 3rd ed. New York, Oxford University Press, 1960.

B. Texts

Alexander, Franz (Ed.) and Ross, Helen (Ed.): *Dynamic Psychiatry.* Chicago, University of Chicago Press, 1952. (Paperback condensation: *The Impact of Freudian Psychiatry.*)

Arieti, Silvano (Ed.): *American Handbook of Psychiatry.* New York, Basic Books, 1959, 2v.

Bleuler, Eugen.: Authorized English Ed. by A. A. Brill. *Textbook of Psychiatry.* New York, Macmillan, 1924.

English, Oliver Spurgeon and Finch, Stuart M.: *Introduction to Psychiatry,* 1st ed. New York, Norton, 1954.

Henderson, Sir David Kennedy and Gillespie, R. D.: *Textbook of Psychiatry for Students and Practitioners,* 9th ed. New York, Oxford University Press, 1962.

Masserman, Jules Hyman.: *The Practice of Dynamic Psychiatry.* Philadelphia, Saunders, 1955.

Noyes, Arthur Percy and Kolb, Laurence C.: *Modern Clinical Psychiatry,* 6th ed. Philadelphia, Saunders, 1963.

Strecker, Edward Adam; Ebaugh, Franklin G. and Ewalt, Jack Richard.: *Practical Clinical Psychiatry,* 8th ed. New York, Blakiston Division, McGraw-Hill, 1957.

II. Neurology, Neuroanatomy, Neurophysiology and Neuropathology

Alpers, Bernard Jacob.: *Clinical Neurology,* 4th ed. Philadelphia, F. A. Davis Co., 1958.

Brain, Sir Walter Russell: *Diseases of the Nervous System,* 6th ed. London, New York, Oxford University Press, 1962.

Merritt, Hiram Houston: *A Textbook of Neurology,* 3rd ed. Philadelphia, Lea & Febiger, 1963.

Ranson, Stephen Walter: *The Anatomy of the Nervous System: Its Development and Function.* Revised by Sam L. Clark, 10th ed. Philadelphia, Saunders, 1959.

III. Psychopathology

A. General

American Psychiatric Association. Committee on Nomenclature and Statistics: *Diagnosis and Statistical Manual for Mental Disorders,* 2nd ed. Washington, D.C., American Psychiatric Association, 1968.

B. Mental retardation

Masland, Richard Lambert; Sarason, Seymour B. and Gladwin, Thomas: *Mental Subnormality: Biological, Psychological, and Cultural Factors.* New York, Basic Books, 1959.

C. Psychotic disorders

1. Affective reactions

Greenacre, Phyllis (Ed.) : *Affective Disorders: Psychoanalytic Contribution to Their Study.* New York, International Universities Press, 1953.

Lewin, Bertram D.: *The Psychoanalysis of Elation.* New York, Norton, 1950.

2. Schizophrenic reactions and psychotherapy of

schizophrenic reactions

Arieti, Silvano: *Interpretation of Schizophrenia.* New York, R. Brunner, 1955.

Bellak, Leopold (Ed.) and Benedict, Paul K. (Ed.) : *Schizophrenia: A Review of the Syndrome.* New York, Logos Press, 1958.

Bleuler, Eugen: *Dementia Praecox: Or, The Group of Schizophrenias.* Trans. by Joseph Zinkin. New York, International Universities Press, 1950.

Brody, Eugene Bloor (Ed.) and Redlich, Frederick Carl (Ed.) : *Psychotherapy with Schizophrenics.* New York, International Universities Press, 1952.

Hill, Lewis B.: *Psychotherapeutic Intervention in Schizophrenia.* Chicago, University of Chicago Press, 1955.

Jackson, Don deAvila (Ed.) : *The Etiology of Schizophrenia: Genetics, Physiology, Psychology, Sociology.* New York, Basic Books, 1960.

Kasanin, Jacob S. (Ed.) : *Language and Thought in Schizophrenia: Collected Papers Presented at the Meeting of the American Psychiatric Association, May 12, 1939, Chicago, Illinois and brought up to date.* Berkeley, Calif., University of California Press, 1944.

Rapaport, David (Ed.) : *Organization and Pathology of Thought: Selected Sources.* New York, Columbia University Press, 1951.

Sechehaye, Marguerite Albert: *Reality Lost and Regained: Autobiography of a Schizophrenic Girl.* New York, Grune & Stratton, 1951.

Sechehaye, Marguerite Albert: *Symbolic Realization, a New Method of Psychotherapy Applied to a Case of Schizophrenia.* New York, International Universities Press, 1952.

D. Psychosomatic disorders

Alexander, Franz: *Psychosomatic Medicine: Its Principles and Applications.* New York, Norton, 1950.

Dunbar, Helen Flanders: *Emotions and Bodily Changes: A Survey of Literature on Psychosomatic Interrelationships,* 1910–1953, 4th ed. New York, Columbia University Press, 1954.

Weiss, Edward and English, Oliver Spurgeon: *Psychosomatic Medicine: A Clinical Study of Psychophysiologic Reactions,* 3rd ed. Philadelphia, Saunders, 1957.

E. Psychoneurotic disorders

English, Oliver Spurgeon and Pearson, Gerald Hamilton Jeffrey: *The Common Neuroses of Children and Adults.* New York, Norton, 1937.

English, Oliver Spurgeon and Pearson, Gerald Hamilton Jeffrey: *The Emotional Problems of Living: Avoiding the Neurotic Pattern.* New York, Norton, 1945.

Fenichel, Otto: *The Psychoanalytic Theory of Neurosis.* New York, Norton, 1945.

F. Personality disorders

Cleckley, Hervey Milton: *The Mask of Sanity: An Attempt to Clarify Some Issues about the So-Called Psychopathic Personality,* 4th ed. St. Louis, Mosby, 1964.

Hunt, Joseph McVicker, (Ed.): *Personality and the Behavior Disorders: A Handbook Based on Experimental and Clinical Research.* New York, Ronald Press, 1944, 2v.

IV. Therapies

A. Interview techniques and psychotherapy

1. Individual

Colby, Kenneth Mark: *Primer for Psychotherapists.* New York, Ronald Press, 1951.

Deutsch, Felix and Murphy, William F.: *The Clinical Interview.* New York, International Universities Press, 1955, 2v.

Fromm-Reichmann, Frieda: *Principles of Intensive Psychotherapy.* Chicago, University of Chicago Press, 1950.

Gill, Merton M.: Newman, Richard, and Redlich, Frederick Carl: *The Initial Interview in Psychiatric Practice.* New York, International Universities Press, 1954.

Levine, Maurice: *Psychotherapy in Medical Practice.* New York, Macmillan, 1942.

Menninger, Karl Augustus: *Manual for Psychiatric Case Study,* 2nd ed. New York, Grune & Stratton, 1962.

Sullivan, Harry S.: *The Psychiatric Interview.* Ed. by Helen Swick Perry and M. L. Gawel. New York, 1954.

Wolberg, Lewis Robert. *The Techniques of Psychotherapy.* New York, Grune & Stratton, 1954.

2. Group

Powdermaker, Florence B.; Frank, Jerome D. and Abrahams, Joseph: *Group Psychotherapy: Studies in Methodology of Research and Therapy. Report of a Group Psychotherapy Research Project of the U. S. Veterans Administration.* Cambridge, Mass., Harvard University Press, 1953.

Slavson, Samuel Richard: *An Introduction to Group Therapy.* New York, Commonwealth Fund, 1943.

B. Hospital psychiatry and milieu therapies

Jones, Maxwell Shaw: *The Therapeutic Community: A New Treatment Method in Psychiatry.* New York, Basic Books, 1953.

Linn, Louis: *A Handbook of Hospital Psychiatry: A Practical Guide to Therapy.* New York, International Universities Press, 1955.

Stanton, Alfred H. and Schwartz, Morris S.: *The*

Mental Hospital: A Study of Institutional Participation in Psychiatric Illness and Treatment. New York, Basic Books, 1954.

C. Somatic therapies

Kalinowsky, Lothar B. and Hoch, Paul Henry: *Somatic Treatments in Psychiatry: Pharmacotherapy, Convulsive, Insulin, Surgical, and Other Methods.* New York, Grune & Stratton, 1961.

V. Personalogy

A. General

Brenner, Charles: *An Elementary Textbook of Psychoanalysis.* New York, International Universities Press, 1955.

Hall, Calvin Springer and Lindzey, Gardner: *Theories of Personality.* New York, Wiley, 1957.

Mullahy, Patrick: *Oedipus: Myth and Complex: A Review of Psychoanalytic Theory.* New York, Grove Press, 1955.

Monroe, Ruth L.: *Schools of Psychoanalytic Thought: An Exposition, Critique, and Attempt at Integration.* New York, Dryden Press, 1955.

Thompson, Clara M. and Mullahy, Patrick: *Psychoanalysis: Evolution and Development.* New York, Grove Press, 1957.

B. Specific

Abraham, Karl: *Selected Papers on Psychoanalysis.* In Ernest Jones (Ed.). London, Hogarth Press, 1949.

Alexander, Franz: *Fundamentals of Psychoanalysis.* New York, Norton, 1948.

Breuer, Josef and Freud, Sigmund: *Studies in Hysteria.* New York, Basic Books, 1957.

Freud, Anna: *The Ego and the Mechanisms of Defense.* New York, International Universities Press, 1957.

Freud, Sigmund: *The Basic Writings of Sigmund Freud.* New York, Modern Library, 1938.

Freud, Sigmund: *Collected Papers.* New York, Basic Books, 1959, 5v.

Freud, Sigmund: *The Ego and the Id.* Trans. by Joan Riviere. London, Hogarth Press, 1947.

Freud, Sigmund: *A General Introduction to Psychoanalysis: A Course of Twenty-Eight Lectures at the University of Vienna.* Authorized English trans. of the rev. ed. by Joan Riviere. New York, Liveright Pub. Co., 1935.

Freud, Sigmund: *The Interpretation of Dreams.* New York, Basic Books, 1955.

Freud, Sigmund: *New Introductory Lectures on Psychoanalysis.* Trans. by W. J. H. Sprot. New York, W. W. Norton Co., 1933.

Freud, Sigmund: *An Outline of Psychoanalysis.* Trans. by James Strachey. New York, W. W. Norton Co., 1963.

Freud, Sigmund: *The Problem of Anxiety.* Trans. from German by Henry A. Bunker. New York, Norton, 1936.

Freud, Sigmund: *Three Contributions to the Theory of Sex. (1) The Sexual Abberations. (2) Infantile Sexuality. (3) The Transformations of Puberty.* New York, Nervous & Mental Diseases Publishing Co., 1930.

Fromm, Erich: *Escape from Freedom.* New York, Farrar & Rinehart, 1941.

Horney, Karen: *The Neurotic Personality of Our Time.* New York, Norton, 1937.

May, Rollo; Angel, Ernest and Ellenberger, Henry F. (Eds.): *Existence: A New Dimension in Psychiatry and Psychology.* New York, Basic Books, 1958.

Menninger, Karl A.: *The Human Mind,* 3rd ed. New York, Knopf, 1945.

Menninger, Karl A.: *Man Against Himself.* New York, Harcourt Brace, 1938.

Menninger, Karl A.: *The Theory of Psychoanalytic Technique.* New York, Basic Books, 1958.

Meyer, Adolf: *Commonsense Psychiatry: 52 Selected Papers.* In Alfred Lief (Ed.). New York, McGraw-Hill, 1948.

Reich, Wilhelm: *Character Analysis: Principles and Techniques for Psychoanalysts in Practice and Training,* 3rd ed. Trans. by Theodore P. Wolfe. New York, Orgone Institute Press, 1949.

Sullivan, Harry Stack: *Interpersonal Theory of Psychiatry.* In Helen Swick Perry and Mary L. Gawel (Ed.). New York, Norton, 1953.

VI. Child Psychiatry
  A. General
Aichhorn, August: *Wayward Youth: A Psychoanalytic Study of Delinquent Children, Illustrated by Actual Case Histories.* New York, The Viking Press, 1935.

Caplan, Gerald (Ed.): *Emotional Problems of Early Childhood.* New York, Basic Books, 1955.

Eissler, Kurt Robert (Ed.): *Searchlights on Delinquency: New Psychoanalytic Studies.* New York, International Universities Press, 1949.

Finch, Stuart M.: *Fundamentals of Child Psychiatry.* New York, Norton, 1960.

Kanner, Leo: *Child Psychiatry,* 3rd ed. Springfield, Charles C Thomas, 1957.

Pearson, Gerald H. J.: *Emotional Disorders of Children: A Case Book of Child Psychiatry.* New York, Norton, 1949.

  B. Psychotherapy
Allen, Frederick H.: *Psychotherapy with Children.* New York, Norton, 1942.

Bettelheim, Bruno: *Love is Not Enough: The Treatment of Emotionally Disturbed Children.* Glencoe, Ill., Free Press, 1950.

Freud, Anna: *The Psychoanalytic Treatment of Children: Technique, Lectures and Essays.* New York, International Universities Press, 1959.

Witmer, Helen L. (Ed.): *Psychiatric Interviews*

with Children. New York, Commonwealth Fund, 1946.

VII. Community Psychiatry

Joint Commission on Mental Illness and Health: *Action for Mental Health: Final report of the Commission.* New York, Basic Books, 1961.

VIII. Forensic Psychiatry

Davidson, Henry Alexander: *Forensic Psychiatry.* New York, Ronald Press, 1952.

Guttmacher, Manfred S. and Weihofen, Henry: *Psychiatry and the Law.* New York, W. W. Norton Co., 1952.

IX. The Individual, His Family, and His Culture

Ackerman, Nathan Ward: *The Psychodynamics of Family Life: Diagnosis and Treatment of Family Relationships.* New York, Basic Books, 1958.

Benedict, Ruth: *Patterns of Culture.* New York, Houghton Mifflin, 1934.

Deutsch, Helene: *The Psychology of Women: A Psychoanalytic Interpretation.* New York, Grune & Stratton, 1944–45, 2v.

Erikson, Erik Homburger: *Childhood and Society,* 2nd ed. New York, Norton, 1964.

Hollingshead, August de Belmont and Redlich, Frederick Carl: *Social Class and Mental Illness: A Community Study.* New York, Wiley, 1958.

Kallmann, Franz Joseph: *Heredity in Health and Mental Disorders: Principles of Psychiatric Genetics in the Light of Comparative Twin Studies.* New York, Norton, 1953.

Kinsey, Alfred C.; Pomeroy, W. B. and Martin, C. E.: *Sexual Behavior in the Human Male.* Philadelphia, Saunders, 1948.

Kluckhorn, Clyde and Murray, Henry A. (eds.) : *Personality in Nature, Society and Culture,* 2nd ed. New York, Alfred A. Knopf, 1953.

Mead, Margaret: *Male and Female: A Study of the*

Sexes in a Changing World. New York, Morrow, 1949.

X. History, Biography and Autobiography

Ackerkecht, Erwin Heinz: *A Short History of Psychiatry.* Trans. from the German by Sulammith Wolff. New York, Hafner, 1959.

American Psychiatric Association: *One Hundred Years of American Psychiatry.* New York, Published for the American Psychiatric Association by Columbia University Press, 1944.

Beers, Clifford Whittingham: *A Mind that Found Itself: An Autobiography.* Garden City, New York, Doubleday, 1953.

Deutsch, Albert: *The Mentally Ill in America: A History of Their Care and Treatment from Colonial Times.* New York, Columbia University Press, 1937.

Jones, Ernest: *Sigmund Freud: Life and Works.* (Abridged). London, Hogarth Press, 1957.

Zilboorg, Gregory and Henry, George William: *A History of Medical Psychology.* New York, Norton, 1941.

Reference

Woods, J. B., Pieper, S. and Frazier, S. H.: Basic psychiatric literature as determined from the recommended reading lists of residency training programs. *Am J Psychiatry, 124:* 217–224, 1967.

JOURNALS AND PERIODICALS OF INTEREST TO PSYCHIATRISTS

Joseph R. Novello, M.D.

The compendium of professional journals presented in Table XI-I is intended to be a reasonably exhaustive list of periodicals currently available in psychiatry. In addition, journals published in other related fields but of professional interest to many psychiatrists have also been included. While no journal has been purposefully omitted, the author recognizes that oversights invariably occur in projects such as this one. Interested readers are invited to submit information on journals or periodicals that they believe should be included in any future edition of this handbook.

The ninety-one journals referenced in Table XI-I are listed in alphabetical order. The following information, when pertinent, is provided. (1) Name of journal, (2) a brief description of the content, i.e. what subject areas are generally covered in each of the periodicals, (3) when a journal is an official publication of a professional society or group this is noted, (4) cost of annual subscription (Note: many journals provide special discount rates for medical students and residents in training. This is noted in many instances. In other cases the interested reader may contact the various subscription offices.), (5) address of subscription office and (6) address for submitting manuscripts. (Note: prospective authors are cautioned that journals have varying style requirements; before submitting an article to a particular journal, the author is wise to consult the editor or refer to the Information for Authors section that appears in most periodicals. In addition, the prospective author is cautioned that not all professional journals accept unsolicited manuscripts; a short letter of query to the editor, inquiring about publication policies, is often time-saving in the end.)

The author wishes to acknowledge the assistance of Mr. Michael Brachman, University of Michigan.

TABLE XI-I

JOURNALS IN PSYCHIATRY

Journal	Description	Official Publication of	Frequency of Publication	Cost of Subscription	Subscription Information	Send Manuscripts To
Adolescence	"An international quarterly devoted to the physiological, psychological, psychiatric, sociological and educational aspects of the second decade of life."		Quarterly	$10/year	Libra Publishers Inc. P.O. Box 165 391 Willets Rd. Roslyn Heights, N.Y. 11577	% Editor Libra Publishers Inc. same address
Aging and Human Development	emphasizes psychological and social studies of aging and the aged; international.		Quarterly	$20/volume	Greenwood Periodicals Co. 51 Riverside Ave. Westport, Conn. 06880	Dr. Robert J. Kastenbaum, Editor Aging and Human Development Center for Psychological Studies of Death, Dying, and Lethal Behavior MacKenzie Hall Wayne State University Detroit, Mich. 48202
American Journal of Clinical Hypnosis	articles on theory and practical issues in hypnosis.	American Society of Clinical Hypnosis	Quarterly	$8/year	American Journal of Clinical Hypnosis 800 Washington Ave., S.E. Minneapolis, Minn. 55414	Editor, American Journal of Clinical Hypnosis Colgate University Hamilton, N.Y. 13346
Acta Paedopsychiatrica	General child psychiatry; international.	International Association for Child Psychiatry	12 issues/year	68 Sw. francs	Schwabe & Co. Verlag, Basel/Stuttgart	Dr. D. Arn van Krevelen Scheveningseweg 3, s-Gravenhage, Holland

TABLE XI-I Continued

Journal	Description	Official Publication of	Frequency of Publication	Cost of Subscription	Subscription Information	Send Manu-scripts To
Archives of General Psychiatry	Broad in scope. General psychiatry.		Monthly	$12/year ($6/year to residents, students)	American Medical Association 535 N. Dearborn Street Chicago, Ill. 60610	Editor same address
American Journal of Psychoanalysis	Reflects holistic approach.	1. Association for the Advancement of Psychoanalysis. 2. Affiliated with the Karen Horney Psychoanalytic Institute	2 issues/year	$8/year	Editor, *American Journal of Psychoanalysis* 329 E. 62nd Street New York, N.Y. 10021	Same address
American Journal of Psychotherapy	Theory and practical problems in psychotherapy.	Association for the Advancement of Psychotherapy	Quarterly	$16/year	Business Manager, *American Journal of Psychotherapy* 119–21 Metropolitan Ave. Jamaica, N.Y. 11415	Editor, *American Journal of Psychotherapy* 15 West 81st St. New York, N.Y. 10024
Annals of Adolescent Psychiatry	Yearly review of adolescent psychiatry.		1 issue/year	$15/year	*Annals of Adolescent Psychiatry* 741 St. Johns Avenue Highland Park, Ill. 60035	Same address
American Journal of Orthopsychiatry	Focuses on "better understanding of human behavior and effective treatment of behavior disorders." General child psychiatry with many articles dealing with current societal problems.	American Orthopsychiatric Association, Inc.	5 times/year	$16/volume ($10/volume to students)	AOA Publications 49 Sheridan Ave. Albany, N.Y. 12210	*American Journal of Orthopsychiatry* 1790 Broadway New York, N.Y. 10019

Journal	Scope	Publisher/Sponsor	Frequency	Price	Address	Editor
American Journal of Psychiatry	Broad in scope. General psychiatry.	American Psychiatric Association	Monthly	$12/year	American Journal of Psychiatry 1700 Eighteenth St., N.W. Washington, D.C. 20009	Same address
Behavior Genetics	"An international journal devoted to research in the inheritance of behavior in animal and man."		Quarterly	$30/year	Greenwood Periodicals Inc. 51 Riverside Ave. Westport, Conn. 06880	Same address
Behavioral Neuropsychiatry	general psychiatry, interdisciplinary; international.		Monthly	Rates on request	Behavioral Neuropsychiatry Medical Publishers Inc. 17 East 82nd Street New York, N.Y. 10028	Executive Editor, Albert A. Laverne, M.D., same address
Behavior Research and Therapy	international, multidisciplinary journal of behavior modification.		Quarterly	$15/year	Pergamon Press Inc. Fairview Park Elmsford, N.Y. 10523	Editor in chief, Prof. H. J. Eysenck Institute of Psychiatry De Crespigny Park Road Denmark Hill London S.E.5, England
Behavioral Science	"original articles which develop theories of human behavior to explicate basic behavioral concepts and report data specifically oriented toward such theories."		Bimonthly	$15/year	Behavior Science Mental Health Research Institute University of Michigan Ann Arbor, Michigan 48104	Editor same address

TABLE XI-I Continued

Journal	Description	Official Publication of	Frequency of Publication	Cost of Subscription	Subscription Information	Send Manuscripts To
Behavior Therapy	general articles on theory, techniques on behavioral therapy.	Association for Advancement of Behavior Therapy	Quarterly	$9/year (members; others on request)	Academic Press, Inc. 111 Fifth Ave. New York, N.Y. 10003	Editor, Cyril M. Franks The Psychological Clinic Rutgers University New Brunswick, New Jersey 08903
Biological Psychiatry	wide range of psychiatric clinical and research topics; emphasis on biological/organic psychiatry.	Society of Biological Psychiatry	Quarterly	$20/year	Plenum Publishing Co. 227 W. 17th Street New York, N.Y. 10011	Editor, Biological Psychiatry Dr. Joseph Wortis Department of Psychiatry Maimonides Medical Center 4802 Tenth Avenue Brooklyn, N.Y. 11219
British Journal of Psychiatry	General Psychiatry.		Quarterly	$25/year	Cambridge University Press 32 East 57th Street New York, N.Y. 10022	Editor in Chief., R.C. Psychiatry Chandos House 2 Queen Anne Street W 1 M., London, England
Community Mental Health Journal	"devoted to emergent approaches in mental health research, theory and practice as they relate to community, broadly defined."		Quarterly	$20/year (individual professional and students $10)	Behavioral Publications, Inc. 2852 Broadway— Morningside Heights New York, N.Y. 10025	Dr. Lenin Baler Community Mental Health Journal University of Michigan School of Public Health Room M 5108 S.P.H. II Ann Arbor, Michigan 48104

Title	Description	Society/Body	Frequency	Price	Publisher	Editor
Comprehensive Psychiatry	Broad scope. General psychiatry.	American Psychopathological Association	Bimonthly	$16/year	Grune & Stratton, Inc. 111 Fifth Avenue New York, N.Y. 10003	Editor, Comprehensive Psychiatry Fritz A. Freyhan, M.D. 2015 R Street Washington, D.C. 20009
Conditional Reflex	"A Pavlovian journal of research and therapy." Focus on behavioral analysis.	Pavlovian Society of America	Quarterly	$10/year	J.B. Lippincott Co. East Washington Sq. Philadelphia, Pa. 19105	Editor in Chief, Conditioned Reflex Pavlovian Research Lab. V.A. Hospital Perrypoint, Md 21902
Digest of Neurology and Psychiatry	"Abstracts and reviews of selected literature in psychiatry, neurology and their allied fields."	Institute of Living	Monthly	Free of charge on request	Institute of Living Hartford, Conn.	
Diseases of the Nervous System	"A practical journal on psychiatry and neurology."		Monthly	$12/year	Physicians Postgraduate Press 992 Springfield Ave. Irvington, N.J. 07111	
Electroencephalography and Clinical Neurophysiology	Electrical activity of brain is central theme but also publishes studies on spinal and peripheral nervous system and electrophysiology of muscle.	International Federation of Societies for Electroencephalography and Clinical Neurophysiology	Monthly	$40.50/year	Elsevier Publishing Co. P.O. Box 211 Amsterdam, The Netherlands	Editor, The EEG Journal Dept. of Anatomy Brain Research Institute U. of California Medical Center Los Angeles, Calif. 90024

TABLE XI-I Continued

Journal	Description	Official Publication of	Frequency of Publication	Cost of Subscription	Subscription Information	Send Manuscripts To
Excerpta Medica (Psychiatry)	Excerpts from psychiatric articles published monthly throughout the world.		Monthly (plus 6 additional issues)	$40/year	*Excerpta Medica* P.O. Box 1126 Amsterdam-C, The Netherlands	
Experimental Brain Research	"covers brain research in its entirety."		5 issues/year	$40/year	Springer-Verlag N.Y. Inc. 175 Fifth Ave. New York, N.Y. 10010	Experimental Brain Research, Prof. J. C. Eceles Lab of Neurobiology, State University of N.Y. at Buffalo 4234 Ridge Road Amherst, N.Y. 14226
Foreign Psychiatry	translations of material from scholarly journals and books throughout the world.		Quarterly	$15/year	International Arts & Sciences Press, Inc. 901 North Broadway White Plains, N.Y. 10603	
Geriatrics Digest	monthly summary of the world's literature on preventive geriatrics (mostly medical but significant amount of psychiatric material).		Monthly	$15/year (may be available gratis)	*Geriatrics Digest*, Inc. 445 Central Ave. Northfield, Ill. 60093	
Group for the Advancement of Psychiatry	periodic reports on wide-ranging problems and issues by various GAP task forces.	Group for Advancement of Psychiatry	Periodically	$1/issue	Publications Office, GAP 419 Park Avenue South New York, N.Y. 10016	
Group Psychotherapy and Psychodrama	psychodrama, sociodrama; theory and technique.	American Society of Group Psychotherapy and Psychodrama		On request	Beacon House, Inc. P.O. Box 311 Beacon, N.Y. 12508	Same address

Title	Scope	Society	Frequency	Price	Address	Editor/Contact
Humanitas: Journal of the Institute of Man	Existential orientation. Original articles complemented by reprints of classical articles in fields of psychiatry, psychology, philosophy, and sociology.	The Institute of Man	February May, November	$7.50/year	Publication Manager, Institute of Man Duquesne University Pittsburgh, Pa. 15219	Adrian van Kaam, Ph.D. same address
Hospital and Community Psychiatry	broad scope of articles dealing with issues in hospital and community practice.	American Psychiatric Association (for agencies and institutions)	Monthly	$7.50/year ($9 non-members)	*Hospital and Community Psychiatry* 1700 Eighteenth St., N.W. Washington, D.C. 20009	Editor, *Hospital and Community Psychiatry* same address
Human Inquiries	"articles falling within the general area of the phenomenology of man."	Association for Existential Psychology and Psychiatry	3 issues/year	$9/year	*Human Inquiries* Suite 825 1500 Massachusetts Ave., N.W. Washington, D.C. 20005	Same address
International Journal of Child Psychotherapy	"concerned specifically with psychotherapeutic techniques in the treatment of children. . ."		Quarterly	$16/year	International Journal Press 59 Fourth Avenue New York, N.Y. 10003	Richard A. Gardner, Editor in Chief 155 County Road Cresskill, N.J. 07626
International Journal of Clinical and Experimental Hypnosis	wide range of articles, occasional issues are devoted entirely to one specific subject of interest in clinical or experimental hypnosis.	International Society for Clinical and Experimental Hypnosis	Quarterly	$12/year	*International Journal of Clinical and Experimental Hypnosis* 111 North 49th Street Philadelphia, Pa. 19139	Same address

TABLE XI-1 Continued

Journal	Description	Official Publication of	Frequency of Publication	Cost of Subscription	Subscription Information	Send Manuscripts To
International Journal of Psychiatry	"significant topics in psychiatry are presented and then critically evaluated by prominent specialists around the world, authors then reply to discussants."		Quarterly	$16/year	International Journal Press 59 Fourth Ave. New York, N.Y. 10003	Same address
International Journal of Psychoanalysis	"covers the theory and practice of Psychoanalysis."		Quarterly	$12.50/year	Balliere Tindell 7&8 Henrietta Street London W.C.2 England	International Journal of Psychoanalysis Mt. Zion Hospital and Medical Center 1600 Divisadero St. San Francisco, CA 94115
International Psychiatric Clinics	Hard cover. Each issue devoted to a single topic. By leaders in special fields of psychiatry.		Bimonthly	$21.50/year	Little, Brown and Co. 34 Beacon St. Boston, Mass. 02106	
International Journal of Group Psychotherapy	Group therapy: theory, practice, technique.	American Group Psychotherapy Assoc., Inc.	Quarterly	$15/year	International Universities Press 239 Park Avenue South New York, N.Y. 10003	International Journal of Group Psychotherapy P.O. Box 230 150 Christopher St. New York, N.Y. 10014
International Journal of Transactional Analysis	Articles relating to theory and practice of transactional analysis.	International Transactional Analysis Assoc.	Quarterly	$10/year	International Transactional Analysis Association 3155 College Avenue Berkeley, CA. 94705	Same address

Title	Description	Organization	Frequency	Price	Publisher Address	Editor
Journal of the American Academy of Child Psychiatry	articles "relevant to maturational patterns, child development and childhood problems that will serve to increase or integrate knowledge concerning the psychological aspects of childhood."	American Academy of Child Psychiatry	Quarterly	$15/year	Quadrangle Books Room 208 330 Madison Ave. New York, N.Y. 10017	Eveoleen N. Rexford, M.D. 100 Memorial Drive, Suite 2-9 B Cambridge, Mass. 02142
Journal of American Geriatrics Society	contains many psychiatrically-oriented articles.	American Geriatrics Society	12 issues (monthly)	$15/year	American Geriatrics Society 18 Columbus Circle New York, N.Y. 10019	Editor in Chief, *Journal of the American Geriatrics Society* 220 Central Park South New York, N.Y. 10019
Journal of the American Psychoanalytic Association	Psychoanalysis: theory and practice.	American Psychoanalytic Association	Quarterly	$15/year ($9 for candidates)	International Universities Press 239 Park Avenue South New York, N.Y. 10003	Editor of the *Journal of the American Psychoanalytic Association* Dept. of Psychiatry Brookdale Hospital Center Linden Blvd. and Brookdale Plaza Brooklyn, N.Y. 11212
Journal of Applied Behavorial Science	general articles on the practical application of psychological knowledge.	National Training Laboratories	Bimonthly	$15/year	National Institute for Applied Behavioral Science 1201 16th Street N.W. Washington, D.C. 20036	Editor 94 Sparkhill Ave. Tappan, N.Y. 10983

TABLE XI-I Continued

Journal	Description	Official Publication of	Frequency of Publication	Cost of Subscription	Subscription Information	Send Manuscripts To
Journal of Child Psychology and Psychiatry	General child psychiatry and psychology.	Association of Child Psychology and Psychiatry	Quarterly	$13.50/year	Pergamon Press, Inc. Fairview Park Elmsford, N.Y. 10523	Same address
Journal of Individual Psychology	Articles on theory and practice of Adlerian Psychology.	American Society of Adlerian Psychology	2 issues/year	$5/year	H.L. Amsbacher, Editor University of Vermont John Dewey Hall Burlington, Vt. 05401	Same address
Journal of Psychiatric Research	"a medium of communication of research reports in psychiatry."		Quarterly	$10/year	Pergamon Press, Inc. Fairview Park Elmsford, N.Y. 10523	Editor in Chief, Semour Katz, M.D. Psychiatric Research Labs Research-4 Massachusetts General Hospital Boston, Mass. 02114
Journal of Behavior Therapy and Experimental Psychiatry	Interdisciplinary: theory, methods, training. Aim is to overcome the gap in behavioral therapy training for the psychiatrist.		Quarterly	$9/year ($6 to residents and students)	Pergamon Press, Inc. Fairview Park Elmsford, N.Y. 10523	Joseph Wolpe, M.D., Editor Eastern Pennsylvania Psychiatric Institute 3300 Henry Avenue Philadelphia, Pa. 19129
Journal of Nervous and Mental Disease	Broad scope. General psychiatry.		Monthly	$20/year ($12/year for residents and students)	Williams and Wilkins Co. 428 East Preston St. Baltimore, Maryland 21202	Editor in Chief, Eugene Brody, M.D. Institute of Psychiatry and Human Behavior University of Maryland School of Medicine Baltimore, Maryland 21201

Title	Organization	Frequency	Price	Address	Editor	Scope
Journal of Pastoral Care	Association for Clinical Pastoral Education (in cooperation with American Assoc. of Pastoral Counselors)	Quarterly	$8/year	Association for Clinical Pastoral Education Suite 450 475 Riverside Dr. New York, N.Y. 10027	Managing Editor, Dr. Luberta M. McCabe 61 Lexington Avenue Cambridge, Mass. 02138	contains articles pertaining to psychiatry and religion (alcoholism, suicide, etc.) and others.
Journal of Personality Assessment	Society for Personality Assessment, Inc.	Bimonthly	$15/year	Society for Personality Assessment 1070 E. Angeleno Ave. Burbank, CA. 91501	Executive Editor, *Journal of Personality Assessment* 7840 S.W. 51st Ave. Portland, Ore. 97219	articles relating to psychological tests used in assessment of personality: projective and others.
Journal of Psychosomatic Research		Quarterly	$15/year	Pergamon Press Fairview Park Elmsford, N.Y. 10523	Dr. Denis Leigh The Maudsley Hospital London S.E.5, England	general psychosomatic topics: research, theory, treatment; international.
Journal of Religion and Health	Academy of Religion and Mental Health	Quarterly	$8/year	Academy of Religion and Mental Health 16 East 34th Street New York, N.Y. 10016	Editor, Rev. Harry C. Meserve 17150 Maumee Avenue Grosse Pointe, Mich. 48230	Multidisciplinary; "for all who are interested in the indivisibility of human well-being: physical, emotional and spiritual."
Journal of Sex Research	The Society for the Scientific Study of Sex	Quarterly	$12/year	Robert V. Sherwin, Esq. Suite 1104 12 East 41st Street New York, N.Y. 10017	Hugo G. Beigel, Ph.D. 138 East 94th Street New York, N.Y. 10028	interdisciplinary, international: "explanation of factors contributing to or determining sexual behavior."

TABLE XI-I Continued

Journal	Description	Official Publication of	Frequency of Publication	Cost of Subscription	Subscription Information	Send Manuscripts To
Journal of Youth and Adolescence	interdisciplinary. Stressing research reports but also including theoretical papers and comprehensive review articles.		Quarterly	$16/year	Plenum Press 227 West 17th Street New York, N.Y. 10011	Same address
Medical Aspects of Human Sexuality	"A journal for physicians covering the physical, psychological and cultural components of human sexuality and related aspects of family life."		Monthly	$20/year (usually distributed free to interested physicians)	Hospital Publications, Inc. 18 East 48th Street New York, N.Y. 10019	Editor in Chief same address
Medical Insight	articles deal with emotional factors in general medicine.		Monthly	$10/year (may be available free to qualifying physicians)	Medical Insight 150 E. 58th Street New York, N.Y. 10022	Same address
Mental Health Digest	reflects the entire spectrum of mental health; condensations of current literature.	National Clearinghouse for Mental Health Information (NIMH)	Monthly	$3.50/year	Government Printing Office Washington, D.C. 20402	
Mental Hygiene	designed for policymakers in the mental health field; development and improvement of health care delivery systems.	National Assoc. for Mental Health, Inc.	4 times/year	$10/year	Mental Hygiene 49 Sheridan Ave. Albany, N.Y. 12210	Editor, Mental Hygiene 1800 N. Kent Street Rosslyn, Arlington, Va. 22209

Journal	Description	Organization	Frequency	Price	Address	Editorial Address
Mental Retardation	general articles on all aspects of mental retardation.	American Assoc. on Mental Deficiency	Bimonthly	$7/year	AAMD Publication Office 49 Sheridan Ave. Albany, N.Y. 12210	Same address
Merrill-Palmer Quarterly	General psychology. Includes marriage and the family.	Merrill-Palmer Institute of Human Development and Family Life	4 times/year	$8/year	Managing Editor Merrill-Palmer Institute 71 East Ferry Ave. Detroit, Mich. 48202	Editor, Merrill-Palmer Quarterly Department of Psychology University of Michigan Ann Arbor, Mich. 48104
Michigan Mental Health Research Bulletin	"to facilitate communication of mental health and retardation research findings." Publishes in abstract format.	Department of Mental Health, State of Michigan	Quarterly	Free	Office of Public Information Department of Mental Health Lansing, Mich. 48926	
Neuroendocrinology	"International journal for basic and clinical studies on neuroendocrine relationships."		Monthly	$27/year	Albert J. Phiebig, Inc. P.O. Box 352 White Plains, N.Y. 10602	Same address
Neuropharmacology	original studies of drug actions on CNS and peripheral nervous system in animals and man.		Bimonthly	$15/year	Pergamon Press Fairview Park Elmsford, N.Y. 10523	Editor, Laboratory of Preclinical Pharmacology National Institute of Mental Health Wm. A. White Bldg., St. Elizabeth's Hosp. Washington, D.C. 20032

TABLE XI-I Continued

Journal	Description	Official Publication of	Frequency of Publication	Cost of Subscription	Subscription Information	Send Manuscripts To
Neuropsychologia	Basic neurophysiology. Mixed animal experimentation and clinical articles; international.		Quarterly	$15/year	Pergamon Press Fairview Park Elmsford, N.Y. 10523	Prof. H. L. Fevber MIT, Psychology Section Cambridge, Mass.
Omega	"An international journal for the psychological study of dying, death, bereavement, suicide and other lethal behaviors." Multidisciplinary.		Quarterly	$20/year	Greenwood Periodicals Inc. 51 Riverside Ave. Westport, Conn. 06880	Editor, *Omega* Dr. Richard A. Kalish 1521-A Shattuck Ave. Berkeley, CA 94709
Pastoral Psychology	written primarily for clergy; many articles by psychiatrists.		10 issues/year	$5/year	Meredith Corporation 400 Community Drive Manhasset, N.Y. 11030	Managing Editor same address
Psychiatric News	general news items of interest to psychiatrists	American Psychiatric Assoc.	Biweekly	$6/year	*Psychiatric News* 1700 18th Street, N.W. Washington, D.C. 20009	
Psychiatric Opinion	General psychiatry. Each issue is dedicated to a single topic in the field of mental health.		Bimonthly	May be available free of charge	Opinion Publications, Inc. 39 Cochituate Road Framingham, Mass. 01701	Editor, *Psychiatric Opinion* same address
Psychiatry Annual (Medical World News)	annual review of articles and news in general psychiatry.			$12.50 (may be available free of charge)	Medical World News 299 Park Avenue New York, N.Y. 10017	
Psychiatry	"Journal for the study of interpersonal processes." Integrative approach among various disciplines, stressing concepts of Harry Stack Sullivan.		Quarterly	$12.50/year	William Alanson White Psychiatric Foundation 1610 New Hampshire Ave. N.W. Washington, D.C. 20009	Same address

Psychiatry Digest	summary of world-wide psychiatry and neurology literature; occasional original articles.	Monthly	$17.50/year (is available free of charge)	*Psychiatry Digest* 445 Central Avenue Northfield, Ill. 60093	
Psychiatry in Medicine	observational, clinical studies. Focuses on psychiatric consultation in general medical setting: patient care, MD-patient relationship, social and family factors, other special problems such as: transplants, ICU, etc.	Quarterly	$20/year	Greenwood Periodicals Co. 51 Riverside Ave. Westport, Conn. 06889	Editor, *Psychiatry in Medicine* Department of Psychiatry Mount Auburn Hosp. 330 St. Auburn Street Cambridge, Mass. 02138
Psychiatric Quarterly	General psychiatry.	New York State Department of Mental Hygiene	Quarterly	$8/year	*The Psychiatric Quarterly* 44 Holland Avenue Albany, N.Y. 12208	Same address
Psychoanalytic Study of the Child	Collection of outstanding papers in child analysis: theoretical, clinical, other. Hard-cover.	Annual	Approx. $12/volume	International Universities Press 239 Park Avenue South New York, N.Y. 10003	
Psychological Medicine	"A journal for research in psychiatry and the allied sciences."	Quarterly	$11/year	% British Medical Journal 1172 Commonwealth Ave. Boston, Mass. 02134	Editor, *Psychological Medicine* BMA House Tavistock Square London, W.C.1, England

TABLE XI-I Continued

Journal	Description	Official Publication of	Frequency of Publication	Cost of Subscription	Subscription Information	Send Manuscripts To
Psychoanalytic Quarterly	psychoanalysis.		Quarterly	$15/year	*Psychoanalytic Quarterly* 57 West 57th Street New York, N.Y. 10019	Editor, *Psychoanalytic Quarterly* same address
Psychological Issues	integrates psychoanalytical theory with findings and concepts of other disciplines.		Quarterly	$15/year	International Universities Press, Inc. 239 Park Avenue South New York, N.Y. 10003	Same address
Psychology Today	General, popular psychology. Stresses article of social relevance and interviews with leaders in field.		Monthly	$12/year	*Psychology Today* Box 2990 Boulder, Colorado 80302	Editor, *Psychology Today* 317 14th Street Del Mar, CA. 92014
Psychopharmacologia	features articles on effects of drugs on behavior, in broadest sense. Both clinical and animal experimentation. International.		Published at frequent intervals, as material is received.	Approx. $25/year	Springer-Verlag 175 Fifth Avenue New York, N.Y. 10010	Professor Jonathan O. Cole, M.D. Dept. of Mental Health Boston State Hospital 591 Morton Street Boston, Mass. 02124
Psychopharmacology Abstracts	"citations and abstracts of psychopharmacology literature (150–175 abstracts in 17 categories).	National Clearinghouse for Mental Health Information	Monthly	$18/year	Superintendent of Documents U.S. Government Printing Office Washington, D.C. 20402	
Psychopharmacology Bulletin	rapid, informal reporting of work in psychopharmacology that has not yet appeared elsewhere in the literature.	National Institute of Mental Health	Quarterly	$2/year	Superintendent of Documents Government Printing Office Washington, D.C. 20402	Alice Leeds, M.D. Chief, International Reference Center on Psychotropic Drugs N.I.M.H. 5454 Wisconsin Ave, Room 10-D-06 Chevy Chase, Md.,

Journal	Description	Society	Frequency	Cost	Publisher	Editor
Psychophysiology	reports of original research in psychophysiology (experimental, theoretical, clinical, methodological).	The Society for Psychophysiological Research	Bimonthly	$15/year	Psychophysiological Research Society Mt. Royal and Guilford Aves. Baltimore, Md. 21202	Editor, *Psychophysiology* Society for Psychophysiological Research 951 Lafayette Detroit, Mich. 48207
Physiology and Behavior	"original reports of systematic studies in physiology and behavior, in which at least one variable is physiological and the primary emphasis and theoretical context are behavioral." International; mostly animal studies.		Monthly	$24/year	Brain Research Publications, Inc. Highbridge Terrace Fayetteville, N.Y. 13066	Editor in Chief, Brain Research Laboratory Syracuse University 601 University Ave. Syracuse, N.Y. 13210
Psychosomatics	An international journal exploring the role of psychiatry in the daily practice of comprehensive medicine.	Academy of Psychosomatic Medicine	Bimonthly	$15/year ($10/year to residents and students)	Psychosomatics 992 Springfield Ave. Irvington, N.J. 07111	Editor, Wilfred Dorfrom, M.D. 1921 Newkirk Ave. Brooklyn, N.Y. 11226
Psychosomatic Medicine	topics in psychosomatic medicine.	American Psychosomatic Society	Bimonthly	$12/year ($6.50/year for residents and interns)	Harper & Row, Publishers 23 So. Virginia Ave. Hagerstown, Maryland 21740	Morton F. Reiser, M.D., Editor in Chief 265 Nassau Rd. Roosevelt, N.Y. 11575
Psychotherapy and Psychosomatics	international scope; psychosomatics especially as related to psychotherapy.	International Federation for Medical Psychotherapy.	Bimonthly	$13.50/year	Albert Phiebig, Inc. P.O. Box 352 White Plains, N.Y. 10602	Editor, *Psychotherapy and Psychosomatics* Dept. of Psychiatry University of California School of Medicine San Francisco, CA 94122

TABLE XI-I Continued

Journal	Description	Official Publication of	Frequency of Publication	Cost of Subscription	Subscription Information	Send Manuscripts To
Quarterly Journal of Studies on Alcohol	articles dealing with alcohol and wide-ranging aspects of alcoholism.	Rutgers Center of Alcohol Studies	Quarterly	$15/year	Quarterly Journal of Studies on Alcohol Rutgers University New Brunswick, N.J. 08903	Editor, *Quarterly Journal of Studies on Alcohol* Center of Alcohol Studies Rutgers University New Brunswick, N.J. 08903
Schizophrenia Bulletin	"to facilitate the dissemination and exchange of information about schizophrenia." Includes abstracts of recent literature.	Center for Studies of Schizophrenia, National Institute of Mental Health	about once/year	$1/volume	Superintendent of Documents Government Printing Office Washington, D.C. 20402	
Seminars in Psychiatry	entire journal dedicated to a single topic that changes each issue; general psychiatry; articles by leaders in special fields of psychiatry.		Quarterly	$15/year ($12/year for residents, interns, students)	Grune & Stratton 111 Fifth Ave. New York, N.Y. 10003	Dr. Ernest Hartman 591 Morton Street Boston, Mass. 02124
Social Science & Medicine	international journal with contributions from psychiatrists from all parts of the world. Interdisciplinary.		Bimonthly	$12.50/year	Pergamon Press Fairview Park Elmsford, N.Y. 10523	Renee C. Fox University of Pennsylvania Philadelphia, Pa. 19104
Voices: The Art and Science of Psychotherapy	articles revealing personal and professional discoveries which promise to influence, modify, change, transform the reader.	American Academy of Psychotherapists	Quarterly	$15/year	American Academy of Psychotherapists Suite 241 1040 Woodcock Rd. Orlando, Florida 32803	Dr. Vin Rosenthal, Editor Voices 815 Indian Road Glenview, Illinois 60025

Chapter XII

THE PSYCHIATRIST AND HIS POSTGRADUATE EDUCATION

ORMAL RESIDENCY TRAINING in psychiatry is but a beginning. It is but the first step toward a lifetime of professional study and growth.

Newly-trained psychiatrists become quickly aware of the need for continuing education as they prepare for board examinations soon after leaving their residency programs. Yet they learn that even board certification itself is not an end, but rather another point of departure, another beginning.

Professional education following the formal residency training can take several forms. This chapter provides information on ways that the psychiatrist might prepare for board examination (Preparing for Board Examinations), and information concerning various formal postgraduate study programs that are available to psychiatrists (Specialized Training Programs for Psychiatrists). In addition, the reader may refer to Chapter XI, The Psychiatrist's Bookshelf, for a guide to the current literature and to standard reference books in psychiatry. The reading lists cited in Chapter XI are an excellent source of continuing education.

PREPARING FOR BOARD EXAMINATIONS

JOSEPH R. NOVELLO, M.D.

I. The American Board of Psychiatry and Neurology

The American Board of Psychiatry and Neurology,

Inc. (Executive Offices: 1603 Orrington Ave., Evanston, Illinois 60201) is the official certification board for psychiatry and neurology in the United States. It is composed of twelve members (four from the American Psychiatric Association, four from the American Neurological Association, and two each from neurology and psychiatry as elected by the Section on Nervous and Mental Diseases of the American Medical Association). The board has several functions including the responsibility to determine competency of specialists in psychiatry and neurology and to grant certification after proper investigation and examination of qualified applicants.

II. Requirements for Applicants in General Psychiatry
    A. Physician (M.D. or D.O.) with an unlimited license to practice medicine in a state of the United States or its possessions, or a province of Canada, if residing in Canada.
    B. Satisfactory moral, ethical and professional standing.
    C. Satisfactory completion of the Board's specialized training and experience requirements. This requires a total of five calendar years of training and experience, all undertaken in the United States or Canada; three years must be spent in an approved residency program and the applicant must have two years of additional experience. At least two years of the formal training must be taken within a single approved training program.
    D. Other Applicants: The Board is also responsible for certification in three other areas: neurology, child psychiatry and child neurology. Each type of certificate requires certain specific requirements for training and experience. For details, the reader may request the booklet: "Information for Applicants," from the American Board of Psychiatry and Neurology.

III. How and When To Apply

A. Application forms may be obtained by writing to the American Board of Psychiatry and Neurology, Inc., 1603 Orrington Ave., Evanston, Illinois 60201.

B. Completed applications must be received in the executive office no later than October 31 in order to receive consideration for the following May examination. (Part I of the examination, the written test)

    1. Individuals who have recently taken the board exams strongly advise that the application be submitted as early as possible, preferably in the summer. This will guarantee action on the application within six to eight weeks. Also, it is commonly believed by those taking the tests that individuals are subsequently scheduled for Part II (the oral exam) in the order in which their original applications were submitted. Therefore, if a person is one of the early applicants he is more likely to be assigned to a testing center for the orals that is more geographically convenient for him.

C. Individuals who will complete their board eligibility (three years residency plus two years experience) by June 30 can qualify to take the exam in the preceding May. Their application, like all others, must be submitted by October 31 of the preceding year.

D. The present fee for Part I is $175. Part II requires an additional $150 fee. Travel expenses, room and board, incidentals are at the expense of the applicant.

IV. General Format of the Examination

A. Applicants for certification must pass the written exam (Part I) before being admitted to the oral exams (Part II). The written exam is given once each year (April or May) in several locations throughout the country. Applicants are assigned to the testing center closest to their residence.

B. It generally takes six to eight weeks for the Board to notify the applicant of the results. If the applicant passes Part I he is scheduled to take Part II about six months later; the applicant must, in fact, take the orals within one year of passing the written exam. The candidate who fails the written exam may reapply by October 31 and retake the exam the following May ($50 fee). Two failures of Part I require a reapplication and complete re-evaluation by the Credentials Committee. The applicant may fail one or two subjects in the oral exam (Part II) and be said to condition the examination. In this case he is eligible for re-examination in those subjects within one year ($100 fee). If he allows the year to lapse without retaking the exam he must resubmit the entire application, and requalify for the orals by again passing the written examination. Other details re: pass, fail are documented in the "Information for Applicants" booklet.

V. Part I (Written Examination)

A. Description: The Part I exam in general psychiatry is a multiple-choice written examination. It consists of two separate tests; the applicant is given two hours to complete each test. The first test includes a one hour segment in basic psychiatry and a one hour segment devoted to basic neurology. The second test is oriented toward clinical psychiatry and requires two hours for completion.

1. Basic psychiatry (one hour): Topics covered include development, mental retardation, diagnosis, etiology, history of psychiatry, psychodynamics, psychophysiology, psychopharmacology, psychopathology, psychotherapy, social psychiatry (including forensic psychiatry).

2. Basic neurology (one hour): Topics covered include clinical neurology, neuroanatomy, neurochemistry, neuropathology, neuropharmacology, neurophysiology.

3. Clinical psychiatry (two hours) : Questions focusing on clinical issues, utilizes case reports, vignettes, etc.

B. How to prepare

1. The American Board of Psychiatry and Neurology does not recommend or endorse any particular text or course of study. The Board believes that the approved training programs provide the essential information and experience that a candidate needs to pass the examination. Nevertheless most candidates find it necessary to engage in considerable study and preparation. The following suggestions on how to prepare for Part I are derived from recommendations made by several psychiatrists who took the exam in 1972.

2. Texts in psychiatry: As a basic, overall review most candidates select one or more major psychiatric textbooks. The current favorites are: *Modern Clinical Psychiatry,* Noyes and Kolb; *Comprehensive Textbook of Psychiatry,* Freedman and Kaplan.

3. Texts in neurology: The most recommended general textbook in neurology is *A Textbook of Neurology,* Merritt. Two other books that are often found to be valuable are: *Correlative Neuroanatomy and Functional Neurology,* Chusid and McDonald; *Programmed Atlas of Neuroanatomy,* Sidman and Sidman.

4. Other valuable texts: *Glossary of Psychiatric Terms* (American Psychiatric Association) and the official *Diagnostic and Statistical Manual, II Edition.* American Psychiatric Association; reproduced in its entirety in this handbook by courtesy of the A.P.A., Chapter I.

5. Journals: Generally speaking, Part I does not require a knowledge of the most recent literature. In fact, many recent candidates believe

that reviewing recent journal articles in preparing for Part I may actually be self-defeating.
The answers called-for on the test are based on
the most documented and widely-accepted facts:
The kind of information that is found in standard textbooks. Data reported in recent journals
has not yet stood the test of time~and is apt to
be more speculative.

6. A.P.A. Self-Assessment Program: The American
Psychiatric Association offers an examination
(Psychiatric Knowledge and Skills Self-Assessment Program) that tests skills in four broad
categories: Patient Management Problems, Problems in Diagnosis, Problems in Treatment and
Problems of Current Concern to Psychiatry. Applicants receive the test by mail and are fur-
nished with an answer key and bibliography.
The APA also provides norm tables for comparison with how peers have fared on the examination. Results are confidential. Candidates
for board certification in psychiatry have found
this test useful in their preparation for the written exam, particularly in pinpointing areas of
relative strength and weakness in their own
knowledge. Cost for taking the exam varies:
$15 for residents, $25 for APA members, $40
for other physicians. Applications may be obtained by writing: APA-PKSAP, 1700 18th St.,
N.W., Washington, D.C. 20009.

7. Exam guides: Two books that provide candidates with a question and answer type of review
are: *Psychiatry Specialty Board Review* (The
Medical Examination Publishing Co.) and *Neurology Specialty Board Review* (The Medical
Examination Publishing Company). These
books' major value is that they present the questions in the various kinds of multiple-choice for-
mats that are apt to be encountered in an ex-

amination such as Part I. Most candidates are out of practice when it comes to taking a multiple-choice exam. The style in which these questions are asked can be puzzling in itself. It is wise to brush up on the basics of test-taking.

8. Formal courses: Standardized courses designed for the psychiatrist who is preparing for board examinations are offered periodically at the Menninger Clinic (Topeka, Kansas) and the New York State Psychiatric Institute (New York City). Others are also available. Most are advertised in the APA Newsletter.

9. Personal communication: Most candidates have found it worthwhile to discuss the test beforehand with someone who has recently taken it. This is valuable mostly in learning more about the logistics of the testing procedure and may help allay some anxiety. The test itself, of course, is changed each time.

VI. Part II (Oral Examination)

A. Description: The Part II exam for psychiatrists is entirely oral. It consists of three clinical examinations, two in psychiatry and one in neurology. The candidate is then questioned about his findings (and other related information) by a team of examiners. The three separate sections are usually all scheduled for the same day but, because of scheduling conflicts, some candidates may require two days in attendance.

1. The psychiatric examinations: The general format calls for the candidate to interview a patient (under observation) for twenty minutes and then to discuss the case with the examiners for twenty-five minutes. The timing can be a bit flexible depending upon the examiners' prerogative.

2. The neurological examination: The candidate performs a history and neurological exam on a

patient, being given approximately twenty minutes. He is then questioned by the examiners for twenty-five minutes. The same flexibility rule applies.

B. How to prepare for the orals in psychiatry

　　1. Probably the most common mistake made by candidates is to be underprepared. Candidates in psychiatry tend to think: "I have been interviewing patients for five years. There is no need to prepare any further." This can be a costly error. Few psychiatrists are accustomed to conducting an interview in only twenty minutes. It is wise to practice several short interviews prior to the examination. This can usually be arranged in a clinic environment. It is also quite helpful to carry out this practice interview under the observation of another psychiatrist and to discuss the case with him following the interview.

　　2. Practice answering questions out loud. There is a certain skill in doing this that only comes with practice.

　　3. Journals: It was pointed out earlier that journal reading is not especially important (and may be harmful) for the written exam (Part I). The opposite is true for the orals. The candidate will be expected to have a knowledge of recent developments in the field of psychiatry. An adequate preparation for the orals should include a review of the recent literature. Many candidates find it useful to establish a card-catalog system for summarizing their journal reading. The Board does not endorse or recommend any particular journal. Most recent candidates recommend four basic journals of general psychiatry: *Journal of the American Psychiatric Association, Archives of General Psychiatry* (published by the A.M.A.), *Journal of Nervous and*

Mental Diseases and *Diseases of the Nervous System.* In addition, many recommend various abstracting services such as *Psychiatry Digest* ("A Monthly Summary of the World Literature for Psychiatrists").

4. Audio-Digest cassette tapes: Many recent candidates for the boards recommend a subscription to the Audio-Digest service in psychiatry as a handy, convenient way to keep abreast of current literature and recent developments in the field. The subscriber is provided with two cassette tapes each month that summarize the most important journal articles, conferences and seminars. (Cost $75/year.) In addition, the subscriber receives an indexing system and cumulative six-month cross indexes. Portable cassette tape recorders are also available at a discount. Write: Audio-Digest Foundation (Psychiatry), 1250 S. Glendale Avenue, Glendale, California 91205.

C. How to prepare for the orals in neurology

1. Most psychiatrists find it necessary to briefly repeat the review of basic clinical neurology that they had done in preparing for Part I. Since the oral exam is largely limited to clinical neurology there is little premium placed on again reviewing such items as cellular neuropathology, etc.

2. Review the basic neurological examination and know the indications for the ancillary diagnostic tests (brain scan, carotid arteriogram, etc.). It may be especially important to be knowledgeable about the differential diagnosis between certain neurological conditions and psychiatric entities. See Chapter VIII of this handbook, (Neurology for Psychiatrists).

3. Recent candidates report that the most important preparation is to actually practice doing

the complete neurological examination under the guidance of a trained neurologist. Many candidates arrange to spend some time working and observing in a neurology clinic or private neurology practice prior to taking the Part II examination.

4. Journals: Although the neurologists taking the examination must certainly be knowledgeable about the current neurological literature; this is not generally expected of the psychiatrists (just as the neurologists are not expected to be read up-to-the-minute in the psychiatric literature). Yet, if the psychiatrist is so inclined he may review the two major journals in neurology: (1) *Archives of Neurology* and (2) *Neurology*.

References

Information for Applicants, The American Board of Psychiatry and Neurology, Inc., 1971.

Note: The American Board of Psychiatry and Neurology does not recommend or endorse any specific methods, courses, text or other aids in the preparation for board examination. The opinions expressed are solely the author's based on interviews with several recent board candidates (1972).

SPECIALIZED TRAINING PROGRAMS FOR PSYCHIATRISTS

JOSEPH R. NOVELLO, M.D.

In addition to the training in general psychiatry that is offered by approved residency programs (See The Psychiatrist's Address Book, Chapter XIII) there are available, throughout the country, many programs that offer training in specialized areas within psychiatry. While only one such subspecialty, child psychiatry, is recognized as an official subspecialty with its own certification board, these other programs offer valuable training to psychiatrists and present rich alternatives in both philosophical orientation and treatment techniques.

The following listing of specialized training programs for psychiatrists outlines the major features of these training opportunities and offers the reader additional resources that may be contacted for further information.

The programs outlined include:

1. Administrative Psychiatry
2. Adolescent Psychiatry
3. Analytical Psychology (Jung)
4. Behavioral Therapy
5. Child Psychiatry
6. Community Psychiatry
7. Family Therapy
8. Forensic Psychiatry
9. Geriatric Psychiatry
10. Gestalt Psychology
11. Holistic Approach to Psychoanalysis (Horney)
12. Hypnosis
13. Individual Psychology (Adler)
14. Interpersonal Theory of Psychiatry (Sullivan)
15. Psychiatric Consultation
16. Psychoanalysis
17. Psychodrama
18. Psychosomatic Medicine
19. Treatment of Sexual Dysfunction
20. Training Group Laboratories
21. Transactional Analysis

I. Administrative Psychiatry[1]

Basic philosophy and technique: The application of administrative and managerial skills in the practice of psychiatry, includes such subject areas as: social psychology, dynamics of institutional change, organizational psychology, group process, systems planning, budget, communications, public relations, labor relations, forensic psychiatry, political science, public health and epidemiology, fund raising and others.
National headquarters: Interested parties may contact:

Archie R. Foley, M.D.
Chairman, APA Committee on Certification
in Administrative Psychiatry
630 West 168th Street
New York, New York 10032

Training programs available: List of training programs available by contacting party above.

Requirements for entry into training program: Varies. Two or more years of approved psychiatric residency. It is pos-

---

[1] Dr. Novello asknowledges the assistance of Walter E. Barton, M.D., Medical Director, American Psychiatric Association.

sible that in the near future administrative psychiatry will be recognized as an official subspecialty of psychiatry with its own board examinations, etc.

Length of training: Varies.

Description of training program: Varies. Programs provide some administrative experience along with training in many of the areas listed in basic philosophy and technique.

Representative Textbooks: *Administration in Psychiatry,* Barton.

II. Adolescent Psychiatry[2]

Basic philosophy and technique: Training in the special area of adolescent psychiatry. Techniques vary.

National headquarters:

> American Society for Adolescent Psychiatry
> 88-77 Elderts Lane
> Woodhaven, New York 11421

Training programs available: Many fourth year fellowships are available in college mental health at various university-based psychiatric training centers. Relatively few programs are available in adolescent psychiatry (University of Michigan, Michael Reese Hospital in Chicago and others) ; Write to above address for details.

Requirements for entry into training program: Three years in general psychiatry.

Length of training: One or two years.

Description of training program: Supervised psychotherapy of inpatients and outpatients, didactic seminars and clinical conferences, research, community consultation in high schools, etc.

Journals: *Annals of Adolescent Psychiatry*
Journal of Youth and Adolescence

---

[2] Dr. Novello acknowledges the assistance of Daniel Offer, M.D., Editor, *Journal of Youth and Adolescence.*

Representative textbooks: *On Adolescence,* Blos
Wayward Youth, Aichorn
The Age Between, Miller

III. Analytical Psychology[3]
(JUNG)

Founder: Carl Jung

Basic philosophy and techniques: Ego emerges from the inner self and must rerelate to its source. The unconscious is not just a discarded remnant for consciousness but has, as a substrate, the collective unconscious which all people share in common. Individuation (becoming one's own unique self), is the goal of individual therapy. Jungian psychology is also referred to as analytical psychology.

Training programs available:

New York Institute of the C. G. Jung
Foundation
815 Second Avenue
New York, New York 11017

C. G. Jung Institute of San Francisco
2040 Gough Street
San Francisco, California 94109

Requirements for entry into training program: M.D. degree with at least one year of psychiatric residency. Personal analysis of at least 100 hours with qualified Jungian analyst. (Other qualified mental health professionals may be accepted for training.)

Length of training: Varies. Approximately four years.

Description of training program: Personal and control analysis, seminars, tutorial readings, thesis. Special emphasis is placed on the trainee's ability to interpret symbolic material

---

[3] Dr. Novello acknowledges the assistance of the C. G. Jung Institute of San Francisco and Edward C. Whitmont, M.D. of the New York Institute of the C. G. Jung Foundation.

such as dreams, fantasies and to deal appropriately with transference and countertransference phenomena.

Representative textbooks: *The Symbolic Quest: Basic Concepts of Analytical Psychology,* Whitmont

IV. Behavioral Therapy[4]

Basic philosophy and technique: Basic assumption is that a great many unadaptive habits are learned and, in order to eliminate such habits, it is appropriate to make use of experimentally established knowledge of the learning process itself. Behavioral therapy is the systematic application of conditioning and learning theory to research, assessment and treatment of emotional disorders.

National headquarters:

> Behavior Therapy and Research Society
> Temple University Medical School
> c/o Eastern Pennsylvania Psychiatric Institute
> Henry Avenue
> Philadelphia, Pennsylvania 19129

> Association for the Advancement of
> Behavioral Therapy
> 415 E. 52nd Street
> New York, New York 10022

Training programs available: Several available throughout the United States. Contact the addresses listed above for details.

Requirements for entry into training program: Varies. Temple University program requires M.D. degree plus three years of psychiatric residency.

Length of training: One year (Temple), others vary.

---

[4] Dr. Novello acknowledges the assistance of Joseph Wolpe, M.D., Professor of Psychiatry, Temple University School of Medicine, and Dorothy J. Susskind, Executive Secretary of the Association for the Advancement of Behavioral Therapy.

Description of training programs: Didactic seminars, demonstrations, supervised cases.

Journals: *Journal of Behavior Therapy and Experimental Psychiatry*
Behavior Therapy

Representative textbook: *Practice of Behavioral Therapy,* Wolpe.

V.   Child Psychiatry[5]

Basic philosophy and technique: Child psychiatry is the only official subspecialty of psychiatry in the United States. Board certification in psychiatry is a prerequisite to certification in child psychiatry. Philosophy is based upon various theoretical frameworks of childhood psychological growth and development. The psychoanalytic model is the major influence in the United States. Techniques vary.

National headquarters:

American Academy of Child Psychiatry
1800 R. Street N. W.
Suite 904
Washington, D.C. 20009

American Board of Psychiatry and Neurology
Committee on Certification in Child Psychiatry
1603 Orrington Avenue
Suite 490
Evanston, Illinois 60201

Training programs available: Many throughout the United States. See Chapter XIII, Psychiatrist's Address Book, for complete listing.

Requirements for entry into training program: Most programs require a minimum of two years of residency in gen-

[5] Dr. Novello acknowledges the assistance of Saul I. Harrison, M.D., Professor of Psychiatry and Director of Training, Children's Psychiatric Hospital, University of Michigan.

eral psychiatry. Some programs waive this requirement for entry and assume that it can be fulfilled after the residency in child psychiatry.

Length of training: The American Board requires four years which typically consist of two years in general psychiatry and two years in child psychiatry.

Description of training program: Seminars, supervised cases.

Journal: *Journal of the American Academy of Child Psychiatry.*

Representative textbook: Section on Child Psychiatry, *Comprehensive Textbook of Psychiatry,* Freedman and Kaplan *Child Psychiatry,* Finch

VI. Community Psychiatry[6]

Basic philosophy and technique: Essentially a delivery system that brings a comprehensive set of mental health services to a given population. Emphasis is on groups, social and interpersonal interactions, crisis intervention and preventive techniques. Consultations and the training of paraprofessionals are critical tools.

Sources of further information:

> Gerald Caplan, M.D.
> Laboratory of Community Psychiatry
> Harvard Medical School
> 58 Fenwood Road
> Boston, Massachusetts 02115

> National Institute of Mental Health
> 5600 Fishers Lane
> Rockville, Maryland 20852

Training programs available: There are many training programs available throughout the country. For information contact:

---

[6] Dr. Novello acknowledges the assistance of Philip Margolis, M.D., Professor of Psychiatry, University of Michigan.

Walter Shervington, M.D.
Chief of Psychiatry Training
National Institute of Mental Health
5454 Wisconsin Avenue
Chevy Chase, Maryland 20203

Requirements for entry into training program: Usually two years of basic, general psychiatric residency.

Usual length of training: One to two years.

Description of training program: Combination of didactic and anecdotal seminars. Field experience and one-to-one supervision of clinical cases, consultation, administration and politics.

Journals: *Community Mental Health Journal*
Hospital and Community Psychiatry

Representative textbooks: *Handbook of Community Psychiatry and Community Mental Health,* Bellak.
The Theory and Practice of Mental Health Consultation, Caplan.

VII. Family Therapy[7]

Founders: John Bell, Nathan Ackerman, Murray Bowen, Lymon Wynne, Don Jackson, Virginnia Satir

Basic philosophy and technique: Individual psychopathology is the result of familial interactions. Changes in the individual can occur only if the family system changes. Family therapy is any therapeutic intervention technique that has as its major focus the alteration of the family system. Techniques vary: Systems approach, psychoanalytic, transactional analysis, etc.

National headquarters: No official national organization. The journal, *Family Process* (149 E. 78th St., New York,

---

[7] Dr. Novello acknowledges the assistance of the late Nathan W. Ackerman, M.D., Judith Leib, A.C.S.W., Executive Secretary of the Nathan W. Ackerman Family Institute, New York and Andrew Ferber, M.D., Bronx State Hospital, New York.

New York 10021) might be considered an unofficial head-quarters.

Training programs available: There are many family institutes throughout the United States that offer training. Contact Editor, *Family Process* for details.

Requirements for entry into training program: Generally open to fully trained mental health professionals in all disciplines depending on individual qualifications.

Length of training: Varies. Usually two to three years.

Description of training programs: Seminars, workshops, observations, supervised cases.

Journal: *Family Process*

Representative textbooks: *The Psychodynamics of Family Life*, Ackerman.
    Treating the Troubled Family, Ackerman.
    The Book of Family Therapy, Ferber.

VIII. Forensic Psychiatry[8]

Basic philosophy and technique: Utilization of basic psychiatric diagnostic and treatment techniques in the interface between psychiatry and the law. Includes criminal law, workman's compensation, Federal Employee's Liability Act, Civil tort actions, treatment of the mentally ill offender, correctional psychiatry, court clinic work, etc.

National headquarters:

> American Academy of Psychiatry and the **Law**
> Box 2060
> Ann Arbor, Michigan 48106

Training programs available: Programs available at Center for Forensic Psychiatry, Ann Arbor, Michigan; Temple University, Philadelphia, Pennsylvania; UCLA, Los Angeles, California; Boston University, Boston, Massachusetts; USC,

---

[8] Dr. Novello acknowledges the assistance of Ames Robey, M.D., Director, Center for Forensic Psychiatry, Ann Arbor, Michigan.

Los Angeles, California. Other programs are in the stage of early development.

Requirements for entry into training program: Usually requires completion of three years of psychiatric residency.

Length of training: Variable. Three months elective to full two-year fellowships.

Description of training program: Shorter programs consist of didactic seminars with the minimal amount of practical experience. Longer programs contain actual court experience and work in diagnosis, evaluation, treatment of mentally ill offenders.

Journal: *Journal of the American Academy of Psychiatry and The Law.*

Representative textbooks: *Forensic Psychiatry,* Davidson.

Readings in Psychiatry and the Law, Allen, Ferster, and Rubin.

IX. Geriatric Psychiatry[9]

Basic philosophy and technique: Principles of general psychiatry applied to the special problems and needs of the elderly. Recognizes a multiplicity of factors including: psychological, physical, social, economic.

Training programs available: As yet there are few programs devoted exclusively to Geriatric Psychiatry. The interested reader may contact any of the following three programs for information:

> Martin A. Berezin, M.D.
> Boston Society for Gerontologic Psychiatry
> 90 Forest Avenue
> West Newton, Massachusetts 02165

> > Adrian ver Woerdt, M.D.
> > Gero-Psychiatry
> > Duke University Medical Center
> > Durham, North Carolina 27706

---

[9] Dr. Novello acknowledges the assistance of Martin A. Berezin, M.D., Editor, *Journal of Geriatric Psychiatry* and Wolfgang W. May, M.D., Chief, Gerontology Research, Ypsilanti State Hospital (Michigan) .

Wolfgang W. May, M.D.
Gerontology Research
Ypsilanti State Hospital
3501 Willis Road
Ypsilanti, Michigan 48197
(affiliated with University of
Michigan Gerontology Institute)

Requirements for entry into training program: Varies. Positions available to residents in training and to postgraduate psychiatrists.

Length of training: Varies. Electives of several months. Full fellowships.

Description of training program: Contact above programs for details.

Journal: *Journal of Geriatric Psychiatry*

Representative textbooks: Geriatric psychiatry, Goldfarb (In, *Comprehensive Textbook of Psychiatry*, Freedman and Kaplan [Eds.])

> *Psychodynamic Studies on Aging*, Levin and Kahana (Eds.)
> *Behavior and Adaptation in Late Life*, Busse and Pfeiffer

X. Gestalt Psychology[10]

Founder: Fritz Perls

Basic philosophy and technique: Emphasizes the centrality of the existential encounter. Diversity of techniques bound to a clearly delineated frame of reference. Authenticity of personal experience and the here-and-now are stressed. Gestalt practices integrate action with introspection.

Training programs available: Several programs throughout the United States. Many are integrated into transactional analysis and family therapy training programs. For further information, write to:

Gestalt Institute of Cleveland
12921 Euclid Avenue
Cleveland, Ohio 44112

---

[10] Dr. Novello acknowledges the assistance of the Gestalt Institute of Cleveland.

Requirements for entry into training program: Varies. Usually limited to qualified psychiatrists, psychologists and social workers with M.D., Ph.D., or M.S.W. degrees. Psychiatric residents usually admitted.

Length of training: Varies. Some three-year programs available, others provide short-term workshops.

Description of training program: Didactic, group experience, supervised group therapy.

Representative textbooks: *Ego, Hunger, and Aggression,* Perls

   Gestalt Therapy Verbation, Perls

XI. Holistic Approach to Psychoanalysis[11]
(KAREN HORNEY)

Founder: Karen Horney

Basic philosophy and technique: Acknowledges historical debt to Freud and his achievements and recognizes continued need to build upon that foundation. The theory of neurosis and of human growth which has been developed by Karen Horney is based on the belief "that man has the capacity as well as the desire to develop his potentialities . . . . and that man can change and go on changing as long as he lives."

National headquarters:

> American Institute for Psychoanalysis
> 329 East 62nd Street
> New York, New York 10021

Training programs available: American Institute for Psychoanalysis is associated with the Karen Horney Psychoanalytic Institute and Center (same address).

Requirements for entry into training program: M.D. degree and at least one year of psychiatric residency. (Also open to fourth year medical students by special arrangement.)

Length of training: Four years.

---

[11] Dr. Novello acknowledges the assistance of Harry Gershman, M.D., Dean, American Institute for Psychoanalysis.

Description of training program: Twenty-five courses, fifty credits required for certification. Minimum of 500 hours training analysis. Three supervisory analyses of at least fifty hours each.

Journal: *American Journal of Psychoanalysis*

Representative textbooks: *The Neurotic Personality of Our Time,* Horney
New Ways in Psychoanalysis, Horney

XII. Hypnosis[12]

Founders: True founders of hypnosis are lost in antiquity. Among modern psychiatrists who have pioneered the use of hypnosis in treatment are: Mesmer, Charcot, Bernheim, Janet, Freud.

Basic philosophy and technique: Various induction procedures are employed to produce a state of concentrated attention (trance). Suggestions are then preferred, geared toward goals of tension reduction, symptom removal or alleviation, behavior modification or exploration of unconscious conflict. In psychiatry, hypnosis is employed as part of overall psychotherapeutic approach: supportive, educational or analytic.

National headquarters:

> Society for Clinical and Experimental Hypnosis
> 140 West End Avenue
> New York, New York 10023

> American Society of Clinical Hypnosis
> 800 Washington Ave. S. E.
> Minneapolis, Minnesota 55414

Training programs available: The two societies above sponsor periodic seminars and workshops. Also contact Melvin D. Yahr, M.D., Assoc. Dean, Columbia University, College of

---

[12] Dr. Novello wishes to acknowledge the assistance of Lewis P. Wolberg, M.D., Medical Director, Postgraduate Center for Mental Health, New York and Herbert Spiegel, M.D., Associate Clinical Professor of Psychiatry, Columbia University, College of Physicians and Surgeons.

Physicians and Surgeons, 630 West 168th Street, New York, New York 10032.

Requirements for entry into training program: M.D. degree; some programs require psychiatric postgraduate training.

Length of training: Varies. Weekend workshops to full fellowships (individually arranged).

Description of training program: Lectures, seminars, demonstrations, supervised cases. Most training focuses upon induction procedures and trance utilization.

Journals: *American Journal of Clinical Hypnosis*
International Journal of Clinical and Experimental Hypnosis

Representative textbook: *Medical Hypnosis,* Wolberg

XIII. Individual Psychology[13]
(ALFRED ADLER)

Founder: Alfred Adler

Basic philosophy and technique: The assumption of Adlerian psychology (also called individual psychology) is that all human behavior is purposive. The individual is an indivisibly whole organism striving towards a subjectively conceived goal of success. The approach is phenomenological. Diagnosis and treatment are difficult to distinguish since the diagnosis of the subjectively conceived goal is partly a correction of its fictional character.

Training programs available: Several available throughout the United States. For information contact:

American Society of Adlerian Psychology
P. O. Box 17097
Houston, Texas 77031

Requirements for entry into training program: Psychotherapy training requires M.D., Ph.D., M.S.W. or M.A. in clinical psychology.

---

[13] Dr. Novello acknowledges the assistance of Eugen J. McClory, Director, Alfred Adler Institute, Chicago.

Length of training: Varies. Usually two to three years.

Description of training program: 13 courses and 120 hours of practicum plus 30 hours of small group supervision and two case seminars.

Journal: *Journal of Individual Psychology*

Representative textbook: *Fundamentals of Adlerian Psychology,* R. Dreikurs

XIV.   Interpersonal Theory of Psychiatry[14]
(HARRY STACK SULLIVAN)

Founder: Harry Stack Sullivan

Basic philosophy and technique: Anxiety is the focal issue in personality development but unlike Freud who stressed the intrapsychic nature of anxiety, Sullivan saw anxiety as an interpersonal phenomenon. (The focus is on anxiety in the here-and-now since it is less prone to distortion.) Although many techniques of classic psychoanalysis are used, Sullivanian therapists differ from Freudians in that they consider themselves active participant-observers in therapy.

Training programs available:
> William Alanson White Institute
> 20 West 74th Street
> New York, New York 10023
> (Psychoanalytic training that relies heavily on Sullivan's concepts)

> Washington School of Psychiatry
> 1610 New Hampshire Ave. N. W.
> Washington, D.C. 20009
> (Various programs available; not exclusively Sullivanian)

Requirements for entry into training program: M.D. degree from medical school accredited by A.M.A., at least one year of approved psychiatric residency. Must complete three years

---

[14] Dr. Novello acknowledges the assistance of Robert G. Kvarnes, M.D., Director, Washington School of Psychiatry.

of residency training prior to graduation. (Ph.D. psychologists also accepted.)

Length of training: Varies. Personal analysis is required. Curriculum consists of four years of study; personal analysis proceeds simultaneously.

Description of training program: Seminars, personal analysis, four supervised cases.

Journal: *Psychiatry* (Journal for the Study of Interpersonal Processes)
   Contemporary Psychoanalysis

Representative textbooks: *The Interpersonal Theory of Psychiatry,* Sullivan
   The Psychiatric Interview, Sullivan

XV.   Psychiatric Consultation[15]

Basic philosophy and technique: The basic philosophy embodies the principles of comprehensive medicine with an emphasis on ecological concepts and a view of illness as a process. The objective of the consultation is to apply psychiatric knowledge and skills for the benefit of general medical and surgical patients. Various techniques may be used: patient-oriented, consultee-oriented, milieu-oriented.

National headquarters: None

Training programs available: Approximately thirty to forty programs available. Write to chairmen of the various departments of psychiatry for details.

Requirements for entry into training program: Internship or one year of psychiatric residency are minimal requirements.

Length of training: Three to six months is minimum; six months is average; some programs provide a full year of training.

---

[15] Dr. Novello acknowledges the assistance of John J. Schwab, M.D., Professor of Psychiatry, College of Medicine, University of Florida.

Description of training program: Five to ten medical/surgical consultations per week under supervision, work rounds with medical-surgical staff, seminars and conferences in both medicine-surgery and psychiatry.

Representative textbook: *Handbook of Psychiatric Consultation*, Schwab

XVI. Psychoanalysis[16]

Founder: Sigmund Freud

Basic philosophy and technique: The basic philosophy and technique are based upon the work of Sigmund Freud and subsequent psychoanalytic scholars. Fundamental principles include: Theory of the unconscious, free-association, interpretation of dreams, concept of transference. Basic technique is free association and the making conscious of previously unconscious material.

National headquarters:

The American Psychoanalytic Association
One E. 57th Street
New York, New York 10022

Training programs available: There are currently twenty-one institutes approved by the American Psychoanalytic Association. These institutes are scattered throughout the United States. Write to National Headquarters for details. Requirements for entry into training program: Graduation from A.M.A.-approved medical school and completion of one year of residency. (Some institutes offer limited training to nonmedical candidates.)

Length of training: Varies. In general, five to eight years (including the personal analysis).

Description of training program:

1. Personal analysis: A therapeutic analysis to prepare the candidate for the later task of conducting analyses himself.

---

[16] Dr. Novello acknowledges the assistance of George A. Richardson, M.D., Professor of Psychiatry, University of Michigan.

2. Didactic seminar curriculum: A three to four year program which systematically covers basic concepts, psychopathology, continuous cases, etc.

3. Supervised analyses: Candidate conducts analyses under supervision of senior supervising analyst.

Journal: *Journal of the American Psychoanalytic Association*
Representative textbook: *An Elementary Textbook of Psychoanalysis*, Brenner

XVII. Psychodrama[17]

Founder: J. L. Moreno

Basic philosophy and technique: Psychotherapy based on spontaneity-creativity theory. Technique involves drama, role-playing and other group therapy concepts.

National headquarters:

> Moreno Institute
> 259 Wolcott Avenue
> Beacon, New York 12508

Training programs available: Above address.

Requirements for entry into training program: Training is on the graduate level. Interdisciplinary. Professionals in all the helping professions are admitted, if qualified.

Length of training: Total training period, spread over two years, requires sixteen weeks in residence at Moreno Institute. Leads to certification as director.

Description of training program: Every student learns to explore themselves and other group members via psychodrama, sociometry and group dynamics.

Journal: *Group Psychotherapy and Psychodrama*
Representative textbooks: *Psychodrama* (Volume I. II. III), Moreno
Who Shall Survive?, Moreno

---

[17] Dr. Novello acknowledges the assistance of Zerka T. Moreno, Director of Training, The Moreno Institute.

XVIII. Psychosomatic Medicine[18]

Founders: Franz Alexander, Flanders Dunbar

Basic philosophy and technique: Concerned with the application of psychiatric and medical knowledge to: 1. psychological complications of organic disease; 2. psychologic reactions to organic disease; 3. somatic presentations of psychiatric disorders; 4. classical psychosomatic disorders such as asthma, ulcerative colitis, etc.; 5. liaison with medical-surgical services; 6. research into the interrelationship of psychological-physiological-and social factors in the causation of disease.

National headquarters:

> American Psychosomatic Society
> 265 Nassau Road
> Roosevelt, New York 11575

> Academy of Psychosomatic Medicine
> c/o Wilfred Dorfrom, M.D.
> 1921 Newkirk Avenue
> Brooklyn, New York 11226

Training programs available: A list of ten training programs, all based in university-sponsored departments of psychiatry, is available from The American Psychosomatic Society.

Requirements for entry into training program: Varies. M.D. degree with postgraduate work in psychiatry and/or internal medicine.

Length of training: Varies. One year or more.

Description of training program: Varies. Combined experience in psychiatric and medical settings. Consultation experience. Seminars. Case supervision. Some laboratory experience usually included.

Journal: *Journal of Psychosomatic Research*
  Psychiatry In Medicine
  Psychophysiology

---

[18] Dr. Novello acknowledges the assistance of Monica N. Starkman, M.D., Instructor, Department of Psychiatry, University of Michigan and Ms. Joan K. Erpt, Executive Assistant, *Psychosomatic Medicine.*

Psychosomatics
Psychosomatic Medicine

Representative textbooks: *Psychosomatic Medicine: Its Principles and Applications,* Alexander.
Handbook of Psychiatric Consultation, Schwab.

XIX. Treatment of Sexual Dysfunction[19]

Founders: William H. Masters, Virginnia E. Johnson

Basic philosophy and technique: Objective study of physiology of sexual function and dysfunction and application of specific treatment techniques by specially trained male-female therapy teams.

National headquarters:

>Human Reproductive Biology Foundation
>4910 Forest Park Blvd.
>St. Louis, Missouri 63108

Training programs available: The pilot training programs established by Masters and Johnson have been completed. It is anticipated that another training program will be established soon.

Requirements for entry into training program: Male-female teams. One of the team must be a physician, the other must have a degree in one of the behavioral sciences: Psychology, social work, nursing, etc.

Length of training: Original program covered six weeks but newer programs may be of longer duration.

Description of training program: Pilot program consisted of description, indoctrination regarding psychology of program, reviewing tapes, taking role as co-therapist with member of senior staff of opposite sex, then assignment of the trainee team to a couple from the regular patient pool at the Foundation. Supervision is intensive.

Journal: *Medical Aspects of Human Sexuality*

[19] Dr. Novello asknowledges the assistance of Raymond W. Waggoner, M.D., Sr., Director of Continuing Education, Human Reproductive Biology Foundation.

Representative textbooks: *Human Sexual Response,* Masters and Johnson

Human Sexual Inadequacy, Masters and Johnson

XX. Training Group Laboratories

Founders: National Training Laboratory for Applied Behavioral Science

Basic philosophy and technique: NTL seeks to apply existing knowledge of human behavior to the problems of individuals, groups and organizations. In promoting increased sensitivity and openness to growth, it seeks to enhance the range and validity of alternatives and to improve the processes of choice. Technique includes several designs such as T-group, sensitivity training, role playing, nonverbal activities, theory presentations and intergroup exercises.

National headquarters:

> National Training Laboratory
> 1201 Sixteenth Street, N.W.
> Washington, D.C. 20036

Training programs available: Core curriculum is offered at two major training sites which are located at Bethel, Maine and Loretto Heights College, Denver, Colorado. Other workshops and laboratories are held throughout the United States. Write to NTL for details.

Requirements for entry into training program: Varies.

Length of program: Varies from weekend workshops to full program leading to designation as group leader and trainer.

Description of training program: The fundamental training approach is the group laboratory (T-group) method.

Specific programs are available in many subject areas: Individual Development, Group Problem-Solving, Contemporary Organizational Development, Principles of Consultation and Negotiation and others.

Representative textbooks: *Personal and Organization Change Through Group Methods,* Schein and Bennis.

XXI. Transactional Analysis[20]

Founder: Eric Berne

Basic philosophy and technique: Everyone has three parts or persons within himself: a parent, an adult, and a child. By identifying these and the particular script for living that the person is following *(Games People Play)*, the individual is freed to make new, healthier decisions for living. Technique: group treatment.

National headquarters:

> International Transactional Analysis Association
> 3155 College Avenue
> Berkeley, California 94705

Training programs available: Many programs throughout the United States. Write to ITAA for details.

Requirements for entry into training program: Generally open to mental health workers in all disciplines, depending on individual qualifications.

Length of training: Varies from short work-shop sessions to full two-year curricula.

Description of training program: Varies. Workshops, seminars, experience both as group member and leader, supervision, written and oral examinations, etc.

Journal: *International Journal of Transactional Analysis*

Representative textbooks: *Games People Play*, Berne
  Transactional Analysis in Psychotherapy, Berne
  I'm OK, You're OK, Harris

---

[20] Dr. Novello acknowledges the assistance of Thomas A. Harris, M.D. and Stanley J. Woollams, M.D.

PART THREE:

THE PSYCHIATRIST'S ADDRESS BOOK

Chapter XIII

THE PSYCHIATRIST'S ADDRESS BOOK

THE ORGANIZATIONS AND INSTITUTIONS listed by mailing address in this chapter fall into three basic categories: (1) organizations related in some way to psychiatry and with which the psychiatrist may occasionally wish to correspond, (2) treatment centers (adult and child) to which the psychiatrist may wish to refer patients or initiate correspondence for other reasons, (3) approved training centers (adult and child psychiatry).

The first list (Professional Organizations Related to Psychiatry) is a miscellaneous list of organizations frequently contacted by psychiatrists in professional correspondence. It is followed by a complete roster of the National Association of Psychiatric Hospitals and a complete roster of member institutions of the American Association of Psychiatric Services for Children. Finally the reader is provided a complete list of all approved residency programs in both adult and child psychiatry.

The purpose of this *address book* is to make available in this one volume these addresses that are otherwise scattered among many diverse sources and are relatively inaccessible to most psychiatrists.

PROFESSIONAL ORGANIZATIONS
RELATED TO PSYCHIATRY

Academy of Psychosomatic Medicine
Edwin Dunlop, M.D., Exec. Sec.
150 Emory St.
Attleboro, Mass. 02703

Academy of Religion and Mental Health
Rev. James R. MacColl, III, D.D.
Director, Professional Services
16 E. 34 St.
New York, N.Y. 10016

American Academy for Cerebral Palsy
Gerald Solomons, M.D., Sec.
University Hospital School
Iowa City, Iowa 52240

American Academy of Child Psychiatry
Joseph D. Noshpitz, M.D., Sec.
1700 18th St., N.W.
Washington, D.C. 20009

American Academy of Neurology
Stanley A. Nelson, Exec. Sec.
4005 W. 65th St.
Minneapolis, Minn. 55435

American Academy of Psychiatry and the Law
Jonas R. Rappeport, M.D., Pres.
3811 O'Hara St.
Pittsburgh, Pa. 15213

American Academy of Psychoanalysis
Eric D. Wittkower, M.D., Pres.
40 Gramercy Park North
New York, N.Y. 10010

American Anthropological Association
George M. Foster, Ph.D., Pres.
1703 New Hampshire Ave., N.W.
Washington, D.C. 20009

American Association of Community Clinic
and Center Psychiatrists
William McKnight, Pres.
P.O. Box 70
Livingston, N.J. 07039

American Association on Mental Deficiency
John J. Noone, Ed.D., Exec. Dir.
5201 Connecticut Ave., N.W.
Washington, D.C. 20015

American Association of Neuropathologists
S. M. Aronson, M.D., Sec.-Treas.
Dept. of Pathology, State University of N.Y.
Downstate Medical Center, 450 Clarkson
Ave.
Brooklyn, N.Y. 11203

American Association of Psychiatric Services
for Children
1701 Eighteenth St., N.W.
Washington, D.C. 20009

American Association of Suicidology
Avery Weisman, M.D., Pres.
Dept. of Psychiatry, Mass. General Hospital
Boston, Mass. 02114

American Board of Psychiatry and Neurology,
Inc.
Lester H. Rudy, M.D.
Executive Secretary-Treasurer
1603 Orrington Ave.
Evanston, Illinois 60201

American College of Psychiatrists
Melvin Sabshin, M.D., Sec.-Gen.
University of Illinois Medical Center
P.O. Box 6998
Chicago, Ill. 60680

American Group Psychotherapy Association
Emanual Hallowitz, Pres.
1790 Broadway, Rm. 702
New York, N.Y. 10019

American Hospital Association
840 N. Lake Shore Dr.
Chicago, Ill. 60611

American Medical Association
535 N. Dearborn St.
Chicago, Ill. 60610

American Medical Society on Alcoholism, Inc.
Frank A. Seixas, M.D., Sec.
2 Park Ave., Suite 1720
New York, N.Y. 10016

American Medical Women's Association Inc.
Josephine E. Renshaw, M.D., Pres.
1740 Broadway
New York, N.Y. 10019

American Neurological Association
Samuel A. Trufant, M.D., Sec.-Treas.
Cincinnati General Hosp.
Cincinnati, Ohio 45229

American Ontoanalytic Association
Jordan Scher, M.D., Exec. Sec.
520 N. Michigan Ave.
Chicago, Ill. 60611

American Orthopsychiatric Association
Marion F. Langer, Ph.D., Exec. Dir.
1790 Broadway
New York, N.Y. 10019

American Personnel and Guidance Association
Dr. Willis E. Dugan, Exec. Dir.
1607 New Hampshire Ave., N.W.
Washington, D.C. 20009

American Psychiatric Association
Walter E. Barton, M.D., Med. Dir.
1700 18th St., N.W.
Washington, D.C. 20009

American Psychoanalytic Association
Mrs. Helen Fischer, Exec. Sec.
One E. 57th St.
New York, N.Y. 10022

American Psychological Association
Kenneth B. Little, Ph.D., Exec. Officer
1200 17th St., N.W.
Washington, D.C. 20036

American Psychopathological Association
Max Fink, M.D., Sec.
5 E. 102nd St.
New York, N.Y. 10029

American Psychosomatic Society, Inc.
Joan K. Erpf, Exec. Ass't.
265 Nassau Rd.
Roosevelt, N.Y. 11575

American Society for Adolescent Psychiatry
Herman D. Staples, M.D., Sec.
24 Green Valley Rd.
Wallingford, Pa. 19086

American Sociological Association
N. J. Demerath III, Exec. Officer
1001 Connecticut Ave., N.W.
Washington, D.C. 20036

Association for the Advancement of Psychoanalysis
Arnoldo Apolito, M.D., Sec.
329 E. 62nd St.
New York, N.Y. 10021

Association of Medical Superintendents of
Mental Hospitals
Dean Brooks, M.D., Pres.
Oregon State Hospital
Salem, Ore. 97310

Association of Mental Health Administrators
Allen L. Dennis, Pres.
2901 Lafayette
Lansing, Mich. 48906

Association of Mental Health Chaplains
Father Douglas C. Turley, Jr., Pres.
18 Perimeter Park
Atlanta, Ga. 30341

Association for Research in Nervous and
Mental Disease
Rollo J. Masselink, M.D., Sec.-Treas.
710 W. 168th St.
New York, N.Y. 10032

British Medical Association
Miss B. W. Middlemiss, Exec. Officer
Tavistock Square
London, W.C. 1, England

Central Neuropsychiatric Association
David W. Sprague, M.D., Sec.-Treas.
1417 Marlowe Ave.
Lakewood, Ohio 44107

Child Study Association of America
James S. Ottenberg, Exec. Dir.
9 E. 89th St.
New York, N.Y. 10028

Child Welfare League of America, Inc.
Charles Faigin, Admin. Mgr.
44 E. 23rd St.
New York, N.Y. 10010

Eastern Psychiatric Research Association
Arthur Impastato, M.D., Sec. Treas.
Creedmore State Hospital
80-45 Winchester Blvd.
Queens Village, N.Y. 11427

Group for the Advancement of Psychiatry, Inc.
Jack A. Wolford, M.D., Sec.-Treas.
3811 O'Hara St.
Pittsburgh, Pa. 15213

Inter-American Council of Psychiatric Associations
R. J. Weil, M.D., Pres.
5770 South St.
Halifax, N.S., Canada

International Association for Child Phychiatry
and Allied Professions
Dr. S. Lebovici, Pres.
3, avenue du President Wilson
Paris 16e, 75, France

International Federation for Medical Psychotherapy
H. K. Fierz, M.D., Sec.-Gen.
Dolderstr. 107, CH-8032
Zurich, Switzerland

International Society for Social Psychiatry
Jules H. Masserman, M.D., Pres.
8 S. Michigan Ave.
Chicago, Ill. 60603

National Association of Private Psychiatric
Hospitals
Melvin Herman, Exec. Dir.
353 Broad Ave.
Leonia, N.J. 07605

National Association of Psychiatric Information
Specialists
    Joseph N. McCall, Pres.
    2810 Hopkins Ave.
    Lansing, Mich. 48912

National Association for Retarded Children
    Philip Roos, Ph.D., Exec. Dir.
    420 Lexington Ave.
    New York, N.Y. 10017

National Association of Social Workers
    Chauncey A. Alexander, Exec. Dir.
    2 Park Ave.
    New York, N.Y. 10016

National Association of State Mental Health
Program Directors
    Harry C. Schnibbe, Exec. Dir.
    Dodge Hotel, 20 E. St., N.W.
    Washington, D.C. 20001

National Committee Against Mental Illness
    Mr. Mike Gorman, Exec. Dir.
    1028 Connecticut Ave., N.W.
    Washington, D.C. 20036

National Council on Alcoholism
    Frank A. Seixas, M.D., Med. Dir.
    2 Park Ave.
    New York, N.Y. 10016

National Education Association
    Mr. George D. Fischer, Pres.
    1201 16th St., N.W.
    Washington, D.C. 20036

National Guild of Catholic Psychiatrists, Inc.
    Thomas L. Doyle, M.D., Pres.
    P.O. Box 56
    Watertown, Conn. 06795

National Institute of Mental Health
5454 Wisconsin Ave.
Chevy Chase, Md. 20015

National Medical Association, Inc.
P.O. Box 6562, T St. Sta.
Washington, D.C. 20009

Pan American Health Organization, WHO
Rene Gonzalez, M.D.
Regional Advisor in Mental Health
525 23rd St., N.W.
Washington, D.C. 20037

Pan American Medical Association, Inc.
Joseph J. Eller, M.D., Dir. Gen.
745 Fifth Ave.
New York, N.Y. 10022

Psychiatric Outpatient Centers of America
Richard W. Loring, Exec. Sec.
P.O. Box 1048
Oil City, Pa. 16301

Royal Medico-Psychological Association
A. B. Monro, M.D., Gen. Sec.
Chandos House, 2 Queen Anne St.
London, W. 1, England

Sigmund Freud Archives, Inc.
K. R. Eissler, M.D., Sec.
300 Central Park W.
New York, N.Y. 10024

Society for Adolescent Psychiatry
Mio Fredland, M.D., Sec.
215 E. 68th St.
New York, N.Y. 10021

Society for Biological Psychiatry
  Charles Shagass, M.D., Sec.-Treas.
  Eastern Pennsylvania Psychiatric Institute
  Henry & Abbotsford Rd.
  Philadelphia, Pa. 19129

Society of Medical Psychoanalysts
  Alexander Van Daele, M.D., Sec.
  215 E. 68th St.
  New York, N.Y. 10021

Southern Psychiatric Association
  William P. Wilson, M.D., Sec.-Treas.
  Duke University Medical Center
  Durham, N.C. 27706

U.S. Air Force
  Dept. of Psychiatry, U.S.A.F.
  Office of the Surgeon General
  Washington, D.C. 20333

U.S. Army
  Dept. of Psychiatry and Neurology
  Walter Reed General Hospital
  Washington, D.C. 20012

U.S. Navy
  Head, Neuropsychiatry Branch
  Bureau of Medicine and Surgery
  Washington, D.C. 20390

U.S. Public Health Service
  Surgeon General
  Dept. of Health, Education and Welfare
  Washington, D.C. 20201

Veterans Administration
  Psychiatry, Neurology & Psychology Service
  Dept. of Medicine and Surgery
  Washington, D.C. 20420

World Federation for Mental Health
George M. Carstairs, M.D., Pres.
Royal Edinburgh Hospital, Morningside
Park
Edinburgh, 10, Great Britain

World Health Organization
Boris Lebedev, M.D., Chief, Mental Health
Section
Via Appia, 1211
Geneva, Switzerland

World Medical Association, Inc.
Alberto Z. Romualdez, M.D., Sec.-Gen.
10 Columbus Circle
New York, N.Y. 10019

World Psychiatric Association
Denis Leigh, M.D., Sec. Gen.
Maudsley Hospital, Denmark Hill
London, S.E. 5, England

NATIONAL ASSOCIATION OF PRIVATE PSYCHIATRIC HOSPITALS

The following hospitals are members of the National Association of Private Psychiatric Hospitals. Addresses and phone numbers are listed here to aid the reader in making initial contact. Detailed information about each hospital (types of treatment available etc.) can be obtained directly from any of the hospitals or by contacting:

Executive Director
National Association of Private Psychiatric
Hospitals
353 Broad Avenue
Leonia, New Jersey 07605
201-944-4998

Roster of Member Hospitals (1972)

By Permission: Stuart Gould, M.D., President, National Association
of Private Psychiatric Hospitals.

ALABAMA

Hill Crest Hospital
700 5th Avenue So.
Birmingham, Ala. 35212 (205) 836-7201

ARIZONA

Camelback Hospital
5055 N. 34th Street
Phoenix, Ariz. 85018 (602) 955-6200

Palo Verde Hospital
801 S. Prudence Road
Tucson, Ariz. 85710 (602) 298-3363

CALIFORNIA

Alhambra Psychiatric Hospital
4619 N. Rosemead Blvd.
Rosemead, Cal. 91770 (213) 286-1149

Belmont Hills Psychiatric Center
1301 Ralston Ave. (P.O. Box 37)
Belmont, Cal. 94002 (415) 593-2143

Brea Hospital—Neuro-Psychiatric Center
875 No. Brea Boulevard
Brea, Cal. 92621 (714) 529-4963

Calabasas Hospital Neuropsychiatric Center
25100 Calabasas Road
Calabasas, Cal. 91302 (213) 888-7500

Charter Oak Psychiatric Hospital
19757 East Covina Boulevard
Covina, Cal. 91722 (213) 332-2023

Compton Foundation Hospital
820 West Compton Boulevard
Compton, Cal. 90220 (213) 636-1185

Edgemont Hospital
4841 Hollywood Blvd.
Los Angeles, Cal. 90027 (213) 666-5252

Gateways Hospital & Community Mental
Health Center
1891 Effie Street
Los Angeles, Cal. 90026 (213) 666-0171

Everett A. Gladman Memorial Hospital
2633 E. 27th Street
Oakland, Cal. 94601 (415) 536-9455

Glendale Adventist Hospital
Mental Health Unit
1509 Wilson Terrace
Glendale, Cal. 91206 (213) 244-4684

Ingleside Mental Health Center
7500 E. Hellman Ave. (Box 1098)
Rosemead, Cal. 91770 (213) 288-1160

Kern View Community Mental Health Center
and Hospital
3600 San Dimas Street
Bakersfield, Cal. 93301 (805) 327-7621

Kings View Hospital
42675 Road 44 (Box 631)
Reedley, Cal. 93654 (209) 638-2505

Las Encinas Hospital
2900 East Del Mar Blvd.
Pasadena, Cal. 91107 (213) 795-9901

Long Beach Neuropsychiatric Institute
6060 Paramount Blvd.
Long Beach, Cal. 90805 (213) 634-9102

Los Pinos
850 Congress Ave.
Pacific Grove, Cal. 93950 (408) 373-2141

Mesa Vista Hospital
7850 Vista Hill Ave.
San Diego, Cal. 92123 (714) 278-4110

Mission Terrace Hospital
225 30th St.
San Francisco, Cal. 94131 (415) 648-4140

Northside Psychiatric Hospital
1818 West Ashlan Ave.
Fresno, Cal. 93705 (209) 224-0870

Pomona Psychiatric Hospital
566 N. Gordon Street
Pomona, Cal. 91767 (714) 629-4011

Resthaven Psychiatric Hospital and Community Mental Health Center
765 College Street
Los Angeles, Cal. 90012 (213) 626-8241

Santa Ana Psychiatric Hospital
2212 E. 4th St.
Santa Ana, Cal. 92705 (714) 543-8481

Vista Hill Hospital
3 N. Second Ave.
Chula Vista, Cal. 92010 (714) 426-3300

Westwood Hospital
2112 S. Barrington Ave.
Los Angeles, Cal. 90025 (213) 479-4281

Woodview Hospital
6323 Woodman Ave.
Van Nuys, Cal. 91401 (213) 782-2470

COLORADO

Bethesda Hospital and Community Mental
Health Center
4400 E. Iliff Avenue
Denver, Colo. 80222 (303) 757-1231

Emory John Brady Hospital
401 Southgate Road (P.O. Box 640)
Colorado Springs, Colo. 80901 (303) 634-8828

Mount Airy Psychiatric Center
1205 Clermont Street
Denver, Colo. 80220 (303) 322-1803

CONNECTICUT

Elmcrest Psychiatric Institute
25 Marlborough Street
Portland, Conn. 06480 (203) 342-0480

Institute of Living
200 Retreat Avenue
Hartford, Conn. 06106 (203) 278-7950

Natchaug Hospital and Nursing Home
RFD #3
Willimantic, Conn. 06226 (203) 423-2514

Silver Hill Foundation
Valley Road (Box 1177)
New Canaan, Conn. 06840 (203) 966-3561

Yale Psychiatric Institute
333 Cedar Street
New Haven, Conn. 06510 (203) 436-4449

DISTRICT OF COLUMBIA

Psychiatric Institute of Washington, D.C.
2141 K. Street, N.W.
Washington, D.C. 20006 (202) 223-2700

FLORIDA

Anclote Psychiatric Center
Riverside Drive (Box 1224)
Tarpon Springs, Fla. 33589 (813) 937-4211

Coral Ridge Psychiatric Hospital
4545 North Federal Highway
Fort Lauderdale, Fla. 33308 (305) 771-2711

P. L. Dodge Memorial Hospital
1861 N.W. South River Drive
Miami, Fla. 33125 (305) 642-3555

Human Resource Institute of Miami
1660 N.W. 7th Court
Miami, Fla. 33136 (305) 371-5111

Lakeland Manor
2510 N. Florida Ave.
Lakeland, Fla. 33801 (813) 682-6105

GEORGIA

Bradley Center
2000 16th Ave.
Columbus, Ga. 31901 (404) 324-4882

Brawner Hospital
3180 Atlanta St., S.E.
Smyrna, Ga. 30080 (404) 435-4486

College Street Hospital
685 College Street
Macon, Ga. 31201 (912) 745-7944

Metropolitan Psychiatric Center
811 Juniper Street, N.E.
Atlanta, Ga. 30308 (404) 873-6151

Parkwood Hospital
1999 Cliff Valley Way, N.E.
Atlanta, Ga. 30329 (404) 633-8431

Peachtree Hospital
1999 Cliff Valley Way, N.E.
Atlanta, Ga. 30329 (404) 633-8431

ILLINOIS

Fairview Hospital
4840 N. Marine Dr.
Chicago, Ill. 60640 (312) 878-9700

Forest Hospital
555 Wilson Lane
Des Plaines, Ill. 60016 (312) 827-8811

Mercyville Institute of Mental Health
1330 North Lake Street
Aurora, Ill. 60506 (312) 859-2222

Riveredge Hospital
8311 W. Roosevelt Road
Forest Park, Ill. 60130 (312) 771-7000

INDIANA

Oaklawn Psychiatric Center
2600 Oakland
Elkhart, Ind. 46514 (219) 294-3551

Wabash Valley Hospital
2900 N. River Road
West Lafayette, Ind. 47906 (317) 463-2555

KANSAS

C. F. Menninger Memorial Hospital
3617 W. Sixth Ave. (Box 829)
Topeka, Kansas 66601 (913) 234-9566

Prairie View Mental Health Center
P.O. Box 467
Newton, Kans. 67114 (316) 283-2400

KENTUCKY

Our Lady of Peace Hospital
2020 Newburg Road
Louisville, Ky. 40205 (502) 451-3330

LOUISIANA

Brentwood Hospital
1800 Irving Place
Shreveport, La. 71101 (318) 424-6581

DePaul Hospital
1040 Calhoun St.
New Orleans, La. 70118 (504) 899-8282

River Oaks
1800 Jefferson Highway
New Orleans, La. 70121 (504) 835-2661

MAINE

Utterback Private Hospital
31 Kenduskeag Ave.
Bangor, Me. 04401 (207) 947-4555

MARYLAND

Brook Lane Psychiatric Center
P.O. Box 1945
Hagerstown, Md. 21740 (301) 733-0330

Chestnut Lodge
500 W. Montgomery Ave.
Rockville, Md. 20850 (301) 424-8300

Gundry Sanitarium
2 N. Wickham Rd.
Baltimore, Md. 21229 (301) 644-9917

Seton Psychiatric Institute
6400 Wabash Ave.
Baltimore, Md. 21215 (301) 764-2200

Sheppard & Enoch Pratt Hospital
Box 6815
Towson, Md. 21204 (301) 823-8200

Taylor Manor Hospital
College Avenue
Ellicott City, Md. 21043 (301) 465-3322

MASSACHUSETTS

Baldpate
Baldpate Road (Box 156)
Georgetown, Mass. 01830 (617) 352-2131

Bournewood Hospital
300 South Street
Brookline, Mass. 02167 (617) 469-0300

College Mental Health Center of Boston
4360 Prudential Center
Boston, Mass. 02199 (617) 262-3315

Fuller Memorial Sanitarium
231 Washington Street
So. Attleboro, Mass. 02703 (617) 761-8500

Glenside Hospital
49 Robinwood Ave.
Jamaica Plain, Mass. 02130 (617) 522-4400

Human Resource Institute of Boston
227 Babcock Street
Brookline, Mass. 02146 (617) 734-5930

McLean Hospital
115 Mill Street
Belmont, Mass. 02178 (617) 855-2000

Austen Riggs Center
Main Street
Stockbridge, Mass. 01262 (413) 298-5511

Valleyhead Hospital
South Street
Carlisle, Mass. 01741 (617) 369-2600

Westwood Lodge
45 Clapboardtree St.
Westwood, Mass. 02090 (617) 762-0168

Wiswall Hospital
203 Grove St.
Wellesley, Mass. 02181 (617) 235-8400

MICHIGAN

Glen Eden Hospital
6902 Chicago Road
Warren, Mich. 48092 (313) 264-8875

Mercywood Hospital
4038 Jackson Road
Ann Arbor, Mich. 48106 (313) 663-8571

Pine Rest Christian Hospital
6850 S. Division Ave.
Grand Rapids, Mich. 48508 (616) 534-4941

MISSOURI

Robinson Memorial Hospital
2625 West Paseo
Kansas City, Mo. 64108 (816) 421-0623

St. Vincent's Hospital (Division of DePaul
   Community Health Center)
7301 St. Charles Rock Road
St. Louis, Mo. 63133 (314) 726-2700

NEW JERSEY

Carrier Clinic
Belle Mead, N.J. 08502 (201) 359-3101

Christian Sanatorium
301 Sicomac Ave.
Wyckoff, N.J. 07481 (201) 427-2816

Fair Oaks Hospital
19 Prospect St.
Summit, N.J. 07901 (201) 277-0143

NEW MEXICO

Nazareth Hospital
501 Richfield Ave., N.E.
Albuquerque, N.M. 87113 (505) 898-1661

NEW YORK

Brunswick Hospital Center (Louden Hall)
81 Louden Avenue
Amityville, L.I., N.Y. 11701 (516) 264-5000

Craig House
Howland Ave.
Beacon, N.Y. 12508 (914) 831-1200

Falkirk Hospital
Central Valley, N.Y. 10917 (914) 928-2256

Four Winds
Cross River Rd.
Katonah, N.Y. 10536 (914) 763-3141

Gracie Square Hospital
420 E. 76th St.
New York, N.Y. 10021 (212) 988-4400

High Point Hospital
Upper King Street
Port Chester, N.Y. 10573 (914) 939-4420

Linwood-Bryant Hospital
237 Linwood Ave.
Buffalo, N.Y. 14209 (716) 886-8200

Long Island Jewish-Hillside Medical Center
Hillside Division
75-59 263 St.
Glen Oaks, N.Y. 11004 (212) 343-7800

Regent Hospital
115 E. 61st St.
New York, N.Y. 10021 (212) 838-7200

Rye Psychiatric Hospital Center
754 Boston Post Road
Rye, New York 19580 (914) 967-4567

South Oaks Hospital
(The Long Island Home, Ltd.)
Sunrise Highway
Amityville, L.I., N.Y. 11701 (516) 264-4000

Stony Lodge Hospital
Croton Dam Road (Box 591)
Ossining, N.Y. 10562 (914) 941-7400

Twin Elms Hospital
658 W. Onondaga St.
Syracuse, N.Y. 13204 (315) 478-0013

NORTH CAROLINA

Appalachian Hall
Caledonia Road
Asheville, N.C. 28803 (704) 253-5661

Highland Hospital
Division, Duke University Medical Center
Asheville, N.C. 28801 (704) 254-3201

OHIO

Cincinnati Mental Health Institute
(Emerson A. North Hospital)
5642 Hamilton Ave.
Cincinnati, Ohio 45224 (513) 541-0135

Dartmouth Behavioral Sciences Center
1038 Salem Ave.
Dayton, Ohio 45406 (513) 278-7917

Harding Hospital
445 E. Granville Rd.
Worthington, Ohio 43085 (614) 885-5381

Windsor Hospital
115 E. Summit St.
Chagrin Falls, Ohio 44022 (216) 247-5300

Woodruff Memorial Institute
1950 E. 89th St.
Cleveland, Ohio 44106 (216) 795-3700

OKLAHOMA

Coyne Campbell Hospital
2601 Spencer Road
Spencer, Okla. 73084 (405) 427-2441

PENNSYLVANIA

Devereux Foundation
Devon, Pa. 19335 (215) 687-3000

Elwyn Institute
Elwyn, Pa. 19063 (215) 566-8800

Eugenia Hospital
P.O. Box 4313
Philadelphia, Pa. 19118 (215) 247-4344

Fairmount Farm
561 Fairthorn Ave.
Philadelphia, Pa. 19128 (215) 483-0735

Friends Hospital
Roosevelt Blvd. & Adams Ave.
Philadelphia, Pa. 19124 (215) 289-5151

Institute of the Pennsylvania Hospital
111 No. 49th Street
Philadelphia, Pa. 19139 (215) 829-3000

Northwestern Mental Health Center
9801 Germantown Ave.
Philadelphia, Pa. 19118 (215) 247-1600

Philadelphia Psychiatric Center
Ford Rd. & Monument Ave.
Philadelphia, Pa. 19131 (215) 877-2000

Philhaven Hospital
Route 5, Box 345
Lebanon, Pa. 17042 (717) 273-8871

RHODE ISLAND

Emma Pendleton Bradley Hospital
1011 Veterans Memorial Parkway
Riverside, R.I. 02915 (401) 434-3400

Butler Hospital
333 Grotto Ave.
Providence, R.I. 02906 (401) 521-3400

TENNESSEE

Gartly-Ramsay Hospital
696 Jackson Ave.
Memphis, Tenn. 38105 (901) 526-7477

Tranquilaire Mental Health Center
2929 Brunswick Road
Memphis, Tenn. 38128 (901) 388-2723

TEXAS

Arlington Neuropsychiatric Center
701 W. Randol Mill Rd.
Arlington, Tex. 76012 (817) 277-4411

Beaumont Neurological Center
3250 Fannin
Beaumont, Tex. 77701 (713) 835-4921

Belhaven Hospital
6125 Hillcroft
Houston, Tex. 77036 (713) 774-7621

Beverly Hills Hospital
1353 N. Westmoreland Ave.
Dallas, Tex. 75211 (214) 331-8331

Brown Schools
Box 4008
Austin, Tex. 78765 (512) 444-9561

Killgore Children's Psychiatric Center and
   Hospital
1200 Wallace Blvd.
Amarillo, Tex. 79106 (806) 355-9191

Seaview Hospital
1316 Third St.
Corpus Christi, Tex. 78404 (512) 883-0931

Timberlawn Psychiatric Hospital
4600 Samuell Blvd. (Box 11288)
Dallas, Tex. 75223 (214) 381-7181

Villa Rosa
Unit, Santa Rosa Medical Center
5115 Medical Drive
San Antonio, Tex. 78229 (512) 228-2601

VERMONT

Brattleboro Retreat
75 Linden Street
Brattleboro, Vt. 05301 (802) 254-2331

VIRGINIA

Bayberry Psychiatric Hospital
530 E. Queen Street
Hampton, Va. 23369 (703) 722-2504

Saint Albans Psychiatric Hospital
P.O. Box 3608
Radford, Va. 24141 (703) 639-2481

Tidewater Psychiatric Institute
1005 Hampton Blvd.
Norfolk, Va. 23507 (703) 622-2341

Tucker Hospital
212 W. Franklin St.
Richmond, Va. 23220 (703) 648-4481

Westbrook Psychiatric Hospital
1500 Westbrook Ave.
Richmond, Va. 23227 (703) 266-9671

WASHINGTON

Columbia View Hospital
P.O. Box 2276
Vancouver, Wash. 98661 (206) 694-8408

Fairfax Hospital
10200 N.E. 132nd St.
Kirkland, Wash. 98033 (206) 822-6051

WISCONSIN

Milwaukee Psychiatric Hospital
1220 Dewey Avenue
Wauwatosa, Wisc. 53213 (414) 258-2600

Rogers Memorial Hospital
34810 Pabst Road
Oconomowoc, Wisc. 53066 (414) 567-5535

St. Croixdale Hospital
445 Court St. No.
Prescott, Wisc. 54021 (715) 262-3286

St. Mary's Hill Hospital
1445 S. 32nd Street
Milwaukee, Wisc. 53215 (414) 645-4336

PUERTO RICO

Hato Rey Psychiatric Hospital
Stop 31, Ponce de Leon Ave. (Box 789)
Hato Rey, P.R. 00919 (809) 766-0300

AMERICAN ASSOCIATION OF PSYCHIATRIC SERVICES FOR CHILDREN

The psychiatrist who wishes to refer a child for treatment may refer to the following list of institutions throughout the United States that offer such services. Membership in the American Association of Psychiatric Services For Children is on the basis of formal accreditation. Each member organization is certified to meet certain professional standards.

Types of treatment available vary, of course, from institution to institution. The interested psychiatrist may contact the member institution directly for specific information.

Many of the listed institutions are affiliated with established residency programs.

ALABAMA

BIRMINGHAM, 35233
Child Psychiatric Service
University of Alabama
School of Medicine
1919 7th Avenue South
(205) 934-4912

ARIZONA

SCOTTSDALE, 85251
Scottsdale Psychiatric
Center PC
3618 Civic Center Plaza
(602) 946-4225

TUCSON, 85719
Tucson Child Guidance
Clinic
1415 North Fremont
Avenue
(602) 622-4744

CALIFORNIA

COSTA MESA, 92627
Child Guidance Center of
Orange County
171 East 18th Street
(714) 646-7733

FRESNO, 93702
Fresno County Department
of Mental Health Child-
Adolescent Service
4441 East Kings Canyon
Road
(209) 488-3254

LONG BEACH, 90801
Psychiatric Clinic for
Children
2801 Atlantic Avenue
(213) 595-3151

LOS ANGELES, 90027
Division of Psychiatry
Children's Hospital of
Los Angeles
4650 Sunset Boulevard
(213) NO 3-3341, Ext. 681

LOS ANGELES, 90007
The Los Angeles Child
Guidance Clinic and Child
Development Center
746 West Adams Blvd.
(213) 749-4111

LOS ANGELES, 90007
School Guidance Center of
The Mental Health
Program
Los Angeles City Schools
322 West 21st Street
(213) 747-4265

LOS ANGELES, 90048
Thalians Clinic for
Children
Cedars-Sinai
Medical Center
Department of Child
Psychiatry
8720 Beverly Boulevard
(213) 652-5000, Ext. 314

ORANGE, 92668
Children's Psychiatric
Service at Orange County
Medical Center
101 South Manchester
(714) 633-9393

PASADENA, 91105
Pasadena Child Guidance
Clinic
56 Waverly Drive
(213) 795-8471

SACRAMENTO, 95814
Sacramento County Mental
Health Services
2315 Stockton Boulevard
(916) 454-5652

SAN DIEGO, 92123
Child Guidance Clinic
Children's Health Center
8001 Frost Street
(714) 278-0660

SAN FRANCISCO, 94129
Child Psychiatry Service
Letterman General
Hospital
Presidio of San Francisco
(415) 561-4949 or 4388

SAN FRANCISCO, 94115
Mount Zion Hospital
Department of Psychiatry
Children's Service
1600 Divisadero Street
(415) 567-1711

SANTA MONICA, 90404
Kennedy Child Study
Center
1339 20th Street
(213) 829-5465

SYLMAR, 91342
Children's Service
Olive View Community
Mental Health Center
(213) 367-2231

TORRANCE, 90509
Los Angeles County
Harbor General Hospital
Phychiatric Clinic for
Children
1000 West Carson Street
(213) 328-2380

VAN NUYS, 91405
San Fernando Valley
Child Guidance Clinic
7335 Van Nuys Boulevard
(213) 989-5230 or
873-5334

Whittier, 90606
Intercommunity Child
Guidance Center
8106 South Broadway
(213) 692-0383

COLORADO

DENVER, 80220
Department of Psychiatry
University of Colorado
Medical Center
Child Psychiatry Clinic
4200 East Ninth Avenue
(303) 394-7412

CONNECTICUT

BRIDGEPORT, 06604
Child Guidance Clinic of
Greater Bridgeport, Inc.
1081 Iranistan Avenue
(203) 367-5361

HARTFORD, 06112
Albany Avenue Child
Guidance Center
620 Albany Avenue
(203) 566-2433

HARTFORD, 06114
Children's Clinic
Institute of Living
17 Essex Street
(203) 278-7950

HARTFORD, 06105
The Hartley-Salmon Child
Guidance Clinic of Child
and Family Services of
Connecticut, Inc.
1680 Albany Avenue
(203) 236-4511

MANCHESTER, 06040
Community Child Guid-
ance Clinic, Inc.
317 North Main Street
(203) 643-2101

NEW HAVEN, 06510
Child Psychiatry Unit
Yale University
Child Study Center
333 Cedar Street
(203) 436-8220

NEW HAVEN, 06511
Clifford W. Beers
Guidance Clinic, Inc.
One State Street
(203) 772-1270

NORWALK, 06851
Mid-Fairfield Child
Guidance Center, Inc.
74 Newton Avenue
(203) 847-3891

STAMFORD, 06902
Child Guidance Clinic of
Greater Stamford, Inc.
103 West Broad Street
(203) 324-6127

WATERBURY, 06710
Child Guidance Clinic of
Waterbury, Inc.
52 Pine Street
(203) 756-7287

DELAWARE

WILMINGTON, 19802
Wilmington Child
Guidance Center, Inc.
2013 Baynard Boulevard
(302) 654-2414

DISTRICT OF
COLUMBIA

WASHINGTON, 20012
Child Guidance Service
Walter Reed General
Hospital
Forest Glen Section,
Box 301, Building No. 125
(202) 576-5421 thru 5424

WASHINGTON, 20007
Children's Psychiatric
Service
Georgetown University
Hospital
3800 Reservoir Road, N.W.
(202) 625-7351

WASHINGTON, 20009
Hillcrest Children's Center
Children's Hospital of the
District of Columbia
1325 W Street, N.W.
(202) 265-2400

FLORIDA

GAINESVILLE, 32601
  Children's Mental Health
  Unit
  Box 204
  J. Hillis Miller Health
  Center
  University of Florida
  (904) 392-3611

HOLLYWOOD, 33023
  Children's Division
  South Florida State
  Hospital
  1000 Southwest 84th Ave.
  (Post Office Box 4437)
  (305) 983-4321

MIAMI, 33136
  The Children's Psychiatric
  Center, Inc.
  901 N.W. 17th Street
  (305) 377-4036

TAMPA, 33610
  Guidance Center of
  Hillsborough County, Inc.
  5707 North 22nd Street
  (813) 237-3914

ILLINOIS

CHICAGO, 60616
  Child Psychiatry Clinic
  Michael Reese Hospital
  29th & Ellis Avenue
  (312) 791-3900

CHICAGO, 60624
  Department of Child
  Psychiatry
  Ridgeway Hospital
  520 North Ridgeway Ave.
  (312) 722-3113

CHICAGO, 60612
  Institute for Juvenile
  Research
  907 South Wolcott Avenue
  (312) 341-7355

CHICAGO, 60680
  University of Illinois
  Child Psychiatry Clinic
  912 South Wood Street
  Post Office Box 6998
  (312) 996-7721

LA GRANGE, 60525
  Community Family Service
  and Mental Health Center
  23 West Calendar Avenue
  (312) 354-0826

NORTHFIELD, 60093
  North Shore Mental
  Health Association &
  Irene Josselyn Clinic
  405 Central Avenue
  (312) 446-8910

INDIANA

FORT WAYNE, 46802
  Fort Wayne Child
  Guidance Center
  227 East Washington
  Boulevard
  (219) 422-4776

INDIANAPOLIS, 46202
  Child Psychiatry Services
  of Indiana University
  1100 West Michigan Street
  (317) 264-8162

IOWA

DES MOINES, 50309
  DesMoines Child
  Guidance Center
  1206 Pleasant Street
  (515) 244-2267

KANSAS

KANSAS CITY, 66103
  Division of Child
  Psychiatry
  University of Kansas
  Medical Center
  39th & Rainbow Boulevard
  (913) 236-5252, Ext. 431

TOPEKA, 66601
  Children's Division of the
  Menninger Foundation
  Box 829
  (913) 234-9566, Ext. 2676,
  2677

TOPEKA, 66606
  Children's Section
  Topeka State Hospital
  2700 West Sixth Street
  (913) 296-4531

KENTUCKY

LOUISVILLE, 40202
  Bingham Child Guidance
  Clinic
  601 South Floyd Street
  (502) 584-9701

LOUISVILLE, 40223
  Children's Treatment
  Services
  Central State Hospital
  (502) 245-4121, Ext.
  264–267

LOUISIANA

NEW ORLEANS, 70112
  The Morris Kirschman
  Clinic of Child Mental
  Health

Tulane Medical School
Department of Psychiatry
& Neurology
1430 Tulane Avenue
(504) 588-5401

MARYLAND

ROCKVILLE, 20852
  Child Guidance Clinic
  Jewish Social Service
  Agency
  6123 Montrose Road
  (301) 881-3700

TOWSON, 21204
  Department of Child
  Psychiatry
  Sheppard & Enoch Pratt
  Hospital
  (301) 823-2800, Ext. 321
  or 414

MASSACHUSETTS

BELMONT, 02178
  Beaverbrook Guidance
  Center
  115 Mill Street
  (617) 484-5240

BOSTON, 02118
  Department of Child
  Psychiatry
  Division of Psychiatry
  Boston University
  School of Medicine
  82 East Concord Street
  (617) 262-4200, Ext. 5655,
  5654

BOSTON, 02215
Child Psychiatry Unit
Beth Israel Hospital
330 Brookline Avenue
(617) 734-4400, Ext. 654

BOSTON, 02114
Child Psychiatry Unit
Massachusetts General
Hospital
(617) 726-2724

BOSTON, 02116
Douglas A. Thom Clinic
for Children
315 Dartmouth Street
(617) 266-1222

BOSTON, 02111
Judge Baker Guidance
Center
295 Longwood Avenue
(617) 232-8390

BOSTON, 02111
Psychiatric Services for
Children
Tufts-New England
Medical Center
171 Harrison Avenue
(617) 482-2800

BOSTON, 02115
Psychiatry Clinic
The Children's Hospital
Medical Center
300 Longwood Avenue
(617) 734-6000, Ext. 2081
or 2086

CAMBRIDGE, 02138
Cambridge Guidance
Center
5 Sacramento Street
(617) 354-2275

FRAMINGHAM, 01701
The Greater Framingham
Mental Health
Association, Inc.
88 Lincoln Street
(617) 872-6571

LEXINGTON, 02173
Mystic Valley
Mental Health Center
186 Bedford Street
(617) 861-0890

LYNN, 01902
Child Guidance Center
of Great Lynn
56 Baltimore Street
(617) 593-1088

MALDEN, 02148
Tri-City Mental Health
Center
Children's Service
15–21 Ferry Street
(617) 321-1060, 321-3100

NEWTON, 02158
Newton Mental Health
Center
64 Eldredge Street
(617) 969-4925

PITTSFIELD, 01201
The Berkshire Mental
Health Center
Children's Service
741 North Street
Warriner Building
(413) 499-0412

QUINCY, 02169
South Shore Mental
Health Center
77 Parking Way
(617) 471-0350

ROXBURY, 02121
Putnam Children's Center
244 Townsend Street
(617) 427-1715

SOUTH LAWRENCE,
01843
Greater Lawrence
Mental Health Center
581 Andover Street
(617) 683-3128

SPRINGFIELD, 01107
Child Guidance Clinic
of Springfield, Inc.
759 Chestnut Street
(413) 732-7419

WORCESTER, 01604
Worcester Youth
Guidance Center
275 Belmont Street
(617) 791-3261

MICHIGAN

ANN ARBOR, 48104
Children's Psychiatric
Hospital
University Medical Center
1275 North Hospital Drive
(313) 764-0231

DETROIT, 48201
Children's Center of
Wayne County
101 Alexandrine East
(313) 831-5535

SAGINAW, 48602
Saginaw Valley
Child Guidance Clinic
3253 Congress Street
(517) 793-4790

MINNESOTA

SAINT PAUL, 55104
Amherst H. Wilder
Department of Child
Guidance and
Development
919 Lafond Street
(612) 645-6661

MISSOURI

KANSAS CITY, 64108
Department of Child
Psychiatry
University of Missouri
at Kansas City
School of Medicine
600 East 22nd Street
(816) 471-3000

KANSAS CITY, 64112
Family and Child
Psychiatric Clinic
4643 Wyandotte, Suite 203
(816) WE 1-1318

KANSAS CITY, 64108
Section of Child Psychiatry
The Children's Mercy
Hospital
24th & Gillham Road
(816) 471-2026

ST. LOUIS, 63108
Washington University
Child Guidance &
Evaluation Clinic
369 North Taylor Avenue
(314) 361-6884

NEW HAMPSHIRE

CONCORD, 03301
Philbrook Center
for Children's Services
121 South Fruit Street
(603) 224-6531, Ext. 551

NEW JERSEY

EAST ORANGE, 07018
Family Service and
Child Guidance Center of
The Oranges, Maplewood
& Millburn
115 South Munn Avenue
(201) OR 5-3817

EATONTOWN, 07724
Children's Psychiatric
Center
59 Broad Street
(201) 542-2463

HACKENSACK, 07601
Hackensack Hospital
Community Mental Health
Center
66 Hospital Place
(201) 487-4000, Ext. 786-
7-8-9

MONTCLAIR, 07042
Montclair-West Essex
Guidance Center
60 South Fullerton Avenue
(201) 744-6522

MORRISTOWN, 07960
Morris County Guidance
Center
c/o Courthouse
(201) 285-6251

PLAINFIELD, 07060
Union County Psychiatric
Clinic
111 East Front Street
(201) 756-6870

TRENTON, 08618
The Child Guidance
Center of Mercer County
532 West State Street
(609) 695-8542

NEW YORK

ALBANY, 12210
Albany Child Guidance
Center
215 Lancaster Street
(518) 434-5105

BUFFALO, 14222
Child Guidance Clinic
Department of Child
Psychiatry
Buffalo Children's Hospital
219 Bryant Street
(716) 882-3510

BUFFALO, 14214
The Psychiatric Clinic, Inc.
Central Park Plaza
(716) 832-7390

HAWTHORNE, 10532
Hawthorne Cedar Knolls
School
Jewish Board of Guardians
226 Linda Avenue
(914) 769-2790

HAWTHORNE, 10532
Linden Hill School
500 Linda Avenue
(914) RO 9-3206

NIAGARA FALLS, 14301
The Martha H. Beeman
Foundation
Child Guidance Center
650 4th Street
(716) 282-2319

RHINEBECK, 12572
Astor Home for Children
and Astor Child Guidance
Clinic
36 Mill Street
(914) 876-4081
(914) 485-9703

ROCHESTER, 14621
Children and Youth
Division
Rochester Mental Health
Center, Inc.
1425 Portland Avenue
(716) 544-5220

ROCHESTER, 14623
Convalescent Hospital for
Children
2075 Scottsville Road
(716) 436-4442

ROCHESTER, 14620
Division of Child &
Adolescent Psychiatry
Department of Psychiatry
University of Rochester
Medical Center
260 Crittenden Boulevard
(716) 275-3521

SCHENECTADY, 12308
Schenectady County Child
Guidance Center, Inc.
821 Union Street
(518) 346-4296

SYRACUSE, 13202
Onondaga County
Child Guidance Center
423 West Onondaga Street
(315) 477-7261

WHITE PLAINS, 10605
The Center For
Preventive Psychiatry
340 Mamaroneck Avenue
(914) 949-7680

NEW YORK
METROPOLITAN AREA

BRONX, 10461
Child Psychiatry Division
Albert Einstein College of
Medicine & Bronx
Municipal Hospital Center
Pelham Parkway &
Eastchester Road
(212) 430-2264

BROOKLYN, 11201
Brooklyn Psychiatric
Centers, Inc.
189 Montague Street
(212) 875-7510

JAMAICA, 11432
Queens Child Guidance
Center, Inc.
88-29 161st Street
(212) 657-7100

MANHASSET, 11030
North Shore
Child Guidance Center
1495 Northern Boulevard
(516) 627-6671

NEW YORK, 10001
Bureau of Child Guidance
Board of Education
116 West 32nd Street
(212) 594-4720

NEW YORK, 10010
Catholic Charities
Guidance Institute
122 East 22nd Street
(212) OR 7-5000

NEW YORK, 10019
Child Development Center
of the Jewish Board
of Guardians
120 West 57th Street
(212) JU 2-9100

NEW YORK, 10016
Clinic for Children &
Adolescents
Postgraduate Center for
Mental Health
124 East 28th Street
(212) MU 9-7700

NEW YORK, 10019
Madeleine Borg
Child Guidance Institute
Jewish Board of Guardians
120 West 57th Street
(212) 582-9100

NEW YORK, 10026
Northside Center for
Child Development, Inc.
31 Central Park North
(212) 369-6464

STATEN ISLAND, 10301
Staten Island
Mental Health Society, Inc.
657 Castleton Avenue
(212) 442-2225

NORTH CAROLINA

BUTNER, 27509
Children's Psychiatric
Institute
Murdoch Center—
John Umstead Hospital
(919) 575-7768

CHAPEL HILL, 27514
Division of Child
Psychiatry
Department of Psychiatry
University of
North Carolina
School of Medicine
(919) 966-2025

Charlotte, 28211
Children's Division
Mecklenburg County
Mental Health Center
501 Billingsley Road
(704) 374-2023

DURHAM, 27710
Division of Child
Psychiatry
Durham Child Guidance
Clinic
Duke University Medical
Center
402 Trent Street
(919) 286-4456

RALEIGH, 27611
Child Psychiatry Service
Dorothea Dix Hospital
(919) 829-5344

WINSTON-SALEM, 27104
Child Guidance Clinic
of Forsyth County, Inc.
1200 Glade Street
(919) 723-3571

OHIO

AKRON, 44302
Akron Child Guidance
Center
312 Locust Street
(216) 762-0591

CINCINNATI, 45229
Child Psychiatry Division
Department of Psychiatry
University of Cincinnati
Central Psychiatric Clinic
Cincinnati General
Hospital
(513) 872-3346 (In Pt &
Day Care) 872-5803
(Out-Pt)

CLEVELAND, 44118
Bellefaire
22001 Fairmount
Boulevard
(216) 932-2800

CLEVELAND, 44106
Child Psychiatry Division
of University Hospitals
2026 Abington Road
(216) 791-7300

CLEVELAND, 44115
Child Guidance Center
2525 East 22nd Street
(216) 696-5800

COLUMBUS, 43205
Children's Mental Health
Center
721 Raymond Street
(614) 252-5286

COLUMBUS, 43222
Diocesan Child Guidance
Center, Inc.
840 West State Street
(614) 221-7855

DAYTON, 45419
Child Guidance Center for
Dayton & Montgomery
County
141 Firwood Drive
(513) 298-7301

YOUNGSTOWN, 44406
Child and Adult Mental
Health Center
1001 Covington Street
(216) 747-2601

OKLAHOMA

TULSA, 74105
Children's Medical Center
Psychiatric Clinic
4818 South Lewis
Post Office Box 7352
(918) 749-2281

PENNSYLVANIA

ABINGTON, 19001
Abington Hospital Mental
Health/Mental
Retardation Center
1200 Old York Road
(215) 885-4000 Ext. 413

ALLENTOWN, 18102
BETHLEHEM, 18018
Lehigh Valley Guidance
Clinic
1546 Walnut Street,
Allentown
(215) 434-4806
1103 West Broad Street,
Bethlehem
(215) 867-4163

LANCASTER, 17601
Lancaster Guidance Clinic
630 Janet Avenue
(717) 393-0421

MEDIA, 19063
Child Guidance & Mental
Health Clinics of Delaware
County
600 North Olive Street
(215) LO 6-5410

NORRISTOWN, 19401
Montgomery County
Mental Health Clinics, Inc.
1100 Powell Street
(215) 277-4600

PHILADELPHIA, 19133
Child Psychiatry Center at
St. Christopher's Hospital
2603 North Fifth Street
(215) GA 6-5600

PHILADELPHIA, 19107
Children & Adolescent
Services
Thomas Jefferson
University
1127 Walnut Street
(215) 829-6663

PHILADELPHIA, 19129
Children's Unit, E.P.P.I.
Child Psychiatry Division
Medical College of
Pennsylvania
Henry Avenue &
Abbottsford Road
(215) 848-6000

PHILADELPHIA, 19104
Children's & Adolescents'
Psychiatric Clinic
Philadelphia General
Hospital
34th Street & Civic Center
Boulevard
(215) BA 2-1836, Ext. 526

PHILADELPHIA, 19102
Hahnemann Medical
College and Hospital
The Charles Peberdy, Jr.
Child Psychiatry, Inc.
210 North Broad Street
(215) LO 4-5000, Ext. 632,
665

PHILADELPHIA, 19131
The Irving Schwartz
Institute for Children and
Youth
Ford Road & Monument
Avenue
(215) 877-2000

PHILADELPHIA, 19151
Lankenau Hospital
Child Guidance Clinic
City Line & Lancaster
Avenues
(215) MI 9-1400,
Ext. 424, 425

PHILADELPHIA, 19146
Philadelphia Child
Guidance Clinic
1700 Bainbridge Street
(215) KI 5-1836

PITTSBURGH, 15213
Pittsburgh Child Guidance
Center
201 De Soto Street
(412) 683-1825

PITTSBURGH, 15213
Psychiatric Clinic
Children's Hospital of
Pittsburgh
125 De Soto Street
(412) 681-7700

PITTSBURGH, 15234
South Hills
Child Guidance Center
300 Mt. Lebanon
Boulevard
Suite 217A
(412) 343-7166

READING, 19602
Family Guidance Center
57 South 6th Street
(215) 374-5147

WILKES-BARRE, 18702
The Children's Service
Center of Wyoming
Valley, Inc.
335 South Franklin Street
(717) 825-6425

RHODE ISLAND

PROVIDENCE, 02906
Providence Child
Guidance Clinic, Inc.
333 Grotto Avenue
(401) 274-2710

RIVERSIDE, 02915
Emma Pendleton Bradley
Hospital
1011 Veterans Memorial
Parkway
(401) 434-3400

SOUTH CAROLINA

COLUMBIA, 29202
William S. Hall
Psychiatric Institute
Child & Adolescent Service
Box 119
2100 Bull Street
(803) 256-9911, Ext. 778

TENNESSEE

NASHVILLE, 37232
Child Psychiatry Division
(Wills Center)
Department of Psychiatry
Vanderbilt University
Hospital
(615) 322-3463

TEXAS

AMARILLO, 79106
The Killgore Children's
Psychiatric Center and
Hospital, Inc.
Amarillo Medical Center
1200 Wallace Boulevard
(806) 355-9191

DALLAS, 75219
Dallas Child Guidance
Clinic
2101 Welborn
(214) LA 6-7945

EL PASO, 79902
El Paso Guidance Center
1501 North Mesa
(915) 542-1921

GALVESTON, 77550
Division of Child &
Adolescent Psychiatry
University of Texas
Medical Branch
1014 Texas Avenue
(713) SO 5-2417

HOUSTON, 77004
Children's Mental Health
Services of Houston
3214 Austin Street
(713) 522-5196

SAN ANTONIO, 78229
Community Guidance
Center of Bexar County
2135 Babcock Road
(512) 696-7070

UTAH

SALT LAKE CITY, 84103
Children's Psychiatric
Center of Primary
Children's Hospital
363 Twelfth Avenue
(801) 328-1611

SALT LAKE CITY, 84112
Division of Child &
Adolescent Psychiatry
University of Utah
College of Medicine
50 North Medical Drive
(801) 581-7951

VIRGINIA

CHARLOTTESVILLE,
22901
Division of Child &
Adolescent Psychiatry
Department of Psychiatry
University of Virginia
Medical Center
Box 202
(703) 924-2234

FALLS CHURCH, 22044
Fairfax-Falls Church
Mental Health Center
2949 Sleepy Hollow Road
(703) 532-4121

RICHMOND, 23219
Division of Child
Psychiatry
Virginia Treatment Center
for Children
Medical College of
Virginia
515 North 10th Street
(703) 770-3146

RICHMOND, 23220
Lor-Berg Family Guidance
Clinic
2330 Monument Avenue
(703) 355-7496

WISCONSIN

MADISON, 53706
Child Psychiatry Division
University of Wisconsin
Hospitals
427 Lorch Street
(608) 262-9602

MILWAUKEE, 53226
Milwaukee County
Child Psychiatry Clinic
8700 West Wisconsin
Avenue
Floor 8-D
(414) 258-2040

APPROVED RESIDENCIES IN PSYCHIATRY

Adapted from *Directory of Approved Internships and Residencies, 1972–1973*, with permission: American Medical Association

Residency programs in the following hospitals have been approved for three years of training by the Council on Medical Education and the American Board of Psychiatry and Neurology. Applicants intending to qualify for examination by the American Board of Psychiatry and Neurology should refer to the Board requirements that the candidate have had at least two of the three years of his training in a program or programs approved at the two or three-year level.

ALABAMA

Birmingham

University of Alabama Medical Center
University of Alabama Hospitals and
Clinics
619 S. 19th St. 35233

Veterans Administration
700 S. 19th St. 35233

ARIZONA

Phoenix

Arizona State
2500 E. Van Buren St. 85008

Good Samaritan
1033 E. McDowell Rd. 95006

Tucson

University of Arizona Affiliated Hospitals
University
1500 N. Campbell Ave. 85721

Palo Verde
801 S. Prudence Rd., Box 17509
85710

Veterans Administration
3601 South Sixth Ave. 85723

ARKANSAS

Little Rock

Arkansas State
4313 West Markham 72201

University of Arkansas Medical Center
University
4301 West Markham St. 72201

Veterans Administration Consolidated
(North Little Rock Division)
300 E. Roosevelt Rd. 72206

CALIFORNIA

Berkeley

Herrick Memorial
2001 Dwight Way 94704

Camarillo

Camarillo State
Box A 93010

Davis

University of California (Davis)
Affiliated Hospitals

Sacramento Medical Center
2315 Stockton Blvd. 95817

Imola

Napa State Hospital
94558
Napa State
Box A 94558

Loma Linda

Loma Linda University
11234 Anderson St. 92354

Long Beach

    Veterans Administration
    5901 E. 7th   90801

Los Angeles

    Cedars—Sinai Medical Center
    4833 Fountain Ave.   90029

    Cedars of Lebanon Hospital Division
    4833 Fountain Ave.   90029

    Mount Sinai Hospital Division
    8720 Beverly Blvd.   90048

    Los Angeles County—U.S.C. Medical
        Center
    1200 No. State St.   90033

    U.C.L.A.
    Center for the Health Sciences   90024

    Veterans Administration Center,
        Brentwood
    Wilshire & Sawtelle Blvds.,   90073

    Veterans Administration   (Sepulveda)
    16111 Plummer St.   91343

Martinez

    Veterans Administration
    150 Muir Rd.   94553

Norwalk

    Metropolitan State
    11400 St. Norwalk Blvd.   90650

Oakland

    Highland General
    2701 14th Ave.   94606

    Veterans Administration   (Martinez)
    150 Muir Rd.   94553

Orange

> University of California (Irvine)
> Affiliated Hospitals
>
> Orange County Medical Center
> 101 Manchester Ave. 92668

Palo Alto

> Veterans Administration
> 3801 Miranda Ave. 94304

Patton

Patton State
> 26802 Highland Ave. 92369

Sacramento

> Sacramento Medical Center
> 2315 Stockton Blvd., 95817

San Diego

> San Diego County Community Mental
> Health Services
> 345 W. Dickinson St., P.O. Box 3067
> 92103
>
> University of California at San Diego
> 225 W. Dickinson 92103
>
> University Hospital of San Diego County
> 225 W. Dickinson 92103

San Francisco

> Mount Zion Hospital and Medical Center
> 1600 Divisadero St. 94115
>
> Pacific Medical Center—Presbyterian
> Clay and Webster Sts. 94115
>
> St. Mary's Hospital and Medical Center
> 2200 Hayes St. 94117

San Francisco Community Mental Health
  Services
101 Grove St. 94102

University of California Program

Langley Porter Neuropsychiatric Institute
401 Parnassus Ave. 94122

Veterans Administration
4150 Clement St. 94121

San Jose

Agnews State
95114

San Mateo

San Mateo Community Mental Health
  Services
220 W. 20th Ave. 94402

Harold D. Chope Community
222 W. 39th Ave. 94403

Stanford

Stanford University Affiliated Hospitals

Stanford University
94305

Veterans Administration (Palo Alto)
3801 Miranda Ave. 94304

Stockton

Stockton State
510 E. Magnolia St. 95202

Sylmar

Olive View Medical Center
14445 Olive View Dr. 91342

Torrance

Los Angeles County Harbor General
1000 W. Carson St. 90509

COLORADO

Denver

Denver General
W. 6th Ave. and Cherokee St. 80204

Fort Logan Mental Health Center
3520 W. Oxford Ave. 80236

University of Colorado Affiliated Hospitals

University of Colorado Medical Center
4200 East 9th Ave. 80220

Veterans Administration
1055 Clermont St. 80220

Pueblo

Colorado State
1600 West 24th St. 81003

CONNECTICUT

Hartford

Institute of Living
400 Washington St. 06106

University of Connecticut Affiliated
Hospitals

University of Connecticut Hospital—
MC Cook Division
2 Holcomb St. 06112

Hartford
80 Seymour St. 06115

Veterans Administration (Newington)
555 Willard Ave. 06111

Middletown

Connecticut Valley
P.O. Box 351 06457

New Haven

Yale–New Haven Medical Center
Yale–New Haven
789 Howard Ave. 06504

Veterans Administration (West Haven)
West Spring St. 06516

Newington

Veterans Administration
555 Willard Ave. 06111

Newtown

Fairfield Hills
Box W 06470

Norwich

Norwich
Box 508 06360

West Haven

Veterans Administration
West Spring St. 06516

DELAWARE

New Castle

Delaware State
19720

DISTRICT OF COLUMBIA

Washington

Freedmen's
6th and Bryant Streets, N.W. 20001

Georgetown University
1800 Reservoir Rd. N.W. 20001

George Washington University
901 23rd Street, N.W. 20031

FLORIDA

Gainesville

University of Florida Affiliated Hospitals

William A. Shands Teaching Hospital and
Clinics
University of Florida 32601

Anclote Manor (Tarpon Springs)
P.O. Box 1224 33589

Veterans Administration
32601

Miami

University of Miami Affiliated Hospitals

Jackson Memorial
1700 N.W. 10th Ave. 33136

Veterans Administration
1201 N.W. 16th St. 33125

Tampa

University of South Florida Affiliated
Hospitals

Tampa General
Davis Islands 33606

St. Joseph's
3001 W. Buffalo Ave. 33607

Veterans' Administration
13000 N. 30th St. 33612

Tarpon Springs

Anclote Manor
P.O. Box 1224 33589

GEORGIA

Atlanta

Emory University Affiliated Hospitals
Emory University
1364 Clifton Rd., N.E. 30322

Grady Memorial
80 Butler St., S.E. 30303

Central State (Milledgeville)
P.O. Box 325 31062

Georgia Mental Health Institute
1256 Briarcliff Rd. N.E. 30306

Veterans Administration (Decatur)
1670 Clairmont Rd. 30033

Augusta

Medical College of Georgia Hospitals

Eugene Talmadge Memorial
1120 Fifteenth 30902

Veterans Administration
Wrightsboro Rd., 30904

Milledgeville

Central State
P.O. Box 325 31062

HAWAII

Honolulu

University of Hawaii Affiliated Hospitals

Hawaii State (Kaneohe)
Keaahala Rd. 96744

Leahi University of Hawaii
3675 Kilauea Ave. 96816

Queen's Medical Center
1301 Punchbowl St. 96813

Kaneohe

Hawaii State
Keaahala Rd. 96744

ILLINOIS

Chicago

Chicago Medical School Affiliated
Hospitals

Mount Sinai Hospital Medical Center of
Chicago
2755 West 15th St. 60608

Illinois State Psychiatric Institute
1601 West Taylor St. 60612

Chicago-Read Mental Health Center
6500 W. Irving Park Rd. 60634

Michael Reese Hospital and Medical
Center
2929 South Ellis Ave. 60616

Northwestern University Medical Center
Cook County

Chicago Wesley Memorial
250 East Superior St. 60611

Passavant Memorial
303 E. Superior St. 60611

Veterans Administration Research
333 E. Huron St. 60611

Veterans Administration (Downey)
60064

Evanston (Evanston)
2650 Ridge Ave. 60201

Presbyterian—St. Luke's
1753 W. Congress Pkwy. 60612

University of Chicago Hospitals and
Clinics
950 East 59th St. 60637

University of Illinois Hospital
840 S. Wood St. 60612

Veterans Administration (West Side)
820 S. Damen Ave. 60612

Downey

Veterans Administration
60064

Evanston

Evanston
2650 Ridge Ave. 60201

Hines

Madden Mental Health Center
1200 S. First Ave. 60141

Veterans Administration
5th Ave. & Roosevelt Rd. 60141

Maywood

Loyola University Affiliated Hospitals

Loyola University
2160 S. 1st Ave. 60153

Madden Mental Health Center (Hines)
1200 S. First Ave. 60141

Veterans Administration (Hines)
5th Ave. & Roosevelt Rd. 60141

INDIANA

Indianapolis

Indiana University Medical Center

Indiana University Hospitals
1100 West Michigan 46207

Larue C. Carter Memorial
1315 West Tenth St. 46202

Marion County General
960 Locke St. 46202

Veterans Administration
1481 West Tenth St. 46202

IOWA

Cherokee

Mental Health Institute
1200 W. Cedar St. 51012

Independence

Mental Health Institute
50644

Iowa City

State Psychopathic
500 Newton Rd. 52240

KANSAS

Kansas City

University of Kansas Medical Center
39th & Rainbow Blvd. 66103

Veterans Administration (Kansas City, Mo.)
4801 Linwood Blvd. 64128

Topeka

Menninger School of Psychiatry
C.F. Menninger Memorial
3617 W. 6th St., Box 829 66601

Topeka State
2700 West Sixth 66606

Veterans Administration
2200 Gage Blvd. 66622

KENTUCKY

Lexington

University of Kentucky Medical Center
University
800 Rose St. 40506

Veterans Administration
Leestown Pike 40507

Louisville

University of Louisville Affiliated
Hospitals

Central State
40223

John K. Norton Memorial Infirmary
231 West Oak St. 40203

Bingham Child Guidance Clinic
601 S. Floyd St. 40202

Louisville General
323 E. Chestnut St. 40202

Veterans Administration
Mellwood & Zorn Ave. 40202

LOUISIANA

Mandeville

Southeast Louisiana
P.O. Box 3850 70448

New Orleans

> Charity Hospital of Louisiana
>   State University Division
>   1532 Tulane Ave., 70140
>
> Tulane University Affiliated Hospitals
>
> Charity Hospital of Louisiana
>   1532 Tulane Ave. 70140
>
> Veterans Administration
>   1601 Perdido St. 70140
>
> Southeast Louisiana (Mandeville)
>   P.O. Box 3850 70448

Shreveport

> Confederate Memorial Medical Center
>   1541 Kings Highway 71103

MAINE

Portland

> Maine Medical Center
>   22 Bramhall St. 04102

MARYLAND

Baltimore

> Johns Hopkins
>   601 North Broadway 21205
>
> Seton Psychiatric Institute
>   6400 Wabash Ave. 21215
>
> Spring Grove State
>   Wade Ave. 21228
>
> University of Maryland
>   22 S. Greene St. 21201

Crownsville

> Crownsville State
>   21032

Perry Point

Veterans Administration
21902

Sykesville

Springfield State
21784

Towson

Sheppard and Enoch Pratt
York Rd. 21204

MASSACHUSETTS

Belmont

McLean
115 Mill St. 02178

Boston

Beth Israel
330 Brookline Ave. 02215

Boston City
818 Harrison Ave. 02118

Boston State
591 Morton St. 02124

Massachusetts General
Fruit St. 02114

Massachusetts Mental Health Center
74 Fenwood Rd. 02115

New England Medical Center Hospitals
171 Harrison Ave. 02111

University
750 Harrison Ave. 02118

Veterans Administration Hospitals of the
Boston Area

Veterans Administration (Jamaica Plain)
150 S. Huntington Ave. 02130

Cambridge

Cambridge
1493 Cambridge St. 02139

Harding

Medfield State
Hospital Rd. 02042

Hathorne

Danvers State
Box 50 01935

Taunton

Taunton State
Hodges Ave. Ext. 02780

Waltham

Metropolitan State
475 Trapelo Rd. 02154

Worcester

Worcester State
305 Belmont St. 01604

MICHIGAN

Ann Arbor

University of Michigan Affiliated
Hospitals

University
1405 East Ann St. 48104

Veterans Administration
2215 Fuller Rd. 48105

Detroit

Detroit Psychiatric Institute
1151 Taylor 48202

Henry Ford

2799 W. Grand Blvd. 48202

Lafayette Clinic
951 E. Lafayette 48207

Sinai Hospital of Detroit
6767 West Outer Dr. 48235

East Lansing

Michigan State University Affiliated
Hospitals

Michigan State University Health Center
48823

Genesee County Community Mental
Health Services (Flint)
432 N. Saginaw 48503

St. Lawrence Community Mental Health
Center (Lansing)
1201 Oakland 48914

Oakland Medical Center (Pontiac)
140 Elizabeth Lake Rd. 48053

Eloise

Wayne County General
48132

Flint

Genesee County Community Mental
Health Services
432 N. Saginaw 48503

Lansing

> St. Lawrence Community Mental Health
> Center
> 1201 Oakland 48914

Northville

> Northville State
> 41001 West Seven Mile 48167

Pontiac

> Oakland Medical Center
> 140 Elizabeth Lake Rd. 48053

Traverse City

> Traverse City State
> Elmwood & 11th 49684

Ypsilanti

> Ypsilanti State
> 3501 Willis Rd. 48197

MINNESOTA

Minneapolis

> University of Minnesota Affiliated
> Hospitals
>
> University of Minnesota Hospitals
> 412 Union Street, S.E. 55455
>
> Hennepin County General
> Fifth and Portland South 55415
>
> St. Paul-Ramsey (St. Paul)
> 640 Jackson St. 55101
>
> Veterans Administration
> 54th St. & 48th Ave., So. 55417

Rochester

Mayo Graduate School of Medicine
200 First Ave., S.W. 55901

Rochester Methodist
201 West Center St. 55901

St. Mary's
1216 Second St., S.W. 55901

St. Paul

St. Paul-Ramsey
640 Jackson St. 55101

MISSISSIPPI

Biloxi

Veterans Administration Center
39531

Jackson

University of Mississippi Medical Center

University
2500 North State St. 39216

Veterans Administration Center
1500 E. Woodrow Wilson Dr. 39216

Mississippi State (Whitfield)
39193

Whitfield

Whitfield State
39193

MISSOURI

Columbia

University of Missouri Medical Center
807 Stadium Rd. 65201

Kansas City

University of Missouri Residency in
Psychiatry

Kansas City General Hospital and Medical
Center
24th and Cherry 64108

Western Missouri Mental Health Center
600 E. 22nd St. 64108

Veterans Administration
4801 Linwood Blvd. 64128

St. Louis

Jewish Hospital of St. Louis
216 St. Kingshighway 63110

Malcolm Bliss Mental Health Center
1420 Grattan St. 63104

Missouri Institute of Psychiatry—
St. Louis State
5400 Arsenal St. 63139

St. Louis University Group of Hospitals
1402 S. Grand Blvd. 63104

Cardinal Glennon Memorial Hospital for
Children
1465 S. Grand Blvd. 63104

David P. Wohl Memorial Mental Health
Institute
1325 S. Grand Blvd. 63104

Firmin Desloge General
1402 S. Grand Blvd. 63104

Veterans Administration
915 No. Grand Blvd. 63106

Washington University Affiliated Hospitals

Barnes Hospital Group
Barnes Hospital Plaza 63110

NEBRASKA

Omaha

> University of Nebraska Affiliated Hospitals
>
> Nebraska Psychiatric Institute
> 602 South 44th Ave. 68105
>
> Veterans Administration
> 4101 Woolworth Ave. 68105

NEW HAMPSHIRE

Hanover

> Dartmouth Medical School Affiliated
> Hospitals
>
> Mary Hitchcock Memorial
> 2 Maynard 03755

NEW JERSEY

Cedar Grove

> Essex County Hospital Center
> 1 Fairview Ave. 07009

Greystone Park

> Greystone Park Psychiatric
> 07950

Hammonton

> Ancora Psychiatric
> P.O. Ancora Branch 08037

Long Beach

> Monmouth Medical Center
> 3rd & Pavilion Avenues 07740

Flemington

> Hunterdon Medical Center
> Route 31 08822

Hackensack

Hackensack
22 Hospital Pl. 07601

Paramus

Bergen Pines County
East Ridgewood Ave. 07652

Piscataway

CMDNJ-Rutgers Medical School Affiliated
Hospitals

Rutgers Psychiatric Institute
Hoes Lane, University Heights
08854

Hunterdon Medical Center (Flemington)
Route 31 08822

Marlboro

Marlboro Psychiatric
07746

Newark

New Jersey College of Medicine Affiliated
Hospitals

Martland
65 Bergen St. 07107

Princeton

New Jersey Neuropsychiatric Institute
Box 1000 08540

Trenton

Trenton Psychiatric
Station A. 08625

NEW MEXICO

Albuquerque

University of New Mexico Affiliated
Hospitals

Bernalillo County Medical Center
2211 Lomas Blvd. N.E. 87106

Veterans Administration
2100 Ridgecrest Dr. S.E. 87108

NEW YORK

Albany

Albany Medical Center Affiliated
Hospitals

Albany Medical Center
New Scotland Ave. 12208

Veterans Administration
113 Holland Ave. 12208

Binghamton

Binghamton State
425 Robinson St. 13901

Buffalo

Buffalo State
400 Forest Ave. 14213

S.U.N.Y. at Buffalo Affiliated Hospitals

Edward J. Meyer Memorial
462 Grider St. 14215

Central Islip

Central Islip State
Carleton Ave. 11722

Cooperstown

Mary Imogene Bassett
Atwell Rd. 13326

East Meadow

> Nassau County Medical Center—
> Meadowbrook Div.
> P.O. Box 175 11554

Harrison

> St. Vincent's Hospital and Med. Center of
> New York, Westchester Branch
> 240 North St. 10528

Kings Park

> Kings Park State
> Box A 11754

Marcy

> Marcy State
> Box 100 13403

Middletown

> Middletown State
> 141 Monhagen Ave. 10940

New Hyde Park

> Long Island Jewish-Hillside Medical
> Center Program

> Hillside Hospital Division (New York)
> 75-59 263rd St., Glen Oaks 11004

> Queens Hospital Center (New York City)
> 82-68 164th St., Jamaica 11432

New York City

> Albert Einstein College of Medicine
> Affiliated Hospitals

> Bronx Municipal Hospital Center
> Pelham Pkwy. S. & Eastchester Rd.
> 10461

Bronx State
1500 Waters Pl., Bronx 10461

Lincoln
320 Concord Ave., Bronx 10454

Hospital of the Albert Einstein College of
    Medicine
1825 Eastchester Rd., Bronx 10461

Beth Israel Medical Center
10 Nathan D. Perlman Pl. 10003

Brookdale Hospital Center
    Linden Blvd. & Rockaway Pkwy.,
    Brooklyn 11212

Brooklyn State
681 Clarkson Ave., Brooklyn 11203

Catholic Medical Center of South Shore—
    Rockaway Mental Health Center
1600 Central Ave., Far Rockaway 11691

Columbia University Affiliated Hospitals

New York State Psychiatric Institute
722 W. 168th St. 10032

Presbyterian
622 West 168th St. 10032

Mary Imogene Bassett (Cooperstown)
    Atwell Rd. 13326

Creedmoor State
    80-45 Winchester Blvd., Queens Village
    11427

Harlem Hospital Center
532 Lenox Ave. 10037

Hillside Hospital Training Program

Hillside
75-59 263rd St., Glen Oaks 11004

Queens Hospital Center
    82-68 164th St., Jamaica 11432

Maimonides Medical Center
4802 Tenth Ave., Brooklyn 11219

Meyer-Manhattan Psychiatric
Ward's Island 10035

Montefiore Hospital and Medical Center
111 E. 210th St., Bronx 10467

Mount Sinai Hospital Training Program

Mount Sinai
11 East 100th St. 10029

City Hospital Center at Elmhurst
79-01 Broadway, Elmhurst 11373

New York (Payne Whitney Psychiatric
Clinic)
525 East 68th St. 10021

New York Medical College—Metropolitan
Hospital Center
1 East 105th St. 10029

Unit 1—Flower and Fifth Avenue
Hospitals

Unit 2—Metropolitan

New York University Medical Center
550 First Ave. 10014

University
550 First Ave. 10014

Bellevue Hospital Center
First Ave. & 27th St. 10016

Queens Hospital Center
82-68 164th St., Jamaica 11432

Staten Island Mntl. Hlth. Society—
St. Vincent's Med. Ctr. of Richmond

Staten Island Mental Health Society
657 Castleton Ave., Staten Island 10301

St. Vincent's Medical Center of Richmond
355 Bard Ave., Staten Island 10310

Roosevelt
428 W. 59th St. 10019

St. Luke's Hospital Center
Amsterdam Ave. & 114th St. 10025

St. Vincent's Hospital and Medical Center
of New York
153 West 11 St. 10011

St. Vincent's Hsp. & M.C. of New York,
Westchester Br. (Harrison)
240 North St. 10528

State University—Kings County Hospital
Center

Kings County Hospital Center
451 Clarkson Ave., Brooklyn 11203

State University
445 Lenox Road, Brooklyn 11213

Veterans Administration (Bronx)
130 W. Kingsbridge Rd., Bronx 10468

Veterans Administration (Manhattan)
First Ave. at E. 24th St. 10010

Ogdensburg

St. Lawrence State
Station A 13669

Pomona

Rockland County Comm. Mental Health
Center
10970

Orangeburg

Rockland State
10962

Poughkeepsie

    Hudson River State
    Branch B 12601

Rochester

    Rochester General
    1425 Portland Ave. 14621

    Rochester State
    1600 South Ave. 14620

    Strong Memorial Hospital of the
    University of Rochester
    260 Crittenden Blvd. 14642

Syracuse

    S.U.N.Y. Upstate Medical Center
    766 Irving Ave. 13210

    State University
    750 E. Adams St. 13210

    Syracuse Psychiatric
    708 Irving Ave. 13210

    Veterans Administration
    Irving Ave. and Univ. Pl. 13210

Utica

    Utica State
    1213 Court St. 13502

Valhalla

    Grasslands
    10595

West Brentwood

    Pilgrim State
    Box A 11717

White Plains

New York Hospital—Cornell Medical
Center (Westchester Div.)
21 Bloomingdale Rd. 10605

NORTH CAROLINA

Butner
John Umstead
12th St. 27509

Chapel Hill

North Carolina Memorial
Pittsboro Rd. 27514

Durham

Duke University Affiliated Hospitals

Duke University Medical Center
27706

Veterans Administration
508 Fulton St. 27705

Raleigh

Dorotha Dix
Station B 27611

Winston-Salem

North Carolina Baptist
300 S. Hawthorne Rd. 27103

OHIO

Cincinnati

Rollman Psychiatric Institute
3009 Burnet Ave. 45219

University of Cincinnati Hospital Group

Cincinnati General
3231 Burnet Ave 45229

Veterans Administration
3200 Vine St. 45220

Cleveland

Cleveland Clinic
2020 E. 93rd St. 44106

Cleveland Psychiatric Institute
1708 Aiken Ave. 44109

Fairhill Mental Health Center
12200 Fairhill Rd. 44120

University Hospitals of Cleveland
2065 Adelbert Rd. 44106

Veterans Administration
10701 East Blvd. 44106

Columbus

Columbus State
1960 W. Broad St. 43223

Ohio State University Hospitals
410 W. 10th Ave. 43210

Cuyahoga Falls

Fallsview Mental Health Center
330 Broadway East 44222

Toledo

Medical College of Ohio at Toledo
Affiliated Hospitals
P.O. Box 6190 43614

St. Vincent Hospital and Medical Center
2213 Cherry St. 43608

Toledo Mental Health Center
930 S. Detroit Ave. 43603

Worthington

    Harding
    445 E. Granville Rd. 43085

OKLAHOMA

Norman

    Central State Griffin Memorial
    Box 151 73069

Oklahoma City

    University of Oklahoma Medical Center

    University of Oklahoma Hospitals
    800 Northeast 13th 73104

    Veterans Administration
    921 N.E. 13th St. 73104

OREGON

Portland

    University of Oregon Affiliated
        Hospitals

    University of Oregon Medical School
        Hospitals and Clinics
    3181 S.W. San Jackson Park 97201

Salem

    Oregon State
    Station A 97310

PENNSYLVANIA

Bridgeville

    Mayview State
    15017

Coatesville

Veterans Admin.
19320

Norristown

Norristown State
Stanbridge & Sterigere Sts. 19401

Philadelphia

Albert Einstein Medical Center
York & Tabor Rds. 19141

Eastern Pennsylvania Psychiatric Institute
Henry Ave. & Abbotsford Rd. 19129

Hahnemann Medical College and
Hospital
230 N. Broad St. 19102

Hospital of the Medical College of
Pennsylvania
3300 Henry Ave. 19129

Hospital of the University of
Pennsylvania
3400 Spruce St. 19104

Institute of the Pennsylvania Hospital
111 N. 49th St. 19139

Philadelphia General
Civic Center Blvd. at 34th St. 19104

Philadelphia Psychiatric Center
Ford Rd. & Monument Ave. 19131

Philadelphia State
Roosevelt Blvd. & Southampton Rd.
19114

Temple University
3401 N. Broad St. 19140

Thomas Jefferson University
11th & Walnut Sts. 19107

Pittsburgh

Hospitals of the University Health
Center of Pittsburgh
3550 Terrace St. 15213

Western Psychiatric Institute and Clinic
3550 Terrace St. 15213

Warren

Warren State
Jamestown Rd. 16365

PUERTO RICO

Bayamon

Puerto Rico Institute of Psychiatry
P.O. Box 127 00619

San Juan

University of Puerto Rico School of
Medicine (Department of Psychiatry)
Puerto Rico Medical Center 00935

Veterans Admin. Center
G.P.O. Box 4867 00936

RHODE ISLAND

Howard

Rhode Island Medical Center—Institute
of Mental Health
Box 5 02834

SOUTH CAROLINA

Charleston

Medical University of South Carolina
Teaching Hospitals

Medical University of South Carolina
80 Barre St. 29401

Veterans Admin.
109 Bee St. 29403

Columbia

William S. Fall Psychiatric Institute
2100 Bull St. 29202

TENNESSEE

Memphis

University of Tennessee Affiliated
Hospitals

City of Memphis Hospitals
860 Madison Ave. 38103

Tennessee Psychiatric Hospital and
Institute
865 Poplar Ave. 38105

Veterans Administration
1030 Jefferson Ave. 38104

Nashville

George W. Hubbard Hospital of the
Mebarry Medical College
1005 18th Ave. N. 37208

Vanderbilt University Affiliated Hospitals

Vanderbilt University
1161 21st Ave., South 37203

Veterans Admin.
1310 24th Ave., South 37203

TEXAS

Austin
Austin State
4110 Guadalupe 78751

Dallas

Timberlawn Psychiatric
4600 Samuell Blvd. 75223

University of Texas Southwestern
Medical School Affiliated Hospitals
5323 Harry Hines Blvd. 75235

Parkland Memorial
5201 Harry Hines Blvd. 75235

Presbyterian Hospital of Dallas
8200 Walnut Hill Ln. 75231

Veterans Admin.
4500 S. Lancaster 75216

Terrell State (Terrell)
Box 70 75160

Galveston

Univeristy of Texas Medical Branch
Hospitals
8th & Mechanic Sts. 77550

Houston

Baylor College Affiliated Hospitals

Ben Taub General
1502 Taub Loop 77025

Methodist
6516 Bertner 77025

Texas Research Institute of Mental
Sciences
1300 Moursund Ave. 77025

Veterans Administration
2002 Holcombe Blvd. 77031

San Antonio

University of Texas at San Antonio
Teaching Hospitals

Bexar County Teaching
4502 Medical Dr. 78229

Temple

Scott and White Memorial
2401 S. 31st St. 76501

Terrell

Terrell State
Box 70 75160

UTAH

Provo

Utah State
1500 East Center 84601

Salt Lake City

University of Utah Affiliated Hospitals

University
50 North Medical Dr. 84112

Veterans Administration
500 Foothill Dr. 84113

Utah State (Provo)
1500 East Center 84601

VERMONT

Burlington

Medical Center Hospital of Vermont
Colchester Ave. 05401

VIRGINIA

Charlottesville

University of Virginia
Jefferson Park Ave. 22903

Falls Church

> Northern Virginia Mental Health
> Institute
> 3302 Gallows Rd. 22048

Petersburg

> Central State
> Box 271 23803

Richmond

> Virginia Commonwealth University
>
> M.C.V. Affiliated Hospitals
> 1200 E. Broad St. 23219
>
> Medical College of Virginia Hospitals
> 1200 E. Broad St. 23219

Williamsburg

> Eastern State
> Drawer A 23185

WASHINGTON

Fort Steilacoom

> Western State
> 98494

Seattle

> University of Washington Affiliated
> Hospitals
>
> Harborview Medical Center
> 325 Ninth Ave. 98104
>
> University
> 1959 N.E. Pacific St. 98105
>
> Veterans Administration
> 4435 Beacon Ave. S. 98108

Sedro Woolley

> Northern State
> Box 309 98284

WEST VIRGINIA

Morgantown

> West Virginia University Medical Center
> Medical Center 26506

WISCONSIN

Madison

> University of Wisconsin Affiliated
> Hospitals
>
> University Hospitals
> 1300 University Ave. 53706
>
> Mendota State
> 301 Troy Dr. 53704

Milwaukee

> Medical College of Wisconsin Affiliated
> Hospitals
>
> Milwaukee Psychiatric (Wauwatosa)
> 1220 Dewey Ave. 53213
>
> Milwaukee Children's
> 1700 W. Wisconsin Ave. 53233
>
> Milwaukee County Mental Health Center
> 9191 Watertown Plank Rd. 53226
>
> Veterans Administration Center (Wood)
> 5000 W. National Ave. 53193

Wauwatosa

> Milwaukee Psychiatric
> 1220 Dewey Ave. 53213

Winnebago

Winnebago State
54985

UNITED STATES AIR FORCE

Texas

Wilford Hall U.S.A.F. Medical Center,
San Antonio

UNITED STATES ARMY

California

Letterman General, San Francisco

District of Columbia

Walter Reed General, Washington

UNITED STATES NAVY

California

Naval, Oakland

Maryland

Naval, Bethesda

Pennsylvania

Naval, Philadelphia

DEPARTMENT OF HEALTH, EDUCATION, AND WELFARE

District of Columbia

St. Elizabeths, Washington

APPROVED RESIDENCIES IN CHILD PSYCHIATRY

(Adapted from *Directory of Approved Internships and Residencies, 1972–1973,*
with permission: American Medical Association)

ALABAMA

Birmingham

University of Alabama Hospitals and
Clinics
619 S. 19th St. 35233

CALIFORNIA

Berkeley

City of Berkeley Mental Health Services
2515 Milvia St. 94704

Camarillo

Camarillo State
Box A 93010

Davis

University of California (Davis)
Affiliated Hospitals

Sacramento Medical Center (Sacramento)
2315 Stockton Blvd. 95817

Imola

Napa State
Box A 94558

Irvine

University of California (Irvine) Affiliated
Hospitals

Orange County Medical Center (Orange)
101 Manchester Ave. 92668

Los Angeles

Cedars-Sinai Medical Center

Mount Sinai Hospital Division
8720 Beverly Blvd. 90048

Los Angeles County—U.S.C. Medical
Center
1200 No. State St. 90033

Reiss-Davis Child Study Center
9760 West Pico Blvd. 90035

U.C.L.A.
Center for the Health Sciences 90024

Orange

Orange County Medical Center
101 Manchester Ave. 92668

Pasadena

Pasadena Child Guidance Clinic
56 Waverly Dr. 91105

Sacramento

Sacramento Medical Center
2315 Stockton Blvd. 95817

San Diego

Community Mental Health Services
of San Diego County

Child Guidance Clinic
8001 Frost St. 92123

San Francisco

Children's Hospital and Adult Medical
Center
3700 California St. 94119

Mount Zion Hospital and Medical
Center
1500 Divisadero St. 94115

St. Mary's Hospital and Medical Center
2200 Hayes St. 94117

University of California Program

Langley Porter Neuropsychiatric Institute
401 Parnassus Ave. 94122

Stanford

Stanford University Affiliated Hospitals

Stanford University
94305

Torrance

Los Angeles County Harbor General
1000 W. Carson St. 90509

Van Nuys

San Fernando Valley Child Guidance
Clinic
7335 Van Nuys Blvd. 91405

COLORADO
Denver

University of Colorado Medical Center
4200 East 9th Ave. 80220

CONNECTICUT
Hartford

Institute of Living-Children's Clinic
400 Washington St. 06106

New Haven

Yale University Child Study Center
333 Cedar St. 06511

DISTRICT OF COLUMBIA
Washington

Children's Hospital of the District
of Columbia
2125 13th St., N.W. 20009

Georgetown University Medical Center
3800 Reservoir Rd., N.W. 20007

FLORIDA

Gainesville

William A. Shands Teaching Hospital
and Clinics

University of Florida 32601

Miami

University of Miami Affiliated Hospitals

Jackson Memorial
1700 N.W. 10th Ave. 33136

Tampa

University of South Florida Affiliated
Hospitals

Tampa General
Davis Islands 33606

St. Joseph's

3001 W. Buffalo Ave. 33607

GEORGIA

Atlanta

Emory University Affiliated Hospitals

Georgia Mental Health Institute
1256 Briarcliff Rd., N.E. 30306

Grady Memorial
80 Butler St., S.E. 30303

HAWAII

Honolulu

University of Hawaii Affiliated Hospitals

University of Hawaii, Leahi
3675 Kilauea Ave. 96816

Diamond Head Mental Health Clinic
3675 Kilauea Ave. 96816

ILLINOIS

Chicago

Children's Memorial
2300 Children's Plaza 60614

Institute for Juvenile Research
907 South Wolcott Ave., 60612

Michael Reese Hospital and Medical
Center
2929 South Ellis Ave. 60616

Presbyterian-St. Luke's
1753 W. Congress Pkwy. 60612

University of Chicago Hospitals and
Clinics
950 East 59th St. 60637

INDIANA

Indianapolis

Indiana University Medical Center

Indiana University Hospitals
1100 West Michigan 46207

Larue D. Carter Memorial
1315 West Tenth St. 46202

IOWA

Iowa City

State Psychopathic
500 Newton Rd. 52240

KANSAS
Kansas City

University of Kansas Medical Center
39th & Rainbow Blvd. 66103

Topeka

Children's Division, the Menninger
Foundation
3617 W. 6th St. 66601

KENTUCKY
Lexington

University of Kentucky Medical Center

University
800 Rose St. 40506

Children's Treatment Center
(Anchorage) 40223

Louisville

Bingham Child Guidance Clinic
601 S. Floyd St. 40202

LOUISIANA
New Orleans

Louisiana State University Medical
Center
1542 Tulane Ave. 70112

Tulane University Affiliated Hospitals

Southeast Louisiana (Mandeville)
P.O. Box 3850 70448

MARYLAND
Baltimore

Johns Hopkins
601 North Broadway 21205

University of Maryland
22 S. Greene St. 21201

Towson

Shepard and Enoch Pratt
York Rd. 21204

MASSACHUSETTS

Belmont

Beaverbrook Guidance Center
115 Mill St. 02178

Boston

Beth Israel
330 Brookline Ave. 02215

Boston University Medical Center,
Children's Ambulatory Serv.
82 E. Concord St. 02118

Children's Hospital Medical Center
300 Longwood Ave. 02115

Douglas A. Thom Clinic for Children
315 Dartmouth St. 02116

James Jackson Putnam Children's Center
244 Townsend 02121

Judge Baker Guidance Center
295 Longwood Ave. 02115

Massachusetts General
Fruit St. 02114

Massachusetts Mental Health Center
74 Fenwood Rd. 02115

New England Medical Center Hospitals
171 Harrison Av. 02111

Cambridge

Cambridge Guidance Center
5 Sacramento St. 02138

Quincy

South Shore Mental Health Center
77 Parkingway 02169

Waltham

Metropolitan State
475 Trapelo Rd. 02154

Worcester

Worcester Youth Guidance Center
275 Belmont St. 01604

MICHIGAN

Ann Arbor

University
1405 East Ann St. 48104

Detroit

Lafayette Clinic
951 E. Lafayette 48207

Northville

Hawthorn Center
18471 Haggerty 48167

Pontiac

Oakland Medical Center
140 Elizabeth Lake Rd. 48053

Ypsilanti

York Woods Center
Box A 48197

MINNESOTA

Minneapolis

University of Minnesota Hospitals
412 Union Street, S.E. 55455

Rochester

> Mayo Graduate School of Medicine
> 200 First Ave., S.W. 55901

St. Paul

> Wilder Dept. of Child Guidance and
> Development
> 919-A Lafond Ave. 55104

MISSOURI

Columbia

> University of Missouri Medical Center
> 807 Stadium Rd. 65201

Kansas City

> Grtr. Kansas Cty. Mntl. Hlth. Fndn., U.
> Mo. Sch. Med., Kans. City Div.
> 600 E. 22 St. 64108

> Malcolm Bliss Mental Health Center
> 1420 Grattan St. 63104

St. Louis

> William Greenleaf Eliot Div. of Child
> Psych.—Wash. U. Sch. of Med.
> 369 N. Taylor Ave. 63108

NEBRASKA

Omaha

> Nebraska Psychiatric Institute
> 602 South 44th Ave. 68105

NEW HAMPSHIRE

Hanover

> Dartmouth Medical School Affiliated
> Hospitals

> Dartmouth-Hitchcock Mental Health
> Center 03755

Mary Hitchcock Memorial
2 Maynard 03755

NEW JERSEY

Plainfield

Union County Psychiatric Clinic
111 E. Front St. 07060

Trenton

Child Guidance Center of Mercer County
532 W. State St. 08618

NEW YORK

New Hyde Park

Long Island Jewish-Hillside Medical
Center Program

Hillside Hospital Div. (New York City)
75-59 263rd St., Glen Oaks 11004

Queens Hospital Center (New York City)
82-68 164th St., Jamaica 11432

New York City

Albert Einstein College of Medicine
Affiliated Hospitals

Bronx Municipal Hospital Center
Pelham Pkwy. S. & Eastchester Rd.
10461

Brookdale Hospital Center
Linden Blvd. & Rockaway Pkwy.,
Brooklyn 11212

Brooklyn Psychiatric Centers
189 Montague St., Brooklyn 11201

City Hospital Center at Elmhurst
79-01 Broadway, Elmhurst 11373

Columbia University Affiliated Hospitals

New York State Psychiatric Institute
722 W. 168th St. 10032

Presbyterian
622 West 168th St. 10032

Harlem Hospital Center
532 Lenox Ave. 10037

Hillside Hospital
75-59 263rd St., Glen Oaks 11004

Madeleine Borg Child Guidance Institute
120 West 57th St. 10019

Maimonides Medical Center
4802 Tenth Ave., Brooklyn 11219

Mount Sinai
11 East 100th St. 10029

New York (Payne Whitney Psychiatric
Clinic)
525 East 68th St. 10021

Queens Hospital Center
82-68 164th St., Jamaica 11432

New York Medical College-Metropolitan
Hospital Center
1 East 105th St. 10029

Unit 1—Flower and Fifth Ave. Hospitals

Unit 2—Metropolitan Hospital Center

Unit 3—Bird S. Coler Memorial Hospital
and Home

New York University Medical Center

Bellevue Hospital Center
First Ave. & 27th St. 10016

University
550 First Ave. 10016

Postgrad. Ctr. for Mntl. Hlth., Clin. for
Children and Adolescents
124 E. 26th St. 10016

Roosevelt
428 W. 59th St. 10019

St. Luke's Hospital Center
Amsterdam Ave. & 114th St. 10025

Staten Island Mntl. Hlth. Society—St.
Vincent's Med. Ctr. of Richmond

Staten Island Mental Health Society
657 Castleton Ave., Staten Island
10301

St. Vincent's Medical Center of Richmond
355 Bard Ave., Staten Island 10310

State University—Kings County Hospital
Center

Kings County Hospital Center
451 Clarkson Ave., Brooklyn 11203

State University
445 Lenox Road, Brooklyn 11213

Rhinebeck

Astor Home for Children
36 Mill St. 12572

Rochester

Strong Memorial Hospital of the U.
of Rochester
260 Crittenden Blvd. 14642

Schenectady

Schenectady County Child Guidance
Center
821 Union St. 12308

NORTH CAROLINA
Butner

Murdoch Center, Children's Psychiatric
Institute 27509

Chapel Hill

> North Carolina Memorial
> Pittsboro Rd. 27514

Durham

> Durham Child Guidance Clinic, Duke U.
> Medical Center
> 402 Trent St. 27705

OHIO

Cincinnati

> University of Cincinnati Hospital Groups
>
> Central Psychiatric Clinic
> Cincinnati General Hospital 45229
>
> Children's Psychiatric Center of the
> Jewish Hospital
> 3140 Harvey Ave. 45229

Cleveland

> Case Western Reserve University Affiliated
> Hospitals
>
> University Hospitals of Cleveland
> 2065 Adelbert Rd. 44106
>
> Cleveland Guidance Center
> 2525 E. 22nd. St. 44115

Columbus

> Ohio State University Hospitals
> 410 W. 10th Ave. 43210

Dayton

> Dayton Children's Psychiatric Hospital—
> Child Guidance Center
> 141 Firwood Dr. 45419

Toledo

Medical College of Ohio at Toledo
P.O. Box 6190 43614

OKLAHOMA

Oklahoma City

University of Oklahoma Health Sciences
Center
P.O. Box 26901, 800 N.E. 13th St.
73190

Tulsa

Children's Medical Center
4818 South Lewis, P.O. Box 7352 74105

OREGON

Portland

University of Oregon Affiliated Hospitals

University of Oregon Medical School
Hosps. and Clinics
3181 S.W. Sam Jackson Park 97201

PENNSYLVANIA

Norristown

Montgomery County Mental Health
Clinics
1122 Powell St. 19401

Philadelphia

Albert Einstein Medical Center
York & Tabor Rds. 19141

Hahnemann Medical College and
Hospital
230 N. Broad St. 19102

Irving Schwartz Inst. for Children & Youth
of the Phila. Psych. Center
Ford Rd. and Monument Ave. 19131

Medical College of Pa.—Eastern
   Pennsylvania Psychiatric Inst.
   Henry Ave. and Abbotsford Rd. 19129

Philadelphia Child Guidance Clinic
   1700 Bainbridge St. 19146

Philadelphia General
   Civic Center Blvd. at 34th St. 19104

St. Christopher's Hospital for Children
   2600 N. Lawrence St. 19133

Pittsburgh

Hospitals of the U. Health Center of
   Pittsburgh

Western Psychiatric Institute and Clinic
   3550 Terrace St. 15213

Wilkes-Barre

Childrens Service Center of Wyoming
   Valley
   335 S. Franklin St. 18702

PUERTO RICO
San Juan

Univ. of Puerto Rico School of Medicine
   (Dept. of Psychiatry)
   Puerto Rico Medical Center 00935

RHODE ISLAND
Riverside

Emma Pendleton Bradley
   1011 Veterans Meml. Pkwy. 02915

SOUTH CAROLINA
Columbia

William S. Hall Psychiatric Institute
   2100 Bull St. 29202

TENNESSEE

Memphis

University of Tennessee Affiliated
Hospitals

City of Memphis Hospitals
860 Madison Ave. 38103

Gailor Mental Health Center
42 North Dunlap St. 38103

Tennessee Psychiatric Hospital and
Institute
865 Poplar Ave. 38105

Nashville

Vandelbilt University
1161 21st Ave. South 37203

TEXAS

Dallas

University of Texas Southwestern
Medical School

Dallas Child Guidance Clinic
2101 Welborn 75219

Galveston

University of Texas Medical Branch
Hospitals
8th & Mechanic Sts. 77550

Houston

Baylor College of Medicine Affiliated
Hospitals

Texas Research Institute of Mental
Sciences
1300 Moursund Ave. 77025

San Antonio

University of Texas at San Antonio
Teaching Hospitals

Community Guidance Center of Bexar
County
2135 Babcock Rd. 78229

UTAH

Salt Lake City

University of Utah Affiliated Hospitals

University
50 North Medical Dr. 84112

VERMONT

Burlington

Medical Center Hospital of Vermont
Colchester Ave. 05401

VIRGINIA

Charlottesville

University of Virginia
Jefferson Park Ave. 22903

Falls Church

Fairfax-Falls Church Mental Health
Center
2949 Sleepy Hollow Rd. 22044

Richmond

Virginia Treatment Center for Children
515 North 10th St. 23219

WASHINGTON

Seattle

University of Washington Affiliated
Hospitals

University
1959 N.E. Pacific St. 98105

WISCONSIN

Madison

University of Wisconsin Affiliated
Hospitals

University Hospitals
1300 University Ave. 53706

Children's Treatment Center
3814 Harper Rd. 53704

Milwaukee

Milwaukee Children's
1700 W. Wisconsin Ave. 53233

INDEX

A

Abducens nerve, 304–305
Ackerman, N., 212, 491
Acoustic nerve, 306
Acting out, 63, 71
Activity program
  in hospital psychiatry, 251
Adaptive regression, 52
Addison's disease
  psychiatric manifests, Table VII-II, 272
Adie's syndrome, 304
Adjustment reaction
  of adolescence, 17
  of adult life, 17
  of childhood, 17
  of infancy, 16
  of late life, 17
Adler, A., 497
Administrative psychiatry
  training programs, 485–486
Admission criteria, 240–243
Adolescence
  behavior disorders, diagnostic classification, 17
  stages of, 182–183
Adolescent patient
  evaluation of, 181–186
Adolescent psychiatry
  training programs, 486–487
Aerosols, 421
Affect, 7, 27
  flat, 20
  inappropriate, 21
Affective disorders
  diagnostic classification, 11–12
After care, 255
Aim inhibition, 62
Akathisia, 336
Akinetic seizures, 321
Akineton, 338
Alcohol
  simple drunkenness, 10

Alcohol abuse, 410–420
  treatment, 416–420
Alcoholic epilepsy, 411, 413–414
Alcoholic hallucinosis, 411–413
Alcoholic indulgence
  as defense mechanism, 67
Alcoholic psychosis
  diagnostic classification, 9
Alcoholics Anonymous, 256, 420
Alcoholic Screening Test
  Michigan, 108, 110–111, 420, Table III-V, 110–111
Alcoholism
  diagnostic classification, 15
Aldomet
  psychiatric manifestations, Table VII-I, 271
Alexander, F., 502
Alzheimer's Disease, 8, Table VII-II, 273
Ambivalence, 19
American Association of Psychiatric Services for Children, 535–549
American Board of Psychiatry and Neurology, 475–476
American Law Institute's Model Penal Code, 140
Amnesia, 68
  differential diagnosis, Table VIII-III, 314
Amphetamine intoxication
  differential diagnosis, Table I-V, 26–28
Amphetamine overdose, 379
Amphetamine poisoning, 397–398
Amphetamine psychosis
  differential diagnosis, 24, Table I-III, 23
Amphetamines
  abuse of, 150
  and military service, 150
Amphetamine withdrawal, 398
Amytal, 355
Amytal interview, 111–116
Anacephaly, 8